The Complete Guide to Pregnancy after 30

by Carol Winkelman

Adams Media Corporation
Avon, Massachusetts

Published by
Adams Media Corporation
57 Littlefield Street, Avon, MA 02322. U.S.A.
www.adamsmedia.com

ISBN: 1-58062-619-X

Printed in Canada.

J I H G F E D C B

Library of Congress Cataloging-in-Publication Data
Winkelman, Carol.
The complete guide to pregnancy after 30: from conception to delivery--all
you need to know to make the right decisions / by Carol Winkelman.
p. cm.   Includes index.
ISBN: 1-58062-619-X
1. Pregnancy in middle age. 2. Pregnancy. 3. Childbirth. I. Title.
RG556.6   .W55 2002
618.2'4--dc21   2001055208

This publication is designed to provide accurate and authoritative information with regard to the subject matter covered. It is sold with the understanding that the publisher is not engaged in rendering legal, accounting, or
other professional advice. If legal advice or other expert assistance is
required, the services of a competent professional person should be sought.
—From a *Declaration of Principles* jointly adopted by a Committee of the
American Bar Association and a Committee of Publishers and Associations

Cover illustration ©Norbert Schafer/The Stock Market.
Illustrations on pages 435–447 and 564 by Howard Petote.
Illustrations on pages 395, 405, 514, 522, 526, 575, and 590 reprinted
from *The Management of Labor and Delivery,* Creasy, ed., 1997, with
permission of Blackwell Science Inc.

This book is available at quantity discounts for bulk purchases.
For information, call 1-800-872-5627.

Contents

Dedication

This book is dedicated to my own late-in-life parents, Edith Spiegel Winkelman and Cassius Jacob Winkelman.

* * *

Acknowledgments

I'd like to thank my agent, Maxine Berger, for going the extra mile for this book and for her continuous energy, insight, and faith in this project. I also appreciate the efforts of my editors at Adams Media Corporation. My thanks to Anne Weaver who acquired the book and enthusiastically supported it; to Dawn Thompson, my encouraging "book doula" and interim editor; Jennifer Lantagne, my primary editor and project manager, who gracefully saw the manuscript through the editing process; and to Claire Gerus, Sandy Smith, and Laura MacLaughlin for ushering the book through its final stages.

My thanks go to Dr. Susan Porto and Dr. Allen Killam for all those long interviews, for carefully reading and commenting on my manuscript, and for offering valuable insights into pregnancy, childbirth, and the practice of obstetrics. Thanks to midwives Laraine Guyette and Pam Spry for their understanding of pregnancy and birth as a natural process, for teaching me about the important "fourth power" of childbirth, and for adding a much-needed midwifery dimension to the book. I'd also like to thank Dr. Donna Kirz, Dr. Mark Sauer, and Dr. David Walmer for their contributions as primary medical consultants and the time they spent talking to me about fertility, pregnancy, and birth.

I am very grateful to Dr. Murray Enkin for his warmth, his encouragement, his "bible" on evidence-based medicine, and his inspiring commitment to delivering effective and compassionate medical care. I am also grateful to Dr. Brooks Ranney for long talks about obstetrics and the "gentle art" of turning breech babies and to Dr. Edward Quilligan for his thoughts on breech babies, cesarean section, and the practice of medicine.

Numerous midwives and childbirth educators have significantly contributed to the text of this book and to my understanding of pregnancy and birth. I am grateful to midwives Marion McCartney and Lisa Summers from the American College for Nurse Midwives; to midwives Leah Albers, Louise Aucott, Ceal Bacom, Nancy Wainer Cohen, Shelly Gerard, Kathy Herschderfer, Eileen Hutton, Susan Moray, and Mary Sommers; to childbirth educators and doulas Connie Banack, Elizabeth Bing, Michelle Brill, Kathleen Ray Farthing, and Penny Simkin; and to genetics counselor Melissa Trant. My appreciation also goes to sociologist Barbara Katz-Rothman for talking with me about her personal and professional experience with home birth.

Additional appreciation goes to scientists Dr. Lovell Jones and Dr. Richard Hajeck for their willingness to explain hormonal feedback loops and receptor sites and teach me about the impact of hormones on fetal development; Dr. John McLaughlin, the "mouse doctor," who first enlightened me about exposures to hormones during pregnancy; Debra Wiener, my friend and biostatistician, for walking me through difficult epidemiological research and offering helpful editorial feedback on parts of my manuscript; Dr. Alice Whittemore, Dr. Mary Anne Rossing, and Dr. Baruch Modan for carefully explaining their research on fertility drugs; Drs. Louise Brinton, Patricia Hartge, Robert Spirtas, Elaine Ron, Gerry Cunha, and Bruce Stadel for giving me a sense of the larger picture on fertility drugs; Dr. Sandra Kweder for thought-provoking interviews on pharmaceutical drug exposure during pregnancy; and Dr.

Howard Bern for his research on diethylstilbestrol (DES), his knowledge of hormonal drugs in pregnancy, and his enduring commitment to public health.

I also am grateful to Dr. Lousie Kirz for her candid discussion of anesthesia options; Dr. Yi Pan and Dr. Z. J. Chen for their clinical experience in both eastern and western medicine; Dr. Raul Artal Mittelmark; Dr. Margaret Bates; Dr. Gertrude Berkowitz; Dr. Watson Bowes Jr.; Dr. Leslie Boyce; bioethicist Arthur Caplan; Dr. Luis Cibils; Dr. Mark Dwight; Dr. Peter Fisher; Dr. Larry Goldman; Dr. Murph Goodwin; Dr. Arthur Herbst; Dr. Robert Israel; the late Dr. Irwin Kaiser; Dr. Roger Kaufman; Dr. Louis Keith; Dr. Arthur Kohrman; the late Dr. Irving Kushner; Dr. David Meldrum; Dr. Margaret Nusbaum; Dr. John Rogers; and Dr. Katherine Shaw.

Special thanks to Eileen Finnegan for arranging all those interviews; Carolyn and Jim Hougan for reading early stages of the manuscript and offering good advice and enduring friendship; Jim and Bev Cusimano for their feedback and simpatico; Edith, Arcie, Joan, Marie, Linda-Carol, Julie, Donna, Suzanne, Susan, Sally, Mary Ellen, Ellen, Nikos, and Ben for moral support; and to Richard Hart and Ted Vaden for standing behind my newspaper series on egg donation and thus opening the door for this book. You all have been my much-appreciated "book doulas."

To the women and their partners who have shared with me their stories of pregnancy and birth, my deepest appreciation. Thanks to Amanda, Anna, Auben, Carla, Cathy, Cheryl, Claudia, Dion, Eileen, Gretchen, Holly, Jennifer, Jessica, Jim, Joanne, Kathleen R., Kathleen S., Kevin, Leda, Leslie, Linda S., Linda-Carol, Louise, Lucy, Mary, Miriam, Pete, Reyn, Rhonda, Sarah, Sharlene, Sharon, Stacy, Susan G., Susan H., Susan P., Suzanne R., and Thelma.

Disclaimer

The author of this book is a medical writer. Although she has interviewed leading physicians, scientists, and midwives and summarized medical and scientific research, she is neither physician, midwife, nor scientist. Consequently, the information in this book should not be taken as medical advice. Readers should consult their physician or midwife before acting on any of the information contained in this book. While the information in this book is believed to be accurate to date, neither the author nor the publisher can accept any legal responsibility for any errors or omissions that may have been made. The publisher makes no warranty with respect to the material contained in this text. Readers are advised to seek medical advice from their care providers and to stay informed about advances in pregnancy care and reproductive medicine.

Foreword
by Dr. Susan Porto

I often remember a former patient who was outraged when one of my associates marked on her prenatal record that she was "high risk" because of her "advanced maternal age." She was thirty-nine years old. I hope this book will reassure women in their thirties and forties that they are not too old to become pregnant. They are young enough to create life, and they are capable of the natural process of birth.

As a woman who had her first pregnancy at age thirty-nine and her second at forty-one, I joined the ranks of women who had postponed childbearing. With both my children—Lorelei and Emilio—my early phase of labor lasted all day but my active and pushing stages of labor were short and relatively easy.

What I especially like about this book is that it offers a fully rounded view of pregnancy and birth and provides women with the differing perspectives—and combined wisdom—of physicians, midwives, and mothers. The book brings together the medical, emotional, and natural aspects of childbearing, always balancing the medical explanations with the personal experiences of the women whose "voices" are heard throughout the following chapters.

This book is much more than a reference book. It is an excellent resource, a "pregnancy companion," and a source of encouragement to any woman currently pregnant or contemplating pregnancy. When women read the real-life "stories" in the following chapters, they may find anecdotes that apply to their own circumstances and feelings. Many women will get a much-needed boost from hearing about someone else's experiences and learning how another woman "rode the waves of labor," modified her exercise program, "wore her baby in a sling" at work, breastfed twins, struggled with postpartum depression, recovered from a cesarean, or balanced motherhood and a career. Whether the experience is easy or challenging, the anecdotes reaffirm placing your trust in the *natural process* of pregnancy and birth.

For me, practicing obstetrics is a constant struggle between trusting that Mother Nature has a way of leading each pregnancy to a normal outcome and sweating over when—or if—medical interventions are useful. I always try to give my patients a balanced view of pregnancy and birth, providing them with optimism about the normal process of childbearing while, at the same time, making suggestions about maintaining a healthy lifestyle and managing any problem that might arise.

When I was a young resident in a hospital with a busy obstetrical service, we managed a high volume of patients, ranging from normal to extremely high risk. We were always running on high adrenaline. Because the unit was so busy, our main goal was to get women in labor delivered as quickly and safely as possible. Unfortunately, we were never encouraged to slow down and spend time with a single laboring woman and to witness the unfolding of the normal process of childbirth. When I finished my residency, the only approach to labor I knew was an "actively managed" or interventionist approach that sped up labor. I spent eight years in a successful private obstetrics practice honing my expertise in this art of medical management.

However, I eventually learned to practice medicine in a way that worked *with nature* rather than by medically intervening to control nature. I came to realize that the true art of obstetrics is allowing nature to do its own work, while intervening only when necessary. Pregnancy and labor are natural, physiologic body functions. If a woman sees childbirth as normal in this way, she is more likely to accept the changes her body is going though and to find childbirth more understandable and therefore less intimidating.

Four years ago, I began working in a program that is based on a midwifery model of childbirth. The midwives have confidence in the natural process of labor and birth. They help expectant mothers keep themselves healthy, which generally leads to good pregnancy outcomes. The midwives also do a lot of prenatal education, which promotes healthy attitudes towards pregnancy, labor, and breastfeeding. They trust the process of labor to progress on its own with the help of "natural interventions" such as relaxation techniques, positional change, and good labor support. They use medical interventions only when absolutely necessary.

I serve as their consultant and as the provider of obstetrics care to the high-risk patients. I left private practice to join this new midwifery-based practice because I thought that I would broaden my experience to work with midwives who have a strong faith in the natural process of birth. What I did not expect was that I would come to share this faith—and to relearn obstetrics! What has remained constant for me, however, throughout my years of practicing medicine is the privilege of watching the process of creating new life; with each pregnant woman, I am constantly reminded of this privilege.

The Complete Guide to Pregnancy after 30 brings together under one cover the medical and midwifery approaches to pregnancy and childbirth. The book honors the idea that childbirth is a natural, normal event for which women's bodies are well designed while acknowledging that the contributions of modern medicine are sometimes necessary to help nature along.

—Dr. Susan Porto
Attending Obstetrician and Clinical Faculty, Mercy Hospital, Chicago
September, 2001

Author's Foreword

In 1948, when my mother, Edith, was six months short of her fortieth birthday, she had her first baby. During the pregnancy, her obstetrician (and brother), Dr. Manuel Spiegel, neither told her that she was high risk nor expressed concern about possible complications. Instead, Dr. Spiegel calmly went about doing what he felt good obstetricians did: work with nature to facilitate healthy pregnancy and birth.

Everything went well. Edith's pregnancy was normal. She didn't even develop stretch marks. However, because she received a spinal anesthetic, her labor contractions were not efficient enough to push her baby out into the world. Luckily, her doctor was able to use forceps (then in vogue) to artfully guide her baby through the birth canal. Mother and child were fine.

Had my mother been pregnant between 1958 and the mid-1980s, she may automatically have been labeled an "elderly primigravida"—a term defined in 1958 by the Council of International Federation of Obstetrics as "one aged 35 or more" when birthing her first baby. Other loaded and similarly unflattering terms such as "geriatric," "senescent," or "pre-menopausal" appeared in the obstetrics literature from the fifties to the 1980s to describe women pregnant over thirty-five or forty. Such terms were not only pejorative; they were also discouraging since they implied "too old," "too ridiculous," or "too risky."

Fortunately, both Edith and her doctor believed that childbirth was normal and took in stride healthy women having babies in midlife.

I wrote this book to give healthy women the good news: They are neither too old nor too high risk to have babies in midlife. I also wrote it to help women gain a realistic—and often reassuring—perspective on pregnancy after thirty-five, to inform them of up-to-date medical approaches to pregnancy and birth, to alert them to current debates about the safety and effectiveness of infertility drugs and procedures, and to help them find experienced, appropriate doctors and midwives.

This book is written for women thirty-something to fifty-something who are already pregnant, are trying to become pregnant, or are considering becoming pregnant. It is also written for women in their twenties who are assessing their childbearing options and weighing the pros and cons of postponing pregnancy.

The book is inspired by the experiences of mature women who became mothers when they were thirty to fifty-five years of age and the caregivers who supported these women through pregnancy and birth. Many of the women I interviewed told me uplifting stories about midlife pregnancy, birth, and motherhood midlife. For Auben, forty-five, pregnancy was a breeze and motherhood "amazing." Miriam, thirty-eight, an otherwise no-nonsense New Yorker, found childbirth an intense mystical experience. Sarah, forty-six, fell in love with her egg-donor baby while he was still in utero, and Dion, forty-five, was smitten when she first saw the donor embryos that would later become her twin boys. Joanne, at forty-nine, says pregnancy and motherhood increased her energy.

Some women told stories of caregivers who gave them confidence in their ability to birth a healthy baby. One of Joanne's obstetricians responded with glee to her pregnancy at age forty-nine, calling up all his patients whom he had told were "too old" to get pregnant to tell them of Joanne's good news. The doctor who did Joanne's amniocentesis told her that since there were no statistics on birth defects or other pregnancy complications for women at age forty-nine, she might as well assume the best. When Joanne's amnio results were reassuring, she brought her doctors roses. Kathleen R., age thirty-nine, felt calmed by the presence of a doula (labor companion) and midwife who stayed up all night with her, offering her continuous encouragement and comfort through a long labor.

However, becoming a midlife mother is not always easy or euphoric, and many of the women I talked to had faced obstacles imposed by their own bodies, by medical myths, or by discouraging medical and social attitudes.

Some women had been frightened out of all proportion by age-related statistics on infertility, Down's syndrome, and pregnancy complications. Some felt frustrated as they tried to find an emotionally satisfying way of giving birth within a high-tech and often impersonal medical system.

Numerous women I interviewed had been told by their doctors to "forget" pregnancy. Joanne was only thirty-three when an obstetrician told her that she needed a hysterectomy to "cure" her uterine fibroids and that she would never have children because she didn't currently have a boyfriend. Rhonda was told that pregnancy was unlikely because she had only one fallopian tube. Auben, at forty-five, was told she was in menopause and that her fertility was "all over"; she got pregnant within a year of that pronouncement. Some of the women were informed that they were too old at age forty-two or forty-three for in vitro fertilization or other assisted reproduction, or they were presented with conflicting and confusing advice about high-tech procedures such as in vitro fertilization (IVF), gamete intrafallopian transfer (GIFT), and zygote intrafallopian transfer (ZIFT) in "older" women.

I realized that a surprising number of women—even those who were scientists—had felt perplexed by the maze of medical options. Their struggle to inform themselves about numerous (and sometimes controversial) options, make good choices for themselves and their babies, and navigate a complex medical system consumed considerable time and emotional energy. Consequently, I decided to write a book that women and their partners could *use* as a resource to help them sift through conflicting medical opinions, weigh their benefits and risks of midlife pregnancy, consider the appropriateness of infertility medications and surgeries, and make informed decisions. I wanted to provide them with an up-to-date, in-depth, comprehensive guide tailored to their midlife health and lifestyle concerns.

To write this kind of book, I brought in a spectrum of expert opinion in several medical and scientific disciplines. I consulted with prominent obstetricians, surgeons, infertility specialists, developmental biologists, epidemiologists, midwives, and childbirth educators. I consulted two authoritative sources for evidence-based medicine: The Cochrane Library (*www.cochranelibrary.com*) and *A Guide to Effective*

Care in Pregnancy and Childbirth by Dr. Murray Enkin and his coauthors.

I also interviewed women and their partners. The end result is a guide shaped by scientific studies and clinical expertise but brought to life by the real experiences of women, their partners, and their caregivers.

The Cast of Characters

In *The Complete Guide to Pregnancy after 30,* my consultants, whose "voices" are heard throughout the book, are nationally known authorities in obstetrics, midwifery, childbirth preparation, infertility, and assisted reproduction.

My other "characters," of course, are the women I interviewed and their partners. The majority of these women had their first or second babies between the ages of thirty-three and forty-seven. A few had second babies in their fifties. Most had postponed childbearing for one or more of the following reasons: to pursue education and career, establish financial stability, or find the right partner. A few, finding themselves with a stable career but no partner, decided to have babies on their own. Several women became pregnant in their late thirties only a month or two after they started trying. Some attempted to become pregnant in their early thirties but were unable to achieve a successful pregnancy until many years later—after fertility treatments, surgeries, or both.

What impressed me as I talked to these midlife parents was the resourcefulness and humor they brought to pregnancy, birth, and parenthood. My hope is that their stories will offer you a helpful perspective and provide you with strategies that you can use to make good choices, find appropriate medical care, and integrate pregnancy and motherhood with your career and personal life.

I refer to the midlife mothers and their partners by their first names. Most of these people allowed me to use their real names. Six did not; they changed their names to protect their privacy.

The Physicians

Primary Medical Consultants

Dr. Allen Killam, Professor Emeritus and recently retired Chief of Maternal-Fetal Medicine at Duke University Medical Center, has reviewed drafts and offered valuable suggestions, encouragement, and insights. He has also provided a candid and wise perspective on the practice of obstetrics, for which I am very grateful.

Dr. Susan Porto, an obstetrician at Mercy Hospital in Chicago, has patiently reviewed drafts of my manuscript and provided valuable medical information, suggestions, and encouragement. She also has offered both her clinical and personal understanding of birth as a natural process.

Dr. Mark Sauer has been a pioneer in assisted reproduction since the 1980s. He is Professor and Vice Chairman of Obstetrics and Gynecology at Columbia University and Director of the Division of Reproductive Endocrinology at Columbia Presbyterian Medical Center. An international authority on assisted reproduction and one of the "fathers" of egg donation, Dr. Sauer is frequently quoted in *The New York Times* and has been interviewed on television and radio in the United States and Europe.

Dr. Donna Kirz is a high-risk pregnancy specialist and the Chair and Program Director of the Department of Obstetrics and Gynecology at Mercy Hospital, Chicago. In her influential 1985 article entitled, "Advanced Maternal Age: The Mature Gravida," published in *The American Journal of Obstetrics and Gynecology,* Kirz renamed midlife pregnancy as "mature" rather than "elderly," "geriatric," or "dangerous." Dr. Kirz had two children in midlife.

Dr. David Walmer is a Professor of Reproductive Endocrinology at Duke University Medical School.

Additional Consultants

Dr. Margaret Bates and **Dr. Mark Alan Dwight** are partners in an obstetrics and gynecology office at Good Samaritan Hospital in Los Angeles.

Dr. Watson Bowes Jr., recently retired Professor of Obstetrics and Gynecology at the University of North Carolina School of Medicine, has offered innumerable insights on the practice of evidence-based medicine in addition to good common sense and an admirable sensitivity to the needs of pregnant women. He has published widely in medical journals and textbooks.

Dr. Leslie Boyce is a pediatric neurologist at the University of North Carolina, Chapel Hill.

Dr. Z. J. Chen, LIC.AC, and Diplomat of the National Certification Commission for Acupuncture and Oriental Medicine, is a Chinese medical doctor who has practiced acupuncture in both China and the United States.

Dr. Luis Cibils, Professor Emeritus and Mary Campau Ryerson Professor of Obstetrics and Gynecology at the University of Chicago, is a widely published physician.

Dr. Murray Enkin is Professor of Obstetrics at McMaster University in Canada and one of the authors of *A Guide to Effective Care in Pregnancy and Childbirth,* a well-respected book among physicians and midwives. Enkin looks at major issues in childbirth and pregnancy from the point of view of "evidence-based medicine." Both editions of his book are frequently cited throughout the following chapters.

Dr. Peter Fisher is an Assistant Clinical Professor in the

Department of Family Medicine at the University of North Carolina School of Medicine in Chapel Hill, North Carolina.

Dr. Murph Goodwin, a specialist in high-risk pregnancy, is Professor of Maternal and Fetal Medicine at the University of Southern California.

Dr. Arthur Herbst, a gynecological oncologist, is Chairman of Obstetrics and Gynecology at the University of Chicago and coauthor of *The Developmental Effects of DES in Pregnancy.*

Dr. Robert Israel, Professor of Obstetrics and Gynecology at the University of Southern California School of Medicine, is a nationally known gynecological surgeon.

Dr. Louis Keith, an obstetrician specializing in twin and "super-twin" pregnancies, teaches obstetrics at Northwestern University.

Dr. Valery King is Medical Director of the Piedmont Birth Center in Chapel Hill, North Carolina.

Dr. Louise Kirz is an anesthesiologist in Oregon who has considerable experience in obstetrical anesthesia. She is the mother of two children.

Dr. Arthur Kohrman, a pediatrician, is Professor of Pediatrics and Public Health at Northwestern University.

Dr. David Meldrum, a former UCLA Professor of Obstetrics and Gynecology, is a leading national expert on infertility. He practices in Redondo Beach, California.

Dr. Raul Artal Mittelmark, a specialist in high-risk pregnancy, is the author of *Pregnancy and Exercise.* He coined the term "chronologically privileged" to apply to women pregnant over thirty-five.

Dr. Margaret Nusbaum is an Associate Professor in the Department of Family Medicine at the University of North Carolina School of Medicine, Chapel Hill. She has extensive experience delivering babies.

Dr. Yi Pan holds degrees in western and oriental medicine and has practiced oriental medicine in Shanghai, New York City, and Los Angeles. He uses acupuncture and herbs to treat infertility and hormonal imbalances and to facilitate labor and delivery.

Dr. Edward J. Quilligan is Director of the Center for Health Education and Professor Emeritus of Obstetrics and Gynecology at the Medical School of the University of California at Irvine. He is also the author of numerous books and articles.

Dr. Brooks Ranney, an Emeritus Professor of Obstetrics and Gynecology at the University of South Dakota School of Medicine, has delivered thousands of babies. Dr. Ranney is the author of an often-cited article entitled, "The Gentle Art of Cephalic Version" (the art of turning breech babies to the normal, head-down position).

Dr. Katherine Shaw, former Assistant Professor of Maternal-Fetal Medicine at the University of Southern California, now practices obstetrics at White Memorial Hospital in East Los Angeles.

The Midwives

Primary Midwife Consultants
Leah Albers, CNM, Dr. PH., is a Professor of Nursing at the University of New Mexico. She is a well-known researcher who has published medical journal articles on the duration of labor.

Laraine Guyette, CNM, Ph.D., is an Assistant Professor of Nursing at the University of Colorado.

Pam Spry, CNM, Ph.D., is an Assistant Professor of Nursing at the University of Colorado at Denver.

Additional Midwife Consultants
Louise Aucott, CNM, was formerly a lay midwife (and

Bryn Mawr graduate) and has done home and hospital births for fifteen years. She recently attended a home birth that appeared on a CBS network morning show.

Ceal Bacom, CNM, is a certified nurse-midwife at the Alivio Clinic in Chicago.

Nancy Wainer Cohen is a lay midwife who specializes in home birth and maternal positions in labor that facilitate childbirth. She is the author of *Silent Knife.*

Shelly Girard, CPM (Certified Professional Midwife), **LM** (Licensed Midwife), and **MPH** (master's degree in public health), has been a midwife for thirty years.

Kathy Herschderfer is a Dutch midwife and researcher. She is pursuing a Ph.D. degree.

Marion McCartney, CNM, is author of *A Midwife's Pregnancy and Childbirth Book,* and Director of Professional Services, the American College of Nurse-Midwives (ACNM) in Washington, D.C.

Susan Moray, CPM, LM, practices midwifery in Portland, Oregon.

Mary Sommers, CNM, is a midwife at the Alivio Clinic in Chicago.

Lisa Summers, CNM, Dr. PH., is a certified nurse-midwife and Senior Technical Advisor for Professional Services at the ACNM in Washington, D.C.

Doulas and Childbirth Educators

Connie Banack is a the president of the board of directors of ICAN (the International Cesarean Awareness Network), and the executive director of the Canadian Programs for Childbirth and Postpartum Doula Association.

Elizabeth Bing is a childbirth educator, physical therapist, author, and Lamaze expert. She is Emeritus Director for Lamaze International.

Michelle Brill, MPH, is a health educator and doula in New Jersey.

Linda Carol Davis became a La Leche leader after she had her second baby.

Kathleen Gray Farthing is a doula and childbirth educator who lives in Indiana.

Michelle Trant is a genetics counselor at the Perinatal Alliance Medical Group in Los Angeles.

The Research Scientists

Dr. Gertrude Berkowitz, an epidemiologist at the Mt. Sinai School of Medicine in New York City, has conducted studies on pregnancy outcomes in older women.

Dr. Howard Bern is an international authority on the effects of DES. He is coauthor of *The Developmental Effects of DES in Pregnancy* and Professor Emeritus of Integrative Biology and Research Endocrinologist in the Cancer Research Lab at the University of California, Berkeley.

Dr. Richard Hajek is an instructor in gynecologic oncology at the University of Texas and a cancer researcher at the M.D. Anderson Cancer Center in Houston.

Dr. Patricia Hartge is Deputy Director of the Epidemiology and Biostatistics Program at the National Cancer Institute.

Dr. Lovell Jones, Professor of Gynecological Oncology, Biochemistry, and Molecular Biology at the University of Texas and Director of Experimental Gynecology and Endocrinology at the M.D. Anderson Cancer Center in Houston, has conducted research on the effects of progesterone on animals.

Dr. Baruch Modan is a physician and cancer researcher at Chaim Sheba Medical Center and the Stanley Steyer Institute for Cancer Epidemiology and Research (Israel).

Dr. John Rogers is a developmental biologist and reproductive toxicologist who studies environmental endocrine disrupters.

Dr. Mary Anne Rossing is a research associate professor in the Department of Epidemiology at the Fred Hutchinson Cancer Research Center in Seattle. She conducted an NIH-funded study to investigate the possible relationship between taking fertility drugs and developing ovarian cancer.

Dr. Alice Whittemore is a cancer researcher and Professor of Epidemiology and Health Policy at the Stanford University Medical School. In a 1993 study, Dr. Whittemore and her colleagues suggested that the use of fertility drugs may increase a woman's risk of developing ovarian cancer.

* * *

Lengthy discussions over the last five years with the following scientists and physicians have also informed this book:

Dr. Arthur Caplan is Director, Center for Bioethics, University of Pennsylvania. Dr. Caplan is a national authority on bioethics. He has appeared on TV and radio talk shows and is frequently quoted by the national media.

Dr. Bernadine Healy was an editor of *The Journal of Women's Health* and former Director of the National Institutes of Health (NIH).

Nancy King is a lawyer, medical ethicist, and Associate Professor in the Department of Social Medicine, the University of North Carolina at Chapel Hill.

Dr. Robert Spirtas is Chief of the Contraceptive and Reproductive Evaluation Branch, National Institute of Child Health and Development, National Institutes of Health.

Dr. Bruce Stadel is a Medical Officer/Epidemiologist with the Division of Metabolism and Endocrine Drug Products, at the U.S. Food and Drug Administration (FDA).

Other helpful sources:

Peter Kaiser is the son of Dr. Irwin Kaiser. Dr. Irwin Kaiser was a professor of obstetrics and gynecology at the Albert Einstein School of Medicine and coauthor (with Dr. Alan Guttmacher) of the book *Pregnancy, Birth, and Family Planning.*

Dr. Manuel Spiegel, my late uncle, taught me that obstetrics should be practiced "with art, not with force."

The Women

Amanda, age thirty-four and thirty-eight when her children were born, developed gestational diabetes (GD) in the third trimester of her pregnancy with her second child. Her GD was easily managed with diet, and she gave birth to Ben, a healthy nine-pound baby boy.

Anna became pregnant at age forty—much to her surprise. She never relaxed during her pregnancy, since she was told that she was high risk due to her age. Although Anna developed a mild case of pregnancy-induced diabetes, the condition was managed easily with diet, and the pregnancy was normal. Her baby girl, Julia, was delivered by cesarean section.

Auben's doctor told her she was menopausal when she was forty-five, but at age forty-six she gave birth to a baby girl. For Auben, the most stressful part of the pregnancy was deciding whether to risk chorionic villaus sampling (CVS) instead of amniocentesis.

Carla, age thirty-three, felt an exhilarating sense of achievement after she gave birth to her daughter.

Cathy had her first baby at age thirty-three and her second at age thirty-seven. Both labors were difficult. Her first birth required pain medications and a forceps delivery and her second a cesarean section.

Cheryl, a single mom, had her first baby at age twenty-five by artificial insemination. After several unsuccessful attempts at a second pregnancy, she took fertility drugs and eventually became pregnant with twins when she was thirty-one.

Claudia, at age forty-three, underwent an unsuccessful GIFT procedure but became pregnant via artificial insemination with her husband's sperm later that year. She had a healthy pregnancy and birth.

Dion became pregnant with egg-donor twins when she was forty-five. Her pregnancy was normal, and her two boys were healthy, full term—and large. Dion plans to tell her boys of their egg-donor origins when they are older. She is the author of a book on assisted reproduction and a member of a mothers of twins support group. Dion's egg donor remains anonymous.

Eileen was thirty-five when her son, Neil, was born.

Holly became pregnant with her first baby at age thirty-six—the first month she stopped using birth control. Although she had uterine fibroids, they did not interfere with conception, pregnancy, or birth. Holly's son, Soren, was delivered by forceps. She returned to her job as a lawyer three months after his birth. Although she became pregnant at age thirty-nine with a second child, the pregnancy ended in miscarriage

Jean became pregnant with twins when she was thirty-six and pregnant with a single baby when she was thirty-nine. She created the Center for Loss in Multiple Birth (CLIMB) after she lost one of the twins. The remaining twin and her youngest baby are fine. Jean suggests that all women pregnant with twins seek the care of a physician experienced in twin pregnancies.

Jennifer, a single mom at age thirty-four, became pregnant via artificial insemination. She had a healthy pregnancy and a natural birth. The birth was followed by postpartum depression that lasted over a month. When she turned thirty-nine, Jennifer became pregnant with her second child. Her pregnancy and birth were normal, and her baby boy was healthy.

Jessica, when she was forty, was told by her doctor that she was too old to have a baby. However, at age forty-seven, after several miscarriages, surgery for uterine fibroids, and Chinese herbal and acupuncture treatments, she had a baby girl (a result of IVF with her own eggs). Jessica returned to her university teaching position and biology fieldwork carrying her baby in a basket or a sling.

Joanne, at age forty-nine, surprised her doctors—and her-self—by becoming pregnant. Her pregnancy was healthy. However, she had a planned cesarean birth because previous surgery for numerous fibroid tumors had left scars in her uterine walls. Joanne stayed home for six weeks and then brought her son to work—and to administrative meetings—for six months.

Kathleen R. finished a Ph.D. in biology before she started trying to get pregnant at age thirty-three. After surgery to repair blocked tubes and numerous rounds of fertility drug treatments, Kathleen finally became pregnant at age thirty-nine. Her son was delivered with the help of a doula (female birth support person) and midwife. After several months back on the job, Kathleen gave up a promising career as a scientist to become a stay-at-home mom.

Kathleen S., a New York City business woman in her late thirties, balanced motherhood with a demanding career.

Leda, a DES daughter, had several miscarriages due to DES-related abnormalities of her cervix and uterus. After five years of trying to have a baby, she got pregnant at age thirty-eight, spent months in bed to save the pregnancy, and gave birth to a healthy daughter.

Leslie, at age thirty-nine, had her first and only child, a daughter named Anna. Leslie had a normal pregnancy. She chose to stay home and not return to her work.

Lucy had her first baby at age thirty-four and her second at age thirty-nine. Although she gave birth in a hospital, Lucy returned home four hours after her second baby was born.

Mary had her first baby when she was age thirty-six, her second baby at age thirty-eight, and her third baby at age forty-two. She says after the third baby was born, motherhood was "a piece of cake."

Miriam, age thirty-eight, climbed a mountain during her eighth month of pregnancy. She had a healthy pregnancy and a quick, easy labor when she gave birth to her daughter.

Rhonda got pregnant at age thirty-seven, but she had a tubal pregnancy. After one fallopian tube was removed in an emergency surgery, she became pregnant again three months later and gave birth to a healthy boy. When she was forty-two, Rhonda and her husband adopted a Guatemalan baby girl.

Sarah gave birth at age forty-six with the help of donor eggs. Both the pregnancy and birth were normal, although she developed mild preeclampsia during her last weeks of pregnancy. Several weeks later, she returned to work. At age forty-eight, Sarah gave birth to her second child—the product of another egg donor (who is a friend of the first donor). Sarah knows both donors and sees them from time to time.

Sharlene, at age forty-eight, became pregnant with her first baby, conceived using a donor egg. Her pregnancy and birth were normal. At age fifty-two, Sharlene became pregnant with another child (using embryos frozen and stored from the original egg donation). She does not know how, or if, she will tell her children of their egg-donor origins.

Sharon became pregnant with twins when she was forty-three. Pregnancy and birth were normal, but the babies were small and spent four weeks in a neonatal intensive care unit.

Stacy had twin girls when she was twenty-eight and another daughter when she was thirty-one. For both pregnancies she took fertility drugs and underwent IVF and intracytoplasmic sperm injection (ICSI) procedures to become pregnant.

Susan H., at age thirty-five, lost her first baby when he was five months gestational age. During her second pregnancy, at age forty, Susan spent months on bed rest and gave birth to a healthy boy.

Susan Porto had her first baby when she was thirty-nine and her second at forty-one. She is an obstetrician.

The Husbands and Birth Partners

Jim, a scientist, was fifty-four years old when his first son was born, fifty-six when his second son was born, and fifty-eight when his daughter was born. He is a very active father.

Kevin, a scientist, was thirty-five when his first daughter was born and thirty-eight when his second was born.

Pete was thirty-seven when his first child was born and forty-two when his second child was born.

Reyn, Joanne's husband, had children from his first marriage and already had grown boys when at age forty-five he married Joanne. He was forty-nine when their son was born.

Introduction

The Possibilities of Pregnancy in Midlife: The Prime of Life

How old is too old to have a baby? More to the point in recent decades, how old is too old to have a first baby?

My great-grandmother had her eighth baby as she turned fifty. She was surprised but not astonished, since in her time, some women had babies until the very end of their reproductive years. But in the first part of the twentieth century, when women had babies as late as age forty-eight or fifty, the babies were usually not their *first*.

Nowadays, increasing numbers of women in western countries are choosing to postpone having a first or second child into their late thirties, their forties, and even their fifties. In the United States between 1970 and 1990, the rate of first births increased by more than 100 percent for women thirty to thirty-nine years old and by 50 percent for women forty to forty-four, according to a March 8, 1990, article by Dr. Gertrude Berkowitz and her colleagues in *The New England Journal of Medicine.*

If your friends were in their twenties when they had their babies, you may feel out of sync with your generation by having a baby in midlife. But you are not. In the United States, over 1,200 babies are born every day to women between thirty-five and forty-four years old. According to *National Vital Statistics,* 83,090 women aged forty to forty-four gave birth to live babies in 1999, the last year for which final statistics are available. Over 4,000 women aged forty-five to forty-nine had babies—the highest recorded number in thirty years. Due to the assisted reproductive technologies (ART), women are having babies in their early fifties and creating a new category of late-in-life mothers and a new frontier for medical and social research. As we enter a new millennium, that trend continues.

The Complete Guide to Pregnancy after 30 targets the most important issues of midlife or "mature" pregnancy (whether it is a first or a subsequent pregnancy) between ages thirty-five and fifty-five in order to help you realistically plan for future pregnancies or manage your current one.

Midlife, in this context, is a positive thing: It refers to the *prime of life* when you are at your intellectual and emotional peak. It also means that in the half of your life that lies before you, you want to have and raise a child.

Many physicians now see thirty-five as young. Some (though definitely not all) physicians' attitudes toward women over forty-five are also gradually becoming more positive, as doctors are beginning to gain experience with women pregnant in their forties and fifties due to increasingly successful treatments for infertility. However, it is only very recently that medical opinions toward postponing pregnancy have changed dramatically. In the last five years, some fertility clinics have stretched their age limits for in vitro fertilization (IVF) from age forty-two to forty-five. The age cutoffs for recipients of donor eggs have, at some clinics, been pushed from forty-five to fifty, depending upon a woman's overall health. Success rates for egg donation/recipience programs are sometimes as high as 35 to 65 percent.

The Good News

If you are choosing to have a baby after age thirty-five, the news is mostly good. Although getting pregnant may become more difficult in your late thirties and early forties, pregnancy is still possible. It may take a little longer or require some help from modern technology, but you need not give up on conceiving or giving birth to a healthy baby. In fact, as more and more women are refusing to give up on pregnancy, they are dispelling previous myths that midlife pregnancies are either unlikely or unsafe. Their tenacity and optimism have changed medical opinion—and national statistics.

The last decade of medical research on these midlife mothers has found that pregnancy in healthy women in midlife is safe for both mother and child.

But is it a good idea? Does it make social, psychological, and ethical sense? Physicians' answers to these questions vary according to the individual doctor's experience and philosophy. However, many of the mothers whom I interviewed for this book say, "Yes, it's a great idea." They feel that midlife, for them, is the *best* time to have a baby. Instead of feeling too old, they feel "chronologically privileged"—equipped with the perspective, maturity, and stability to make them better, calmer mothers than they might have been at twenty-five.

For Holly, an attorney who was pregnant at thirty-seven, her late thirties was the best time to have a baby. "I felt very ready—very settled in my life. I felt much calmer and knew more about myself and was better able to provide emotionally and financially for a child." Being parents gave Holly and her husband a new zest for the future. "Now we have all sorts of things to look forward to: our son's milestones—all those things add a lot. Having a child keeps you younger."

Joanne, a schoolteacher and administrator, got pregnant at forty-nine when she and her husband were thinking about adoption. Joanne "sailed through" her pregnancy, nursed her baby, and enjoyed mothering a toddler: "I haven't felt any downside of being older. Not one. I know I'm a better mother now than I would have been ten years ago. I feel like I have more capacity now than I ever did."

Are You "High Risk"?

In 1989 when Anna became pregnant, her doctor told her she was "high risk" because she was over thirty-five. Anna took the term to heart. She felt anxious and fragile during much of her pregnancy. However, by the mid-1990s, many doctors' perceptions of pregnancy risk had changed, because medical and epidemiological studies done in the 1980s and 1990s found consistently "good pregnancy outcomes" for women over thirty-five.

Several medical studies have shown that healthy pregnant women between the ages of thirty-four and forty-four have *almost* the same odds as twenty-five-year-olds for bearing healthy babies. Thus, when it comes to safety for the baby, healthy older woman do almost as well as younger women.

Experts in high-risk pregnancy say there are low-risk forty-year-olds and high-risk ones. Preexisting medical conditions such as high blood pressure, kidney disease, or diabetes—not chronological age—are what make the difference when it comes to pregnancy risks. Such illnesses become more prevalent in women over age thirty-five, and they bring with them greater risks of complications for both mother and child. However, even women with diabetes or hypertension can have healthy babies and can minimize their potential risks by obtaining prepregnancy screening and counseling by an experienced obstetrician and getting their diabetes, hypertension, or other illness under control before becoming pregnant.

If you have no preexisting conditions, your pregnancy risks are not significantly elevated. Although women over thirty-five do tend to have a higher incidence of pregnancy-induced medical problems such as hypertension, preeclampsia, or gestational diabetes (GD), these conditions are temporary and usually treatable with diet, medication, bed rest, or delivery of the baby. Many potential complications can be successfully managed or avoided altogether.

Some age-related pregnancy risks are extremely *rare;* even if risks of a rare complication may triple for women over age thirty-five or forty, the actual risk to mother and child may be very, very small. Due to advances in modern medicine, "it is safer for a woman to have a baby at forty-five now" than it was for her mother or grandmother to give birth at age twenty, according to Dr. Allen Killam, Professor Emeritus of Maternal-Fetal Medicine at Duke University.

Interestingly, one of the advances in modern technology that has made pregnancy safer for women is becoming an increasingly common mode of birth in the United States. I am speaking of cesarean section. Although cesarean section is often beneficial, the high rate of cesarean section in the United States has become a cause for concern. Between 1970 and 1998, the national cesarean section rate rose from 7.8 percent to 21.2 percent, according to the March 28, 2000, *National Vital*

Statistics Reports. By the year 2000, the cesarean rate rose to 22.9 percent, according to preliminary national birth statistics. Although the average national rate for women of all ages is high, for women over age thirty-five, cesarean rates nearly double, even though the reasons for cesarean births (such as failure to progress in labor and fetal distress) do not double. Some doctors speculate that women over thirty-five may labor differently than younger women. Others believe that increased anxiety in both women and their doctors may lead to more cesarean deliveries, especially in older women whose "premium pregnancies" are viewed as a last chance at motherhood. Part 7 of this book discusses some ways to increase your odds of a vaginal birth, and Part 8 offers a comprehensive discussion of cesarean surgery and recovery.

Because medical studies have shown that continuous labor support by a doula or midwife decreases cesarean section rates, this book includes considerable information on doulas and midwives. Even if you feel most comfortable having an obstetrician supervise your care and deliver your baby, you may still have a doula at your side to give you emotional support and to help you find labor positions that enhance the progress of your labor.

Is Your Baby at Risk?

A decade of medical research shows that most healthy women over the age of thirty-five, if they do not drink, smoke, or take certain drugs during pregnancy, will have healthy babies.

The odds are in your favor. For instance, at age thirty-nine, you have a 90 to 95 percent chance of having a healthy baby, even though the risk for Down's syndrome and other chromosomal disorders increases dramatically.

However, some genetic disorders and medical problems can pose risks to your baby. If you have severe diabetes, heart disease, or kidney ailments, you may need specialized medical care by perinatologists (high-risk pregnancy physicians) to help ensure the safety of your baby. During pregnancy you will need to become an active participant in your own health care by becoming informed about signs or symptoms that may indicate problems for your baby and seeking appropriate medical care. This book will help you shop for the doctor most appropriate for your baby's needs.

Fertility and Older Eggs: Yes, You Can Conceive

The reality is that some women are fertile well into their forties, and some are not. It's a matter of luck, good genes, and biology, since eggs will age and lose their viability with time.

But there is hope after forty, even after forty-five, says Dr. Margaret Bates, an obstetrician at the Hospital of the Good Samaritan in Los Angeles: "You probably narrow your opportunities as you grow older—but it never means that they're not there."

When I began the research for this book, I was discouraged by the fertility statistics. The numbers showed me a decline in fertility after age thirty-eight and then another precipitous drop after forty-two or forty-three. However, as I interviewed more and more women, I found that it is smart to take note of biological odds without becoming discouraged by them. It is useful to come to terms with the reality that your eggs will age as you age and become less fertile with time. Postponing pregnancy beyond age thirty-eight involves taking some chances. Even if you are in your early thirties, age-related problems such as endometriosis, tubal blockage, infertility, previous infections, and uterine fibroids may make getting or staying pregnant more difficult. The best strategy for pregnancy success is to factor age into your pregnancy plan and, when possible, give yourself an optimal window of opportunity.

To achieve a positive but realistic perspective on such statistical averages, keep in mind that the inevitable ebb in fertility is different for every woman. Some women are biologically younger than their years. If you are over forty-three, you need not give up on becoming pregnant, although you may need to adjust your expectations. Many women in their forties will eventually become pregnant, but it may take some time and a little help from reproductive medicine.

For some of you, none of these warnings will apply. You will fall happily outside the bell curve of statistical averages. As I interviewed women whose names were given to me by friends, relatives, and doctors, I found, to my surprise, numerous women who fell well outside this bell curve. Holly, at thirty-seven, was amazed when she became pregnant the first month she stopped using birth control. Anna, at thirty-nine, assumed that her fertility had diminished, but became pregnant despite the use of a diaphragm. Rhonda, also thirty-nine, became pregnant although she had only one fallopian tube. Although natural conception after age forty-six is relatively uncommon, Joanne became pregnant at forty-nine—a year after giving up on fertility treatments. Jessica had an IVF baby—using her own eggs—at age forty-seven.

I was impressed by these women who had beaten the fertility odds, especially by those who had conceived healthy first babies with their own forty-five-plus-year-old eggs. Though they clearly fall outside the norm—and outside the clinical experience of most obstetricians and infertility specialists—Joanne and Jessica can give hope to women over forty-five.

Interestingly, both Joanne and Jessica are optimists who believed that women could conceive in their forties and had been given such hope by the example of aunts, mothers, and grandmothers. Joanne saw her own mother, at age forty-five, successfully give birth and breastfeed a healthy baby. Jessica comes from a long line of women having their children after the age of forty-two. It is because of these examples that they even dared to try to become pregnant—despite discouraging words from some of their doctors. Some physicians maintain a bleak view of fertility after age forty-three and tell such patients that pregnancy is impossible. At age forty-three, Susan H. was told by her HMO doctor that, when it came to getting pregnant, her HMO "could do nothing for her."

Because medicine has given up on them, women frequently give up on themselves. Some never try to become pregnant. Some try and fail. And a few become pregnant.

The sanest strategy is to keep a positive attitude, but don't count on beating the odds. It is unwise to assume that because you feel young and healthy that your opportunity to become pregnant with your own eggs is guaranteed or open-ended. Scaling mountains, running marathons, and building a career are feats within your control. Ovulating fertile eggs is not.

As Leda, a DES daughter who started trying to get pregnant at thirty-three and finally succeeded five years later, cautions: "If you wait until the career is perfect, you might as well wait for world peace. All you need is to be ready in your head. If you put it off, if you run into problems, time might be one of the problems. Time should be on your side, not against you."

Assisted Reproduction

As you enter the world of assisted reproduction, your choices become tantalizing and often mind-boggling. From Day 1, your head may be swimming from the diagnostic choices alone: the postcoital exams, swim-up tests, hamster tests, endometrial biopsies, laparoscopies, hystosalpingograms. Where do you start—and why?

When you finish with diagnosis, you face IVF and an array of options with confusing acronyms: GIFT, ZIFT, ICSI. You may choose from an assortment of fertility drugs offered alone or in various combinations. Then there are the "high-tech" options of egg donation, embryo "adoption," and assisted hatching, or the "low-tech" options involving intrauterine insemination and ovulation prediction. Even more overwhelming are the numerous fertility clinics with seductive "take-home baby" statistics and heartwarming stories of miracle babies.

Many of these stories are both miraculous and real. Impressive numbers of women between thirty-five and fifty-five years of age have achieved successful pregnancies thanks to assisted reproduction. According to the American Society for Reproductive Medicine (ASRM), in the years between 1985 and 1996 the new assisted reproductive technologies brought 90,000 "miracle babies" into the world—enough people for a small city. The number of miracle babies has steadily increased since then.

Because a growing number of women and men are flocking to fertility clinics only to find themselves overwhelmed with information they can neither assess nor fully comprehend, I have devoted several chapters of this book to assisted reproduction. A stranger in this technological universe needs a road map as well as strategies for evaluating statistics, drugs, procedures, and physicians.

This book is designed to guide you through the myriad choices and to provide strategies for evaluating the benefits, the risks, and the appropriateness *for you* of the various fertility drugs and procedures. It is intended to help you objectively evaluate your options instead of jumping at any promise of pregnancy and investing in the costly, and sometimes lengthy, process of making a baby the high-tech way.

Fertility Drugs

While *The Complete Guide to Pregnancy after 30* tells the optimistic story of successful pregnancies and "miracle" babies, it also discusses the potential dangers to mother and developing baby of some of the "drugs of pregnancy"— fertility drugs and miscarriage-preventing drugs. Most books on the subject of late-in-life pregnancy do not address the possible negative consequences of these drug therapies. Some of the results are splendid, but taking the drugs also involves potential risks that should be clearly presented to you in order for you to make informed choices in your best interest and to minimize your risks.

Ethical and Social Issues

Since the early 1980s, the advent of the new reproductive technologies and the implantation of three to six embryos at a time have dramatically increased the numbers of multiple births. Between 1980 and 1998, the incidence of twin births has risen 49 percent, and the number of triplets and quadruplets has increased by 423 percent, according to the final data on births in the March 28, 2000, *National Vital Statistics Reports*. Women who undergo IVF or who receive donor eggs must contend with such daunting dilemmas as "reducing down to twins" (in the case of triplets or more), discarding or keeping "extra" frozen embryos, choosing an egg donor, or deciding whether or not to tell a child of his or her egg-donor origins.

Finding Strategies and Solutions

In this book, I tell the stories of women who meet the challenges of midlife pregnancy. Through personal anecdotes of midlife mothers, interviews with prominent doctors and research scientists, and a summary of current medical opinion,

I hope to provide mothers-to-be with useful strategies for dealing with everything from preconception planning to the first weeks of motherhood.

The Complete Guide to Pregnancy after 30 is divided into nine parts. Parts 1 and 2 focus on gearing up for pregnancy in terms of attitude, exercise and diet, medical care, and lifestyle. These sections also help you become your own health advocate; select qualified, supportive health care providers; and choose an appropriate birth setting (home, birth center, hospital).

Part 3 provides information on getting pregnant. This section will help you understand and come to terms with your biological clock; assess the benefits and risks of infertility treatments; sort through the medical and emotional issues involved with donor eggs; and cope with possible obstacles to pregnancy such as fibroid tumors, endometriosis, and hormonal imbalances.

Parts 4 and 5 focus on how you can take good care of yourself and your baby during pregnancy and manage or prevent potential risks. Part 5 also offers information on choosing genetic tests, finding an appropriate doctor and hospital if you are "high-risk," coping with pregnancy loss, managing bed rest, and recognizing potential medical emergencies.

Part 6 addresses the ups and downs of pregnancy and parenthood with twins, triplets, or more. Part 7 focuses on labor and birth as a normal process, while Part 8 explains childbirth variations or complications such as breech birth, prolonged labor, forceps deliveries, and cesarean section. Parts 7 and 8 offer strategies for labor and birth in mothers over age thirty-five, and Part 8 includes a comprehensive discussion of how to prepare for and recover from cesarean birth.

Part 9, "Motherhood," offers strategies for planning the first weeks and months of motherhood, recognizing that there is no "right way" to be a mother. Although mothering is a highly individual thing, women can gain from the experience of other midlife mothers. Because many of the women I spoke to had plunged into motherhood in their forties or fifties with few role models, I wrote this chapter to provide the uninitiated with numerous strategies for meshing motherhood with the rest of life: integrating a baby with career and primary relationships—or giving up a career to become a stay-at-home mom.

Part One

Changing Times, Changing Options

Chapter 1
Changing Perspectives: Midlife Mothers and Fathers

With older women, their desire for a baby is great. Their heart is in it, they are socio-economically well off, and their careers are in a better place to carve out plenty of time. They have the intention to love a child, the money to do it, and the time to do it.
—Dr. Mark Sauer, Professor and Vice Chairman of Obstetrics and Gynecology at Columbia University and Director of the Division of Reproductive Endocrinology at Columbia Presbyterian Medical Center in New York City

• • •

I haven't felt any downside of being older. Not one. I feel more connected than I was at thirty-five. I know I'm a better mother now than I would have been ten years ago. Not one time have I thought that I wished I'd had him ten years ago. My husband feels the same way. Being older, I have more perspective. I don't have to prove anything to anybody. I feel like I have more capacity now than I ever did. I don't have the anxieties that younger women have.
—Joanne, age fifty-three, mother of a four-year-old boy

• • •

The example set by more and more women becoming pregnant for the first time or second time at age thirty-five, forty-five, or fifty is changing attitudes not only about midlife pregnancy, but also about age in general. The biological clock is simply not what it used to be. Not only are women over thirty-five no longer considered "elderly," "geriatric," or "senescent" from an obstetrical point of view, but they are now barely middle-aged. Nowadays, from the point of view of many obstetricians and infertility specialists, thirty-five is young. For a growing minority, so is forty.

"I don't think forty is middle-aged anymore. Sixty is. My sister helped keep my mother [who gave birth in her forties] young," says Dr. Donna Kirz, Chairperson and Program Director of the Department of Obstetrics and Gynecology at Mercy Hospital, Chicago. Kirz, who directs the Residency Program in Maternal-Fetal Medicine, had two babies when she was in her forties. Kirz's confidence in midlife pregnancy developed early as she witnessed her mother's healthy pregnancy at age forty. "I saw what could be," says Kirz.

Nowadays, the term "middle age" conjures up associations that vary dramatically from the old stereotypes. Over the last two decades, middle age has gradually shifted from thirty-five to fifty or fifty-five. Retirement has become an equally fluid concept that now applies to a wider range of age groups—anywhere from forty to seventy-five.

In this context, the question, "How old is too old to have a baby?" elicits new answers. The clichés about getting older—becoming "set in your ways" and sedentary—are being challenged by the reality of women pregnant in their forties and fifties, of astronauts flying into space in their seventies, and of more and more people living into their nineties.

The women who are getting pregnant later in life are neither set in their ways nor sedentary—at least not after their babies are born. In fact, most of these women are flexible, energetic, and adapting to their new role as midlife parents with admirable resourcefulness. Frequently, women who choose to become pregnant in midlife feel that midlife is the best time for them to have a baby; they are more emotionally mature, confident, and financially stable than they were in their twenties or even their thirties.

Many midlife mothers have experienced years of personal freedom and consequently do not feel as constrained by a child as they might have when they were younger. Anna, who at age forty gave birth to her daughter, Julia, feels that her wide range of life experiences has helped her become a better mother. Before she became a mother, Anna had a variety of jobs: singer/songwriter, radio producer, family therapist. "I am more mature. I don't have issues about what I could have been if I weren't a mom. I don't feel I've missed anything," says Anna. For Anna, maturity also brings valuable self-control. "I don't just react. I'm not so impulse-oriented. I think of what I will say to Julia before I say it. I don't know if I would have done that in my twenties."

What comes as a surprise to both doctors and to the women and their partners is that midlife parents learn flexibility and find themselves becoming more adaptable "at their age" than they imagined possible. Miriam was thirty-eight when she gave birth to her first and only child, a daughter, and she believes her age and life experience made her a more giving mother than she would have been as a young mother. "It's nice being older because you've done a lot and you don't second-guess yourself. When you are younger you haven't explored and done what you wanted to do. You get more flexible, too, when you're older. You're at the stage of life where you're ready to be less selfish."

Even women who are accustomed to a large degree of

control over their lives may learn to loosen up and change their routine to include their new baby. Many find creative ways to integrate a baby into their lives without giving up biology field trips, Saturday night movies, or European travel. Some show admirable resourcefulness at juggling career and motherhood. Others surprise themselves—and everyone else in their lives—by walking away from blossoming careers to become full-time mothers.

Surprisingly, older parents often have ample energy for parenting. After Joanne became a mother for the first time at age forty-nine, her energy level increased. "I was energized after the baby was born. He never slept through the night. It didn't exhaust me at all. I was just so excited that it carried me. It's all going by much too fast. I love every second of it," says Joanne, whose son is four years old. Dr. Watson Bowes Jr., a father for the seventh time at age fifty, never lost his zest for child rearing, despite his demanding work as an obstetrician. "I was fifty when our youngest son was born. It was the greatest thing that ever happened to me. I love it. I love to go to baseball games and watch *Sesame Street*." Bowes thinks that keeping up with a toddler "isn't a problem" for a physically healthy person.

Late parenthood has changed the way women see their life stages and their futures. The future becomes simultaneously easier and more difficult: enriched by a developing child and complicated with handling a child's college expenses, one's own retirement, and one's own aging parents—all at the same time. Holly, who at age forty-eight is raising a twelve-year-old, often imagines a rosy future. However, she sometimes fears that she, and her husband, Dick, may become frail before their son Soren becomes settled in his own life. "Would we be able to get him through school and on his feet before he would have to take care of us?" Taking care of young children and their aging grandparents at the same time presents another potential difficulty for midlife parents. "I had a two-year-old and an eighty-four-year-old at the same time," says Leda, who, at age thirty-nine, was caring for both a toddler and an aging parent.

Although some women and medical experts still feel that pregnancy over thirty-five or forty is "too old," American society as a whole has responded well to the growing trend of later-in-life pregnancy. Many women expect negative reactions from family, friends, and strangers only to find themselves the source of inspiration, admiration, and, at worst, curiosity and a sense of being different from one's peers. Says Joanne, who was pregnant—and graying—at age forty-nine: "I expected a lot of negativity because of my age. But people surprised me. Strangers would come up to me and ask, 'How old are you?' I'd tell them I was forty-nine, and they'd say, 'Oh, thank you. You give me such hope.'" Holly was also pleased by other people's reactions. "I expected everyone to be guarded about my pregnancy. Not one person I told was guarded. Instead, people said, 'You know, older people are having babies. How old are you again?'"

Despite a generally positive reaction to her pregnancy by friends and strangers, Holly still felt that she had "different" needs than younger pregnant woman. "Older women need the support of other women in the same position. It's a special situation for older women getting pregnant," says Holly. "Seek out a birthing group or a childbirth preparation class with older women."

Getting pregnant in midlife is, as Holly says, special. If you are already pregnant or considering becoming pregnant, you may have few role models upon which to base your ways of managing your job, your daily workout, your relationship, your aging parents, and your career trajectory. If you feel ready but you haven't figured out all the details yet, this is normal. In fact, you must figure out many of the details as you go along. This is where the flexibility comes in. You are beginning a journey that will include improvisation and surprise. You cannot predict how you will feel in advance. You will not know for sure how you will deal with motherhood until you get there.

Shifting Medical Opinions

More and more literature has accumulated showing that late-in-life pregnancy is reasonable, practical, and safe.
—Dr. Mark Sauer

* * *

By the very act of getting pregnant and birthing babies in midlife, women have changed social stereotypes and medical opinion. Although some doctors remain uncomfortable about pregnancy over thirty-five and appalled at pregnancy over fifty, many doctors have come to respect the maturity, energy, and commitment of women who become later-in-life mothers.

"The new attitudes about pregnancy have been driven by the fact that more women over thirty-five are having babies," says Dr. Watson Bowes Jr., a recently retired professor of obstetrics at the University of North Carolina. The incidence of women over thirty-five successfully getting pregnant and giving birth has dramatically changed medical opinion. As a result, physicians define age and physical capacity differently than they did even ten years ago.

Ten years ago women over thirty-five automatically received the label "high risk," but these women are now treated with increasing medical optimism and nonchalance. However, women contemplating pregnancy in their late forties or their fifties still face a confusing array of conflicting medical opinion.

Some doctors, like Columbia University's Mark Sauer, claim that pregnancy from forty-five to fifty-five is reasonably safe and that the age-related complications that may occur can be managed with medication or bed rest. Over the last decade, Sauer has seen countless healthy pregnancies and babies in a population of fit, well-educated patients. However, Sauer sees the well-publicized pregnancies over age sixty as "setting the tone for unrealistic expectations."

Because pregnancy at forty-nine or fifty is rare, there have been few clinical studies on pregnancy over fifty. In fact, there is very little data on the subject of pregnancy over forty-five, since pregnancy at this age—especially pregnancy with a first baby—is not common enough for doctors to conduct large medical studies on it. According to Dr. Maria Bustillo, some preliminary studies in the mid-1990s at New York's Mount Sinai Hospital showed that physically fit women in their fifties fared as well in pregnancy as women in their forties. It was getting pregnant that posed the difficulty—not the pregnancy itself.

Although women in their forties and fifties are more likely to have preexisting medical conditions such as diabetes and high blood pressure than are younger women, and women in midlife are more likely to develop such complications as pregnancy-induced diabetes and high blood pressure, these conditions are usually treatable. According to recent medical studies, the odds of a woman between thirty-five and forty-five birthing a healthy baby are excellent.

However, although some doctors think pregnancy over forty is reasonably safe, many physicians believe that it is not ideal. Dr. Brooks Ranney, a retired professor of obstetrics and gynecology at the University of South Dakota, takes a conservative point of view: "The best time to have a baby is between the ages of twenty-five and thirty-five. This is ideal for the physiology to work." Dr. Allen Killam encourages women to get pregnant before age forty, since their fertility tends to decline dramatically around their mid- to late thirties. But he believes that the "best time" to get pregnant is different for each individual woman, although there is definitely a time limit. "There is, for each woman, an age after which she should not become pregnant," says Killam. "Deciding on that age is often difficult and complex. Ultimately each woman must decide for herself. Medical professionals should give good advice based on data, not just opinion, and only after a thorough evaluation of an individual's health and expectations."

Part Two

Preparing for Midlife Pregnancy

Chapter 2
Prepregnancy Health Plan

A woman who is forty should get prepregnancy counseling. She should be aware of any medical problem she has.
—Dr. Allen Killam, Professor Emeritus of Obstetrics and Gynecology at Duke University Medical School and former Chief, Division of Maternal-Fetal Medicine, Duke University Medical Center

◆ ◆ ◾

Although you may fear that going to see your doctor will bring "bad news," most of the time the information from your medical exam brings good news: that you are healthy and ready for pregnancy.

Having a thorough physical exam before you become pregnant can help you chart a course for improving your health, preventing possible age-related health problems, or identifying and managing pre-existing health conditions such as diabetes or high blood pressure so they will not interfere with your or your baby's health. In fact, taking care of yourself early on may facilitate your getting pregnant, staying pregnant, and giving birth to a healthy baby.

The preconception period—the weeks or months before

you get pregnant—is an excellent time to take care of any routine health maintenance that is appropriate for you given your age and medical history. Have you had a recent mammogram; pap smear; dental exam; EKG or cardiac stress test; nutrition assessment; blood pressure screening; or blood tests for high cholesterol, diabetes, and anemia? If not, see a good doctor, tell him or her that you wish to become pregnant, and discuss whatever testing or planning you may need to do in advance.

Your Medical Profile

Your medical profile, which includes your current health as well as your medical history, will determine a health plan that is appropriate for you. Tell your health care provider about your reproductive and medical history; pertinent family medical history; infectious disease exposure; and lifestyle concerns such as exercise, stress, smoking, exposure to heat, cold, or extremes of altitude, and exposure to chemicals such as herbicides or industrial chemicals.

Family Medical History

Discuss with your doctor your family medical history. Include a family history of twins, allergies, and conditions such as diabetes, early heart disease or stroke, high blood pressure, breast cancer, other cancers, and genetic abnormalities. If your family has a history of genetic problems, ask your doctor for a referral for genetic counseling (see Chapter 12). If you have had three or more miscarriages, have been exposed to hazardous chemicals or radiation that can affect your baby, or are in a high-risk ethnic group for diseases like sickle cell anemia or Tay-Sachs disease, you may benefit from genetic counseling. Tell your doctor if you have a history of late-in-life motherhood or premature menopause in your family.

If your mother took the drug diethylstilbestrol (DES) when she was pregnant with you (especially if she took the drug during her first trimester of pregnancy), you will need a pelvic exam and pap smear before you become pregnant. You also will need to see your doctor frequently during pregnancy to check your cervix for premature dilation. Women prenatally exposed to DES may face greater risk of miscarriage due to a weak or "incompetent" cervix or a small, T-shaped uterus.

Past Pregnancies and Reproductive Surgeries

Obtain your past medical records of any uterine, ovarian, or tubal surgeries since these reports may determine how your caregiver manages your pregnancy and childbirth. For instance, if you have had fibroids removed from your uterus, it is essential that your doctor know whether or not your uterine cavity was cut through—or "entered"—during the surgery. A surgical incision that goes through certain parts of the uterine muscle to the cavity may weaken your uterus so that cesarean delivery becomes the safest way to birth your baby.

Previous Surgeries or Blood Transfusions

If you have had any blood transfusions or previous surgeries, tell your doctor.

Drinking, Smoking, and Recreational Drug Use

If you are or have been a smoker, drinker, or recreational drug user, tell your doctor, even though you may find such disclosures embarrassing. Alcohol and other drugs can adversely affect your baby's health and lead to preterm labor, mental retardation, physical abnormalities, low birth weight, fetal alcohol syndrome (FAS), or to babies addicted to drugs at birth. Alcohol, smoking, and recreational drug use also may create health complications for you during pregnancy (see Chapter 3).

Infectious Disease Exposures

If you have been exposed to Lyme disease, hepatitis, measles, toxoplasmosis (a disease sometimes carried by outdoor cats), or various tropical diseases or parasites, tell your doctor. Your doctor may also want to test you for exposure to common infectious diseases such as herpes, cytomegalovirus, or chlamydia. Many of these illnesses may be easily treated before you get pregnant but are more difficult to safely treat after you become pregnant. Furthermore, the treatments for some of these illnesses may involve medications that could be harmful to your baby.

Travel

If you have recently spent time in the tropics or in developing countries, ask your care provider if you should be tested for malaria, intestinal parasites, tuberculosis, or other diseases to which you may have been exposed.

Common Preconception and Prenatal Medical Tests

You can't control the course of your entire pregnancy, but you can make the course a smoother, calmer one by taking care of some important medical tasks before you get pregnant. Get a complete physical exam that includes a breast exam, pelvic and cervical exam, height, weight, blood pressure, and appropriate medical tests. Some diseases interfere with getting pregnant or staying pregnant, and treating such problems can help you achieve and maintain pregnancy.

Although some of these medical tests should be done during pregnancy, others should be done before you get pregnant. Are you due for a mammogram within the year? If so, have it done before you get pregnant since exposure to x-rays is best avoided once you are already pregnant. If the mammogram reveals a cyst or other problem, it is best to find it and treat if before you get pregnant and thus save yourself from additional worry or medical procedures during pregnancy. However, if you have breast problems that may require a mammogram during pregnancy, you can protect the baby by using a lead apron over your belly. Consult with your physician before having any x-rays during pregnancy.

If you are nearing fifty and are due for a colonoscopy, schedule the test one or two menstrual cycles before you try to get pregnant. If you need barium colon x-rays or diagnostic x-rays of the abdomen or low back, get these tests done one or two menstrual cycles before you try to conceive. However, if diagnostic x-rays are necessary during the course of your pregnancy, ask your care provider to discuss with you the benefits and risks of the procedure.

Attend to dental problems before pregnancy, especially if you require root canal work, fillings, anesthesia, or any procedure that may cause infection.

Common Prepregnancy and Prenatal Medical Tests

Mammogram—An x-ray exam of the breasts that screens for breast cancer and cysts.

Gynecological exam—Pelvic exam, pap smear, breast exam, routine blood test for syphilis (some care providers also take additional cultures or blood tests to screen for sexually transmitted diseases like HIV, herpes, and chlamydia).

Complete physical examination—Blood pressure, pulse, height, weight, and overall exam of head, neck, thorax, abdomen, reflexes, and so on.

Routine Blood Tests

Rh type and screening for irregular antibodies.
Complete blood count (CBC)—Includes tests to check for anemia, infections, and blood abnormalities.
Rubella titer—For German measles.
Fasting blood sugar or random blood sugar.
Glucose tolerance test—Part of prenatal exam that tests for diabetes or pregnancy-induced diabetes (see Part 5).

Additional Blood Tests for Women at Risk For:

Hepatitis B and C.
High cholesterol—Especially if you are over fifty.
Genetic screening—If you belong to certain ethnic groups that are at risk for genetic conditions, you may need screening for some of the following diseases:

Cystic fibrosis: a serious condition that affects the mucous membranes, especially of the lungs, and is found in many different ethnic groups.
Sickle cell anemia: a painful blood disease found in people of African-American or Mediterranean descent.
Tay-Sachs disease: a serious medical condition found in some Ashkenazi Jews and French Canadians.
Thalassemia: a blood disease found in people of Mediterranean or Asian descent.

Toxoplasmosis screening—This is not routine, although it is recommended if you are exposed to outdoor cats or if you work in a garden frequented by neighborhood cats.

Urine Tests

Protein levels.
Urine culture—For bacteria (part of prenatal exam).

Additional Tests

Tuberculosis screening—Skin tests and/or x-rays if you are at risk.
Group B Strep—Part of prenatal exam to test for the presence of certain bacteria in the vagina.
EKG or cardiac stress test—For preconception exam if you have symptoms of heart problems, are at risk, or are over fifty.

Managing Pre-existing Medical Conditions

The longer you postpone pregnancy, the greater your chances of developing any number of medical conditions before you get pregnant. The most common age-related conditions are diabetes, high blood pressure, heart or artery disease, and obesity. Less serious problems include back pain and arthritis, although both can lead to pain and temporary disability.

Such prepregnancy medical conditions need not keep you from a healthy pregnancy and baby, since most preexisting conditions can be controlled by medication or diet and lifestyle changes. However, it is best for you and the baby if you control your medical condition *before* you conceive.

If you are taking medications for a chronic illness, discuss your plans for pregnancy with your care provider to determine if any of the medications you are taking may pose dangers to your developing baby. Your care provider may change your medications to those that will not endanger your baby. (See the discussion of medications beginning on page 22.)

Diabetes

If you have diabetes, work with your care provider to control your diabetes with a proper diet or a combination of diet and insulin—before you become pregnant. Oral diabetic medications are not recommended during pregnancy (see Part 5).

Heart Disease, Circulatory Problems, High Blood Pressure

If you have heart disease or any medical condition that affects your veins, arteries, or blood flow, consult your doctor before you become pregnant because pregnancy increases your blood volume about 40 percent and puts greater stress on your heart and blood vessels. The decision about whether or not to have a baby is ultimately yours, but to make a truly informed choice you need to understand the ways in which your medical condition can or cannot be managed and the problems you may face during the course of your pregnancy.

If you have high blood pressure, make sure you bring your blood pressure under control before you conceive, since uncontrolled high blood pressure can lead to serious problems for both you and your baby, such as premature labor, bleeding, placental abruption, and emergency cesarean section. Fortunately, high blood pressure often can be controlled with medication. However, since some of these medications are not recommended for pregnant women, you may need to switch to different drugs that are safe to use during pregnancy (see "Medications" on page 23).

The information gathered from a thorough preconception medical exam can help you plan for your pregnancy and anticipate such possibilities as changing your diet, decreasing your workload, taking time off from your job, beginning a moderate exercise program, seeking genetic counseling, or creating a support system of family and friends.

Obesity

Because obesity predisposes you to many health problems including back pain, high blood pressure, and cardiovascular disease, it is important that you manage your weight and your diet before and during pregnancy. Obesity may also pose risks to the baby. Paying attention to your weight, however, does not mean obsessing about a few extra pounds if you are an average weight to begin with. It is normal—and healthy—for a woman of average weight to gain twenty-five to thirty pounds during pregnancy. To grow a healthy baby requires fluid, protein, vitamins, and some fat (see Part 4).

Back and Joint Problems

Pregnancy can aggravate pre-existing back problems, especially degenerative disc problems, sciatica, or inflammations of the sacroiliac joint. When you are pregnant your ligaments loosen, your center of gravity changes, and your back takes on the additional weight load of your pregnant body. However, some of these problems can be minimized or prevented by:

- gentle exercises to strengthen the back and stomach muscles prior to pregnancy
- therapeutic massage
- physical therapy
- good posture and body mechanics at home and at work
- yoga (take a class designed for pregnant women)

Managing Pre-existing Depression

I believe that infertility causes depression and the depression, in turn, contributes to infertility.

—Dr. Alice Domar, Director of the Mind/Body Center for Women's Health at the Mind/Body Medical Institute, Beth

Israel Deaconess Medical Center, Harvard Medical School

❖ ❖ ❖

If you have had trouble becoming pregnant, have had frequent miscarriages, are undergoing stressful treatments for infertility, and are depressed, you may wish to include a support group or a "mind/body" group as a part of your preconception health plan. According to Dr. Alice Domar, a Harvard Medical School researcher and Director of the Mind/Body Center for Women's Health, the impact of stress and depression on the reproductive system "may adversely affect ovulation, fertilization, tubal function, or implantation [of a fertilized egg]."

"There's increasing evidence that depression may contribute to infertility. Women with a history of depression have twice the infertility rates of women without a history of depression," says Domar. Several studies have shown that depressed women who attended support groups or "mind/body" groups experienced increased fertility. Domar's own study, published in the April 2000 edition of the medical journal *Fertility and Sterility,* showed that both support groups and mind/body groups designed to manage depression enhanced a woman's ability to become pregnant and maintain a healthy pregnancy. The study found that women who participated in the ten-week groups had over twice the pregnancy rates of depressed women who did not participate in the groups.

For the purposes of her study, Domar led two different kinds of groups: regular support groups and "mind/body" groups. The mind/body groups were based on the philosophy that the way your mind feels affects your body, and the way your body feels affects your mind. The women assigned to the mind/body groups learned relaxation techniques such as guided imagery and meditation to help mind and body work together to relieve depression and achieve pregnancy. In the regular support groups, women shared their feelings about pregnancy and offered one another understanding and moral support.

Dr. Domar's study showed that both kinds of groups increased pregnancy rates. Pregnancy rates were highest—55 percent—among women in the "mind/body" group, and 54 percent in the standard support group. Of the women not participating in either group, only 20 percent became pregnant.

Medications, Alternative Home Remedies, Vitamins, and Herbal Remedies

In general, drugs are available by prescription because they are powerful chemical substances that cause almost as many problems as they cure. It's only logical that some of these medications could cause trouble for the developing fetus. Pregnant women should be the world's most reluctant consumers of prescription medication . . .
—Joe Graedon and Teresa Graedon, *The People's Pharmacy*

• • •

If you are taking any medications for a chronic illness, make sure you speak with your health care provider before trying to become pregnant. There are definitely women who will need to make changes in their medications and shift over to different medicines. For instance, pregnant women should stay away from ACE inhibitors [enalapril, captropril], muscle relaxants, and all nonsteroidal anti-inflammatory drugs [aspirin, ibuprofen, naproxen].
—Dr. Susan Porto

• • •

You may have self-prescribed your medications for the last fifteen years but don't do it during pregnancy. All your medications should be prescribed through your doctor.
—Dr. Gideon Koren, Director of Motherisk and Professor of Pediatrics and Medical Genetics at the University of Toronto

* * *

Medications

"I think the wise thing is to take the perspective of: don't take anything that you really don't need," advises Dr. Sandra Kweder, the Deputy Director of the Pregnancy Labeling Task Force at the FDA.

If you are healthy and do not need to take medicines, avoid taking medications during pregnancy since few medicines are considered absolutely safe during pregnancy. However, if you have a serious medical condition, avoiding drugs may be riskier than taking them. For instance, if you have epilepsy, high blood pressure, asthma, clinical depression, or chronic diabetes, you may need to take medications during your pregnancy, although your doctor may suggest discontinuing some medications and switching to other ones that are safer for your developing baby. In some cases, your doctor may recommend that you switch drugs *before* you become pregnant. After you are pregnant, your doctor may change your dose of medicine to compensate for the changes in your pregnant body or to protect your baby.

Do not discontinue medications that you take for chronic medical conditions unless your doctor asks you to. Although many medications may pose some risk during pregnancy, the disease for which you are taking medication may also pose risks for you and your baby. For instance, epilepsy and chronic diabetes pose dangers to the developing fetus, and stopping your medicines may create serious problems.

But how do you and your care provider weigh the benefits and risks of taking medicine during pregnancy? Your doctor's solution to this touchy situation will be choosing the drug that poses the least risk to the baby while still effectively treating your medical problem. You can participate in the decision by gathering information from books and articles on drugs during pregnancy or by using Internet Web sites like those of Motherisk or Reprotox (see appendix for references) to find the most recent medical information on drug risks. The ultimate decision about drugs will depend on how you and your doctor view your unique circumstances—your medical condition, your pregnancy, the drug, and the age of the fetus.

Often your doctor's decision will involve "a judgment call" based on what is known about the risks and benefits of various drugs, explains Dr. Kweder. "You compare the toxicity of the drug with what it is you are treating," explains Kweder. "Is it something that's a minor annoyance? Or is it something that the mom really needs to be treated for? To me, that's the crux of the issue in patient and physician decision making. We all look for absolutes—for the magic list that tells us 'no'—and there are very few things that are 'absolute always no' or 'absolute always O.K.'"

One of the few "absolute nevers," says Kweder, is Accutane, an acne medication that is known to cause birth defects. Since acne is not life threatening for the mother, the risks of taking the drug during pregnancy far outweigh the benefits.

Medications that cause birth defects and interfere with the development or function of the baby's organs are called teratogens. These medications must be avoided during critical stages of the baby's development. Some of these medications fall into the "absolute never" category, and some should be taken only when no other good options exist. Many teratogenic medications are most dangerous to a fetus during the first trimester of pregnancy when the baby's organs are forming, although some medications must be avoided in the second and third trimester as well.

According to Dr. Kenneth L. Jones, Professor of Pediatrics at the University of California, San Diego, the majority of medicines have not been adequately tested to know for certain what the risks to a fetus may be. "The teratogenic potential of most agents [drugs] is unknown. Whereas only a few agents have been shown to be teratogenic in humans, the majority have not been adequately tested; this creates an obvious dilemma for the physician attempting to provide optimum care for pregnant women," writes Jones in his chapter on "Effects of Therapeutic Diagnostic, and Environmental Agents" in *Maternal-Fetal Medicine*. Although he adds that "no easy answer seems forthcoming," Jones suggests that doctors include pregnant women in the decision process and "provide all pregnant women with all the facts available regarding the teratogenic potential of any drug, chemical, or environmental agent to which they are exposed."

You can do some of the research yourself by using such resources as *The Physicians' Desk Reference* and Internet sources such as Reprotox and Motherisk.

A Partial List of Drugs Currently Known or Suspected to Be Teratogenic or Fetotoxic in Pregnancy

For a more complete list, contact Motherisk (*www.motherisk.org*), Reprotox (*www.reprotox.org*), or call the Teratology Information Services (TERIS) at 888-285-3410. These organizations are an excellent resource for the latest information on drug risks. Here is a list of drugs with potential toxic or teratogenic effects.

ACE inhibitors (may be safe during first trimester): Kidney problems

Accutane (and other systemic retinoids): Central nervous system, head and face, and cardiovascular defects

Alcohol: Neuro-developmental problems

Androgens: Masculinization

Cancer drugs such as Cyclophosphamide and Methotrexate: Fetal malformations

Carbemazepine (Tegretol): Neural tube defects

Diethylstilbestrol (DES): Vaginal cancer, genital/urinary defects

Lithium: Epstein anomaly (heart defects)

Methimazole: Thyroid-related problems in the fetus

Phenytoin: Central nervous system defects

Tetracycline: Abnormalities of bone and teeth

Thalidomide: Limb reduction defects, internal organ defects

Valproic acid: Neural tube defects

Warfarin: Skeletal and central nervous system defects

Sources: Dr. Sandra Kweder, in *Medical Care of the Pregnant Patient*, Lee (ed), American College of Physicians, 2000; Dr. Gideon Koren, Motherisk.

Pharmaceutical drugs are not responsible for the majority of birth defects. However, few drugs are considered absolutely safe in pregnancy. Sometimes the timing of drug exposure—during which trimester you take the drug—is an important factor in whether a drug can damage your developing baby.

There is ongoing debate among scientists and physicians about what drugs are safe and unsafe during pregnancy. Even those drugs approved by the FDA often have not been thoroughly tested in pregnant women due to possible risks to the baby. However, the FDA does rank drug safety by a system of "categories" (A, B, C, D, and X) that are based on a combination of animal experiments, clinical trials on human subjects, and clinical medical experience. These categories offer some guidance but no absolutes, since new scientific findings often make the rankings out of date.

If you are taking medications for any of the following medical conditions, you will need to talk with your doctor about whether or not you should change medications when you become pregnant.

Blood Pressure and Heart Medications

If you have been taking medication for high blood pressure or heart disease, you probably will need to continue taking medications during pregnancy, although your doctor may want you to change to a different medicine that is safer for your baby. Consult your doctor about whether you should change the drugs or dosage *before* attempting to become pregnant. For instance, certain drugs prescribed for high blood pressure or kidney disease, called ACE inhibitors, are safe for adults but are known to cause kidney damage in the fetus. If you are taking ACE inhibitors such as captopril (Capoten), enalapril (Vasotec), lisinopril (Prinivil, Zestril), quinapril (Accupril), ramipril (Altace), or trandolapril (Mavik), your physician may put you on a different drug during your pregnancy.

If you are taking blood thinners such as Warfarin (Coumadin), you may need to change drugs during pregnancy. Consult your doctor regarding the risks and benefits of different medications for your medical condition.

Diabetes Medications

If you have diabetes and are taking oral hypoglycemic agents such as chlorpropamide, glipizide, glyburide, tolazamide, and tolbutamide, your physician may switch you to insulin before you become pregnant and keep you on insulin throughout your pregnancy, since insulin is safer than the oral drugs currently on the market.

Hormonal Medications

Hormonal medications should be used only after discussing the risks and benefits with your physician and pharmacist. If you get pregnant while taking the following hormonal drugs, call your doctor at once to see if you should discontinue the medication:

- estradiol/norethindrone (Activell, Combi-Patch)
- conjugated estrogens/medroxyprogesterone (Prempro)
- birth-control pills
- Lupron
- estrogens
- progesterones
- other hormonal therapies

Do not take fertility drugs unless you are sure you are *not pregnant*. Never take diethylstilbestrol (DES) during pregnancy (see Chapter 7).

Migraine Medications

You may need to change your migraine medications during pregnancy. If you are taking Imitrex or some of the older ergotamine migraine drugs, you may need to change to Tylenol or to lower doses of other migraine medications. Discuss your headache problem with your doctor to find the best solution for you. In some women, migraines become less problematic during pregnancy, and you may actually require fewer medications. However, if your migraines continue, ask your physician about safe medication during pregnancy.

Epilepsy Medications

If you have epilepsy, you need to continue on medications that keep your epilepsy under control during pregnancy.

However, you need to carefully discuss with your doctor the risks posed by your epilepsy and the drugs taken to control it. Some antiepileptic drugs such as phenytoin (Dilantin), carbamazepine (Tegretol), and valproic acid (Depakene, Depakote, Depacon) have been shown to cause birth defects. For instance, Dilantin has been shown to cause facial abnormalities in babies, and valproic acid has been shown to cause spina bifida in 1 percent to 2 percent of the babies exposed in utero. However, uncontrolled epilepsy may also cause some birth defects since women suffer oxygen deprivation while having epileptic seizures, and the lack of oxygen may adversely affect the baby. Consequently, you will need to work with your doctor to find the safest epilepsy medication that is effective for you, and you will need to be closely monitored during your pregnancy.

Medications for Depression, Anxiety, and Other Psychiatric Problems

If you are taking lithium (Eskalith, Lithobid, Lithonate), or if you are mildly depressed or anxious, talk to your doctor about gradually tapering off your medications during pregnancy. However, if you are prone to severe depression or manic depression, the benefits of taking the drugs may outweigh the risks, and you may need to stay on medication during pregnancy.

Discuss your medications with both your obstetrician and prescribing psychiatrist to carefully evaluate the medications that best suit your needs during pregnancy. You may also benefit by consulting a pediatrician, since a pediatrician may be familiar with drug effects on a newborn infant as well as a fetus. Infants may develop withdrawal symptoms from some antidepressants and other psychiatric medications.

Acne and Skin Medications

Isotretinoin, otherwise known as Accutane, is an acne medication that causes birth defects and is dangerous to your baby. Do not use this drug if you are trying to become pregnant! If you find you are pregnant while taking this drug, discontinue it immediately and consult your doctor.

Pain Medications

Nonsteroidal anti-inflammatory drugs may cause serious problems for your baby. Studies show these drugs can cause closure of the ductus arteriosis, the blood vessel connecting the baby's heart and lungs. Acetaminophen is safer than these drugs and recommended if you need relief for aches and pains. For more severe pain, codeine is relatively safe, although if you take it frequently during pregnancy, the drug may cause withdrawal symptoms in your baby.

Pregnancy Drug Precautions

1. Avoid unnecessary medications during your first trimester of pregnancy.
2. Consult with your physicians regarding medications you should take or avoid when you are trying to conceive or when you become pregnant.
3. Make sure your care provider is aware of *all* the drugs—over the counter, prescription, and herbal—that you are using.
4. For pain relief, seek simple home remedies before you take medication, and consult your doctor about any prescription or over-the-counter medication before taking it.
5. Use all medications in moderation and in the dosages recommended by your care provider.

Alternative Home Remedies

For many simple medical problems such as colds, coughs, headaches, backaches, nausea, heartburn, constipation, muscle aches and pains, and some allergies, you often can find non-medicinal therapies that provide a useful alternative to drugs.

Colds and Coughs, Sinus Problems, Hay Fever

Home remedies can relieve some of the congestion of colds and coughs. To ease the nasal irritation and congestion of a cold or cough, stand in a steamy shower or bathroom or use a humidifier or vaporizer. Drink tea (or hot water) with honey and lemon, and rest—before you turn to systemic medications such as decongestants or antihistamines. If you have chronically congested sinuses, apply saline lavages or nose drops. However, if you think you may have a sinus infection, see your doctor since you may need antibiotics.

Try home remedies to treat allergy symptoms. Some people find acupuncture to be helpful. However, if you have serious allergic reactions such as asthma, talk to your doctor about how to treat your medical condition during your pregnancy.

Headache

Some women find that their headaches diminish during pregnancy, but some experience increased headaches. To stave off a headache before it becomes fierce, try relaxation exercises, meditation, biofeedback, visualization techniques, yoga, a warm (not hot) bath or shower, a heating pad or ice pack wrapped around the back of your neck or shoulders, acupressure points on the top of your hands, or all of the above. For some people, massage, acupuncture, acupressure, yoga, or tai chi are useful in preventing headaches.

If you develop headaches from posture problems or previous neck injuries, your doctor may suggest physical therapy.

Backaches

Backaches are common during pregnancy. To prevent backaches and to keep flexible, try massage, yoga, or a relaxing swim. For back pain, try ice wrapped in a warm cloth or heat (whichever works for you). Sleep with a pillow under or between your knees. Acupuncture and acupressure are useful treatments for back pain, although they may not give relief from more serious orthopedic problems such as slipped or ruptured discs. For persistent back pain or searing sciatic pain that shoots into your hip, leg, or foot, see your care provider.

Sprains

To relieve the pain and swelling of a sprain, apply ice packs (or a bag of frozen peas since it adjusts to the shape of your ankle, shoulder, knee, and so on) and elevate your limb. If pain and swelling persist, see your doctor.

Nausea

Try ginger tea, ginger ale, or crackers. Sometimes nausea worsens when your stomach is empty, so try nibbling crackers or dry cereal throughout the day if necessary. Some women find that antinausea wristbands, acupressure, or hypnosis provide some relief from pregnancy-related nausea.

If you are vomiting, stay hydrated by drinking plenty of water, Gatorade, or 7-Up. For persistent nausea and vomiting, see your doctor.

Some physicians recommend vitamin B_6 for nausea. Before taking any vitamin supplement, consult with your care provider.

Heartburn

Avoid fatty or fried foods and eat several small meals throughout the day rather than three large ones. If heartburn is severe, eat bland foods rather than highly seasoned ones.

Constipation

Eat plenty of fiber-rich foods such as fresh fruit and vegetables, bran, prunes, and prune juice. However, taking in fibrous foods such as prunes without drinking *plenty of water* can turn your stool to stone. Make sure you drink at least eight glasses of water a day, and engage in moderate exercise such as walking.

Insomnia

If you can't sleep, try relaxation exercises, relaxation tapes, or self-hypnosis.

Mild Depression or Anxiety

Exercise has been shown to decrease some forms of depression. If you are depressed, try gentle exercise (walking, swimming), guided imagery, and/or meditation; sometimes, combining two or more of these remedies works best. For depression that persists or interferes with your daily life, join a support group, see an experienced psychotherapist, or both.

Vitamins

You may think of vitamins as healthy and benign, but some vitamins, when taken in high dosages, pose dangers to developing fetuses (e.g., vitamin A). Do not take more than 5,000 IUs of vitamin A per day, since high dosages of vitamin A can cause birth defects.

Herbal Remedies

Herbal remedies are not necessarily safe just because they are "natural." St. John's Wort, for instance, is not safe during pregnancy. Some herbal medicines can cause abortion, and some may be toxic to delicate fetal tissues. Double-check all herbal remedies with your care provider. Western medicine is only beginning to investigate the use of herbs and to identify their beneficial and harmful qualities. Currently, herbs considered *unsafe* during pregnancy include: blue or black cohosh, pennyroyal leaf, yarrow, goldenseal, feverfew, psyllium seed, mugwort, coltsfoot, comfrey, juniper, rue, tansy, cottonroot bark, large amounts of sage, senna, cascara sagrada, buckthorn, male fern, slippery elm, and squaw vine. Avoid them. Do not self-medicate even if you are accustomed to an herbal remedy, since most herbal medicines have not been carefully studied regarding use during pregnancy.

Vaccinations and Immunizations

Avoid "live vaccines" such as the oral polio vaccine or the German measles (rubella), mumps, measles, chicken pox (varicella), and yellow fever vaccines during pregnancy and during the three to four months before you conceive.

Some vaccines, such as influenza, tetanus, and diphtheria, are considered safe during pregnancy. However, consult your doctor before receiving any vaccination to make sure that it is necessary.

If you anticipate becoming pregnant, get a rubella titer (a test to see if you have ever had the German measles); if the test is negative, indicating that you have never had rubella, many care providers recommend that you get vaccinated at least four months *before* you become pregnant. If you are exposed to rubella, mumps, or chicken pox during the course of your pregnancy, consult your doctor immediately.

Chapter 3

Lifestyle

Ask yourself how committed you are to the goal of being pregnant, since you will face some lifestyle changes.
—Dr. Katherine Shaw, high-risk pregnancy specialist, White Memorial Hospital, Los Angeles

* * *

Once you become pregnant, you may need to make significant changes in your lifestyle to ensure the health of the developing baby. If in your life before conception you skipped meals, ate junk food, and slid through your day fueled by caffeine and adrenaline, you will need to make some major adjustments in order to grow a healthy baby.

Your Baby Is What You Eat, Drink, and Smoke

Once you become pregnant it is important to take good care of yourself since what you eat, drink, inhale, and experience may profoundly affect your baby and shape her potential as a human being. The food you eat builds the baby's organs, muscles, and bones. If you smoke, drink, or use drugs, your baby will share with you all substances that manage to get into your blood-stream and cross her placenta. Many of the chemicals in alcoholic drinks, cigarette smoke, and recreational drugs pose dangers to babies in utero.

To grow a healthy baby and prepare yourself for the physical demands of pregnancy, birth, and motherhood you will need to conserve your energy and to minimize stress. Do not underestimate your need for both physical and emotional nurturing during this time, since you are eating for two and, quite literally, "growing" a baby. Although the process of pregnancy and birth is a normal one, you must provide nurturing for two in order for the whole process of pregnancy and birth to work at its optimum.

Include moderate exercise as part of your new pregnancy lifestyle, since exercise increases your blood circulation and thus brings important nutrients and oxygen to your baby's developing body. Exercise can also help you prevent constipation, diminish depression, and increase your stamina for the demands of pregnancy and birth. However, excessive exercise may make you more vulnerable to injury. Some studies in women athletes show that excessively vigorous exercise affects ovulation and menstruation and may decrease fertility.

Include sources of social support in your pregnancy lifestyle. Although you may be active and independent throughout most of your pregnancy, there may be times when you need support from family and friends. Such support people are especially important during labor and the first weeks of motherhood, but you may also need to rely on friends, partners, or family members during periods of morning sickness, bad pain, or bed rest.

Nutrition

"It is before most women know that they're pregnant that

their baby's organs are being formed. I started taking prenatal vitamins several months before I tried to conceive," says Dr. Donna Kirz. Nutrition is important before you get pregnant as well as afterward, since "before" is that murky time between your last ovulation and the implantation of an embryo that will become your baby. Start taking prenatal vitamins when you start trying to get pregnant.

Your nutrition at the time of conception influences the health of your baby. For instance, you can significantly reduce your baby's risk of neural tube defects (spina bifida) if you take about 0.4 mg/day of folic acid.

Alcohol

Most of us have heard about fetal alcohol syndrome (FAS) and the facial abnormalities, growth retardation, behavioral abnormalities, and mental and physical disabilities in babies whose mothers drink even a little too much. The alcohol levels in the baby's blood equal the level in the mother's blood, and as few as two ounces of alcohol a day have been associated with problems for the baby. Dr. Robert Andres, in *Maternal-Fetal Medicine,* cautions pregnant women against drinking: "Although it is generally agreed that heavy alcohol use places the patient at significant risk for a delivery of a low birth weight baby or an infant with FAS, a 'safe' level of alcohol consumption has not been determined. . . . At present, there is no clear minimum threshold for the effects of alcohol on the fetus, and pregnant women should be counseled to abstain from its use."

Researchers have found that a baby's prenatal exposure to moderate amounts of alcohol may result in a variety of problems, including growth deficiencies and central nervous system abnormalities. Women who drink during pregnancy also are more prone to premature delivery and spontaneous abortion than women who don't drink.

Caffeine

Drink only moderate amounts of coffee when you are pregnant. Once you are pregnant, your baby will get a direct hit from the coffee or tea that may be part of your routine two, three, or four times a day.

"Having more than seven to eight cups may be associated with low birth weight, spontaneous abortions, still births, and prematurity," says Dr. Susan Porto. If you are trying to get pregnant or are already pregnant, you may need to modify—though not stop—your intake of caffeine.

Some studies show that drinking more than 300 mg/day of caffeine—which translates to three to four cups of coffee—may increase your baby's risk of fetal growth delay. Other studies give conflicting results about the relationship between coffee and low birth weight and spontaneous abortion. Because no one knows for sure how much coffee is safe during pregnancy, your care provider may recommend limiting your coffee intake to less than seven cups a day.

Smoking

"Smoking and age are a bad combination that can lead to a combination of abruption, placenta previa, or preterm labor. If you can quit smoking, you get around most problems. If you are over thirty-five, stop smoking. Then get pregnant," advises Dr. Allen Killam.

Many women planning pregnancy do not realize that smoking can create serious problems for both mother and child—and even more problems if the mother is over thirty-five. Smoking during pregnancy can lead to premature birth, low birth weight, serious placental problems (see Parts 5 and 8), and sudden infant death syndrome (SIDS).

If your partner or friends smoke, secondhand smoke may also create problems for your baby by contributing to a reduction in placental blood flow and a greater risk for a premature or low birth weight baby.

Smoking produces carbon monoxide that enters the baby's bloodstream, binds to its blood, and reduces the amount of oxygen circulating through the baby's body. In addition, smoking reduces uterine blood flow. The result is that the baby no longer receives the necessary amounts of oxygen and other nutrients, leading to low birth weight and growth retardation. In fact, in a 1980 report, the surgeon general stated that maternal smoking was responsible for 20 percent to 40 percent of all low birth weight infants.

If you quit smoking during your first trimester of pregnancy, your chances of having a low birth weight baby are significantly reduced. Reducing the number of cigarettes per day lowers some of your risks but not as dramatically as stopping smoking. Consequently, if you are a smoker, you may want to stop smoking before you become pregnant and to include a smoking cessation program in your prepregnancy health plan.

Some studies show that both smoking and drinking may decrease male fertility; consequently, your partner may want to decrease his cigarette consumption when you are trying to get pregnant.

Recreational Drugs

Cocaine

"Cocaine is nasty," warns Dr. Susan Porto, referring to the potential damage to mother and child caused by maternal cocaine use during pregnancy. Mothers who use cocaine show an increased risk of placental abruption, which sometimes creates medical emergencies for both mother and baby.

Pregnant women who use cocaine may develop irregular heartbeats and, in extremes cases, they may have strokes.

Cocaine also endangers a woman's pregnancy. The drug constricts uterine blood circulation, limiting the amount of blood going to the placenta and baby; this lack of circulation can trigger a placental abruption (in which the placenta separates from the uterus), preterm labor and delivery, premature rupture of the membranes, or spontaneous abortion.

Maternal cocaine use has been associated with problems for the baby such as low birth weight and fetal growth restriction. Cocaine-exposed babies may also be more prone to SIDS.

Cocaine can damage the baby's central nervous system, causing behavioral abnormalities such as sleeping and feeding problems. Babies exposed to cocaine may be difficult to comfort.

Marijuana

The effects of maternal marijuana use on the fetus is the subject of debate. Although several studies suggest an association between maternal marijuana use and low birth weight babies, other studies show no association between marijuana use and low birth weight babies.

Speed

Women who use amphetamine and methamphetamine face increased risks for having low birth weight babies. Studies also suggest that prenatal exposure to amphetamines may cause central nervous system problems in the baby.

Heroin and Other Opiates

Women who take opiates during pregnancy may give birth to premature babies; these babies may be born with such problems as fetal growth restriction, depressed Apgar scores, decreased head circumference, and neonatal withdrawal. Heroin crosses the placenta, and addiction is common in the babies of heroin-addicted mothers.

Withdrawal in heroin- and methadone-exposed newborns, otherwise known as neonatal abstinence syndrome (NAS), may result in restlessness, sneezing, sleeplessness, sweating, and fever; later in life, the children may develop behavioral problems.

Exercise

Pregnancy is a physical feat, like running a marathon, only it is a normal challenge that your body is designed to meet—even if you are over forty.

When you are pregnant, your blood volume increases by 40 percent to 50 percent, making your heart and cardiovascular system work hard. Consequently, exercise that increases your stamina, strength, and flexibility prepares you for pregnancy just as it prepares you for a strenuous athletic event, like running a marathon.

"My doctor thought I had an easy delivery because I was in good shape," says Miriam, an athletic thirty-eight-year-old and former marathon runner, who ran three miles a day during her pregnancy. Some doctors believe that women who exercise have shorter labors and recover more quickly from labor than women who do not exercise. Other doctors believe that exercise may not shorten labor, but that it increases a woman's stamina and confidence and decreases her anxiety. Thus, starting an exercise program can prepare you for childbirth by strengthening some of the muscles you will use during labor, increasing your stamina and flexibility, and teaching you to shift your focus away from pain.

Some women turn to exercise after they become pregnant in order to stay fit and flexible, keep their weight under control, and feel like their old prepregnant selves. If you are beginning an exercise program for the first time, start slow. Aim for mild to moderate exercise, and stick with activities that are familiar to you, such as swimming or walking. Pregnancy is not a good time to begin running, roller-blading, or downhill skiing for the first time, since you do not want to be nursing athletic injuries and taking pain medications during your pregnancy. If you are a seasoned runner, you may continue to run before and during pregnancy as long as you do not experience back or knee problems.

During your pregnancy, avoid activities that involve dramatic changes in pressure or temperature, like scuba diving. Some physicians recommend that you avoid contact sports and sports that might involve high impact falls (skiing, ice skating, and surfing), while others believe that you may continue to ski or play tennis—if you are experienced at the sport.

Although moderate exercise contributes to a healthy pregnancy, excessive exercise may create orthopedic problems, since your back, hips, legs, and feet are already experiencing additional strain from weight gain and are thus more vulnerable to injury. Moderate exercise will help you avoid injury while bringing you the benefits of increased circulation, strength, and stamina.

Before you become pregnant, avoid workouts so strenuous or prolonged that they deplete much of your body fat. Women runners and gymnasts who have little body fat may become annovulatory—which means they no longer ovulate. You need some body fat to ovulate, and you need to ovulate to get pregnant.

Although scientists debate whether or not excessive exercise interferes with pregnancy in humans, there is evidence that in animals, vigorous exercise can suppress fertility, says Harvard psychologist Dr. Alice Domar.

According to Domar, running and some other forms of exercise may cause the release of the "fight or flight" stress hormones in your body—the same chemicals that are stimulated by fear. These chemicals may interfere with conception. The effect of such "fight or flight" hormones on pregnancy in human beings has not been extensively studied.

"When you run," says Domar, "your body thinks it's being chased by a bear. If a woman is jogging five times a week—even if she's doing it for fitness or weight control—her body still thinks it's being chased by a bear five times a week. In cave-days, the only way a woman would run five times a week is if she were in danger and being pregnant would slow her down, putting her in greater danger. From an evolutionary point of view, if a woman is being chased by a bear five times a week and is clearly surviving, if her body would allow her to get pregnant—which would slow her down—the bear could catch her and eat her. So do you think her body is going to allow her to get pregnant? There is increasing evidence that vigorous exercise can suppress fertility. It certainly does in animals."

Stress Reduction

Reducing your stress levels may be an important factor in *staying pregnant* and carrying your baby to term. Although it has not been established that emotional stress prevents concep-tion in humans, there is animal evidence that stress can interfere with pregnancy. "Animal research clearly shows that stress can induce miscarriage, but it has not been shown in humans," says Dr. Domar. However, in her clinical practice Domar has seen indications that human miscarriage may be associated with stress and that stress reduction may significantly decrease recur-rent miscarriage.

Although you have no guarantee that stress reduction tech-niques will save your pregnancy, learning relaxation techniques certainly cannot hurt you, and the techniques may help you cope with whatever challenges your pregnancy may bring.

Learning to relax during your pregnancy may also improve

your experience of childbirth (since stress can interfere with childbirth by stimulating the production of catecholamines, the "stress hormones," which slow down contractions).

Support Systems: Friends and Family on Call

Our childbirth education class lasted twelve weeks. The facilitator had breaks with refreshments during class so people would get to know each other and support each other. A month after our babies were born we had a reunion . . . We all found we desperately needed to get together after the babies were born. We were all zombies, because we weren't getting any sleep. We'd bounce ideas off each other: "What do you do when this happens?" We'd go to each other's houses and parks. We held our babies, fed our babies, and talked.
—Kathleen R.

* * *

Whether you are part of a couple or a single mother, you will benefit from the support of friends, family, and other mothers during your pregnancy as well as after your baby is born.

If you are pregnant and single, set up support systems and contingency plans early in your pregnancy to help you meet your pregnancy, birth, and postpartum needs. Find friends or family who can be available, if the need arises, to drive you to the doctor or accompany you to genetic counseling, amniocentesis, or your first ultrasound. More importantly, find a childbirth "coach" or doula (a pregnancy support person with experience in childbirth, see Part 7) early in your pregnancy, since knowing you have someone to support you during childbirth can make you feel more relaxed throughout the pregnancy.

Some mothers arrange support systems for labor and birth, but they make no arrangements for help during the first few weeks of motherhood—a time when their lifestyle will change dramatically. In the United States, this absence of support is common, whereas in other cultures, even in Western industrialized countries such as the Netherlands, some postnatal care is offered to new mothers for one to two weeks. Fortunately, some American doulas specialize in "mothering the mother" during the weeks following birth (see "Postnatal Doulas" in the appendix).

Whether you are single or part of a couple, extend your support system *beyond childbirth,* since coming home with a new baby can be overwhelming. Arrange for someone to help you with cooking, shopping, and cleaning while you take care of the baby and yourself. If you have a partner, your partner may also be under stress and thus unable to be your only support person. Ask friends, family, and neighbors to take turns helping out so no one person has to carry too much of the workload. If you can afford it, hire someone to help.

A few lucky parents have a support system of close friends already in place. Sharon relied on her long-standing Berkeley friends for food, companionship, and moral support after she and her husband brought home a set of premature twins. Kathleen R. became part of a community of friends formed during her childbirth education class. The group of women became a source of mutual support and parenting strategies for years after the babies were born.

When creating your support system, anticipate any special needs you may have during pregnancy or after the baby is born. For instance, if you have other children, arrange for their care while you are tending to the needs of your newborn baby. If you know your baby will be born by cesarean section, recruit some help with simple daily tasks such as cooking and cleaning for a week or two after you return from the hospital (see Part 8). After a cesarean, you will need to focus all your energy on healing, taking care of your baby, eating nourishing food (that you do not have to prepare), and taking little walks around the house. The challenges of recovery combined with caring for a newborn increase if you are single, if your partner works long hours, or if your partner is not helpful around the house. Arranging for someone to take care of you for a week or two may make the difference between a peaceful recovery and a miserable one.

If your doctor puts you on bed rest for part of your pregnancy, you will need an extensive support system. Call bed rest support groups for telephone support during your time at home or in the hospital (see appendix).

Emergency Supplies

Stock up on food supplies early in your pregnancy in case you become housebound due to morning sickness, bed rest, or a case of the flu. Pack your freezer and fridge with healthy prepared foods as well as with frozen vegetables, bread, yogurt, milk, meat, and fish. Stack your cupboards with morning-sickness remedies such as soup, ginger tea, canned fruit, crackers, and dry cereals. Include staples such as juices, beans, peas, potatoes, rice, soy products, powdered milk, and canned fruits. If you don't drink the local water, accumulate a supply of bottled water. Collect food delivery flyers from your favorite restaurants, so you can order out if you are too tired to cook.

Chapter 4

Choosing Your Medical Care Provider: The Best Person and Place

Some women shop more carefully for a toaster than a health-care provider.
—Michelle Brill, childbirth educator and doula

. . .

The majority of forty-year-olds need an obstetrician who is willing to follow them carefully and if things change [the woman develops problems], the doctor can consult with a nearby medical school obstetrics department. . . . I don't think any woman, just because of her age, needs to go to a maternal fetal [high-risk] medicine specialist. A specialist becomes necessary only if there are complications. A woman pregnant with twins or triplets needs to go to an obstetrician with ample experience in multiple gestation. Triplets almost always deliver early, and the babies may need to spend time in an intensive care nursery. A good neonatal intensive care doctor also is important.
—Dr. Watson Bowes Jr.

. . .

If you are a woman over age thirty-five, you may wonder what kind of care provider is best for midlife pregnancy. Are you "high risk" due to your age, to pregnancy with multiples, or to preexisting medical conditions? If you are high risk, should you choose a *perinatologist*—a doctor who specializes in high-risk pregnancy, or should you continue with your regular obstetrician?

If your pregnancy is not high risk due to medical problems, but you are over thirty-five, what type of care provider should you choose: perinatologist, obstetrician, family practice physician? What about a midwife? (See Chapter 17.) Answers to these questions will differ, depending more upon your health and your personality than your age.

Advanced Maternal Age Does Not Equal High Risk

If you are over thirty-five, your medical history and current health—not your chronological age—will determine whether or not you are high risk. According to experts in high-risk pregnancy, there are low-risk forty-year-olds and high-risk ones. Says Dr. Watson Bowes Jr.: "Women over forty do not need to go to a high-risk pregnancy specialist before they have a problem. They just need to have a heck of a good obstetrician."

Many doctors now believe that even women over forty-five are not necessarily high risk. When Auben, at age forty-five, asked to see the high-risk pregnancy doctor at her local Kaiser HMO, she was told, "You're not high risk. You're healthy. Women have babies all the time."

Thus, do not assume your pregnancy is a high-risk one. First, seek the care of a good obstetrician and primary care provider, get thorough physical and gynecological exams, and then discuss your risk factors with your physicians to determine what kind of obstetrical care is most appropriate for you. If your pregnancy is low risk, you will have numerous health care providers to choose from. Find a provider who does not view you as a medical oddity, has experience with women of your age group, and is optimistic about your ability to birth and raise a baby.

However, if you are pregnant with twins or more, yours is a high-risk pregnancy whether you are twenty-five or forty-five. Choose a doctor who has extensive experience with multiple births (either an obstetrician or a perinatologist).

Your risk category will also help you determine the type of birth setting that is most suitable for you. Birth centers best serve women whose pregnancies are uncomplicated and low risk. Home births are safest for women who are low risk and who have previously had a baby.

If you have preexisting health problems or certain complications of pregnancy, you will "risk out" (not qualify) for a birth center. If you have risk factors such as high blood pressure, heart disease, kidney disease, twins, placental problems, or a breech baby, a hospital birth is your safest choice.

The Best Person

Fortunately, most women pregnant over thirty can now choose from a variety of options: nurse-midwife, certified midwife (otherwise known as a direct-entry or professional non-nurse midwife), family practice physician, obstetrician, perinatologist, or a combination of two caregivers working together, such as a midwife and obstetrician or an obstetrician and perinatologist. If you live in a small community with only one or two doctors to choose from, you may benefit from the additional support of a *doula* (a pregnancy support person) throughout labor and birth (see Chapter 17).

If you want a nurturing, "childbirth-is-normal" approach, you may feel most at ease with a nurse-midwife who is willing to "labor sit" and support you throughout your entire labor. Most American nurse-midwives work with a backup obstetrician or family practice physician who will take care of you if complications arise. A different type of midwife—a certified, non-nurse midwife—specializes in home or birth center births and usually cannot practice midwifery in a hospital setting. If you are transferred to a hospital while under the care of a non-nurse midwife, you will be placed under a doctor's care when you arrive, although your midwife may accompany you to the hospital, "labor sit," and support you during childbirth. (See "Shopping for a Care Provider" at the end of this section. See appendix for more information on finding a midwife or doula in your area.)

If you prefer a doctor instead of a midwife, find a doctor whose attitudes are akin to yours. Your doctor's professional qualifications are very important but so are empathy and respect for your point of view. Shop for the kind of person you want, whether it is a doctor who will form a "medical partnership" with you and collaborate with you in much of the decision-making or an authoritative doctor who will make decisions for you.

If you want to get pregnant but have not succeeded after trying for six months to a year, see a reproductive endocrinologist—an obstetrician/gynecologist who has completed special training in infertility and hormonal problems.

To find an appropriate doctor, contact a local university obstetrics department, call a labor and delivery ward at a reputable hospital near you and ask the charge nurse for a referral, or call a local birth center for a referral. You can also ask friends or your family doctor for referrals.

After you accumulate a shopping list, find the care provider that "fits" you and your circumstances. Use the questions at the end of this section to help you shop for a doctor or midwife.

Reproductive Endocrinologist

If you have been trying to get pregnant for months or years with no success, you may maximize your chances for getting pregnant by seeing a board certified *reproductive endocrinologist*—a doctor who has had several years of specialized training in infertility and assisted reproduction. A doctor who claims to be a fertility specialist but does not have this additional training is *not* a reproductive endocrinologist and may not have as much knowledge when it comes to performing medical tests and surgeries or prescribing fertility drugs.

When should you seek the opinion of a reproductive endocrinologist? Dr. Mark Sauer offers the following advice: "If you are an average woman in your twenties or thirties, ask yourself: Are you having a period every month? Are you having intercourse regularly—every couple of days [during midcycle]? If so, then give yourself three to six months to get pregnant. Most people who are going to be pregnant are pregnant after six months. If you are a little older . . . seek out educated care. That's when you seek out a reproductive endocrinologist."

Perinatologist

Perinatologists are obstetricians who specialize in pregnancies that are high risk due to maternal illnesses, complications of pregnancy, or pregnancy with multiple babies.

If you are pregnant with multiples, find a doctor who has extensive experience with multiple births. Often this person will be a perinatologist, although some general practice obstetricians are experienced with twins and triplets. Ask your doctor how many women pregnant with multiples he or she has seen through pregnancy and birth.

Since pregnancy and birth with multiples is different than pregnancy with a single baby, you will need someone who is able to anticipate potential problems and closely supervise your pregnancy. Many of the problems can be prevented or well managed, but your doctor will need to see you more frequently, and you will need to have more frequent ultrasounds than a woman who is pregnant with only one baby.

Jean was thirty-seven when she became pregnant with twins. Looking back over her pregnancy, she now believes that her general obstetrician missed subtle signs that something was seriously wrong with one of her babies, and she thinks that a high-risk specialist or an obstetrician experienced with twins and multiples might have recognized her symptoms and saved the baby. Jean works with a mothers of twins organization and counsels other women pregnant with multiples to choose doctors experienced in multiple gestation and birth.

If you have a chronic illness, your pregnancy may be sufficiently high risk to require monitoring by a perinatologist. General obstetricians usually can handle gestational diabetes (GD) or mild preeclampsia, but if you have conditions such as uncontrolled diabetes, seriously high blood pressure, heart disease, kidney disease, or epilepsy, your doctor may either refer you to a perinatologist or call in a perinatologist as a consultant.

If you are a DES daughter (which means that your mother took a drug called DES—diethylstilbestrol—during her pregnancy with you), find a doctor who has experience with DES daughters and DES-related complications: a T-shaped uterus, weakened cervix, recurrent miscarriages, or premature labor and delivery. Not all DES daughters have these problems, but if you do, you need a doctor who can recognize these problems and manage them. For instance, a weakened cervix can be managed by the use of *cerclage* (a method of securing the cervix to prevent it from dilating too early).

Some doctors find pregnancy over age forty-five a potentially risky situation that requires the specialized care of a perinatologist. Although Dr. Mark Sauer believes that late-in-life pregnancy is reasonably safe, he still advises these women to seek specialized care: "For women over forty-five, this is a high-risk pregnancy. Such women need high-risk care."

However, there are many circumstances where your physician's prior experience becomes more important than a specialty in perinatology. For instance, some young perinatologists may not have the same hands-on skills that some older general obstetricians may have.

"In the training of young obstetricians, certain skills disappear," says Dr. Watson Bowes Jr. For instance, young perinatologists may skillfully use high-tech ultrasound and fetal monitoring machines but lack experience in such hands-on techniques as the vaginal delivery of breech babies, cephalic version (turning a breech baby), or forceps delivery—techniques that may provide an alternative to cesarean section. Since research shows that older women have a higher incidence of breech babies and forceps deliveries, you may want a doctor with experience in these techniques. (See Part 8.)

However, do not push your doctor into doing something he or she does not ordinarily do. Cesarean section is still a reasonable, relatively safe, and sometimes preferable mode of delivering babies. "Get what it is your doctor is most comfortable with," advises Dr. Donna Kirz.

General Obstetrician

A board-certified obstetrician who has seen women in their thirties and forties through pregnancy and birth is an appropriate care provider for you, especially if you have no serious preexisting medical problems. Choose an experienced obstetrician.

Jessica, at age forty-seven, went to a general obstetrician because she refused to see herself as high risk due to age. She was healthy and active, and she wanted to be treated like a healthy pregnant woman. Jessica had a normal pregnancy and gave birth to a healthy baby by cesarean section. Although Joanne, age forty-nine, was high risk due to scarring from prior uterine surgery, she chose a group of general obstetricians whose careful monitoring, extensive experience with late-in-life pregnancy, and "you can do this" attitude pulled her through difficult moments and made her feel safe: "I was glad to have doctors that were really on top of things. I had some professionals watching over me twenty-four hours a day. I didn't have to worry about things. It made me feel relieved."

Family Practice Physician

Many women do not realize that some family practice doctors deliver babies and continue to care for both mother and child during their hospital stay. A few family physicians are even trained to deliver breech babies or perform cesarean sections (although most family practice physicians are not).

Family practice physicians offer "a continuity of care," says Dr. Michael Fisher, who teaches family medicine at the University of North Carolina. Fisher delivers between eight and fifteen babies a year and supervises up to fifty births a year. "I see someone when they are pregnant and not pregnant, and I see their family as well. That's one of the joys for me." However, Fisher, like most family doctors, does not do surgery, and he refers women with breech babies or serious complications to obstetricians.

Like many family doctors, Fisher cares for both mother and child after birth, which, for him, means keeping the new family together. "If there's a healthy baby, there is no reason to do anything except give the baby to its mother," says Fisher. Rather than take the baby to the nursery to be weighed and examined, Fisher brings the scale to the mother's room.

The training of family practice physicians often puts them somewhere between midwives and obstetricians in terms of childbirth philosophy. For instance, family practice doctors may be more likely than obstetricians to view birth as a normal process that requires little medical intervention, says Fisher. "I think there is a place between midwives and obstetricians for us. We have a sense of how to keep labor a normal process, and we have experience with some of the illness that may occur during pregnancy and labor and delivery. We don't intervene too frequently. I'll let a woman push longer than the average obstetrician would. I put more power into the woman's decision-making than other providers might."

Dr. Fisher and his partners are the backup doctors who consult with midwives from the Piedmont Birth Center, a freestanding birth center about five minutes by car from the University of North Carolina hospital.

Midwives: Nurse-Midwife and Direct-Entry Midwife

In the United States, there are several types of midwives: nurse-midwives and "direct-entry" midwives. In some states (usually in the rural South), there are also "granny" midwives. A certified nurse-midwife (CNM) is a nurse who has taken additional training in midwifery and has become certified by a national organization such as the American College of Nurse-Midwives (ACNM) or Midwives Alliance of North America (MANA).

The Different Types of Midwives: CNM, CPM, CM, LM

- A certified nurse-midwife (CNM) is a nurse who has taken additional training in midwifery and has become certified by a national organization such as the American College of Nurse-Midwives (ACNM) or Midwives Alliance of North America (MANA). In the case of the ACNM, nurse-midwives must take an exam administered by ACNM Certification

Council (ACC), an arm of the ACNM. A certified nurse-midwife can attend births in a hospital or birth center. She may attend home births if her state laws permit.

- A "direct-entry" midwife, a midwife who is not a nurse, can become a certified midwife (CM) or a certified professional midwife (CPM), depending on which organization certifies her. There are various ways to become a certified direct-entry midwife, which include a course in midwifery, an apprenticeship, and passing marks on a national exam.

  - A certified midwife (CM) has taken the same exam as a CNM (through the American College of Nurse-Midwives and its Certification Council). A CM usually attends out-of-hospital births at home or in a birth center. Although a CM can function as a doula if her patient is transferred to a hospital, she does not provide medical care in a hospital setting, since she is not a nurse.

  - A certified professional midwife (CPM) has taken a different exam, and her midwifery skills have been evaluated through another national organization, MANA (Midwives Alliance of North America) or North American Registry of Midwives (NARM). Although a CPM can function as a doula if her patient is transferred to a hospital, she also does not provide medical care in a hospital setting.

- A licensed midwife (LM) has been licensed by the state in which she practices to practice midwifery. The midwife must quality for a license according to state regulations, which vary from state to state.

The Dutch Model of Midwifery

The Netherlands' system of maternity care depends on direct-entry midwives who serve as primary care providers, attending normal births in both the hospital and the home. Thirty percent of Dutch babies are born at home. Dutch midwives attend a three-year midwifery school, but they are not nurses. In Holland, midwifery is considered to be a medical profession—but one that differs from nursing.

In the United States, some midwifery schools, like the Seattle Midwifery School, resemble the Dutch model by offering extensive course work as well as clinical apprenticeship.

Nurse-Midwife

A nurse-midwife is a specialist in normal pregnancy and birth. Whether you are twenty-five or forty-five, if your pregnancy is normal and your medical history places you at low risk, a certified nurse-midwife (CNM) is a reasonable choice of care provider. Many nurse-midwives work closely with obstetricians or family practice physicians, giving you the option of staying under the midwife's care if your pregnancy proceeds normally and shifting to a doctor's care if problems arise.

Most nurse-midwives tend to normalize birth and view it as a natural event (although not all midwives share this attitude). Many hold a non-interventionist, "birth-is-normal" philosophy, which means that they will not routinely employ medical interventions such as episiotomies, IVs, pain medications, and medicines to strengthen your contractions, and will offer these interventions only if you request them or if they are clearly necessary for you and your baby. Midwives tend to rely on labor support, relaxation techniques, and positional changes to relieve pain and help labor progress. However, because nurse-midwives tend to focus on you as an individual woman with your own beliefs and concerns, they will try to give you the birth you want whether that includes pain medication in a hospital setting or a Jacuzzi in a birth center. On the other hand, some nurse-midwives adhere to the "medical model" just like a doctor and are inclined to rely on medical interventions. Do not assume that all nurse-midwives are the same. You will need to shop for one who is appropriate for you.

Laraine Guyette, a CNM, Ph.D., and Assistant Professor of Nursing at the University of Colorado, sees nurse-midwives as supporting women's choices and as facilitating the normal process of birth: "Midwives are about options and choices. We listen to women. What is it this woman wants in labor and birth? We facilitate it. If she wants an epidural, we aren't going to say 'no, she can't have an epidural.'" Our responsibility to our client is to bring our knowledge and wisdom about birth as a normal process and about how to facilitate that normal process to the best advantage of mother and baby."

Nurse-midwives tend to view childbirth as a collaborative effort involving both mother and care provider and allowing the mother an active role in childbirth. "I describe childbirth as a kind of team thing," says Guyette. "The mother comes with her knowledge and expertise about herself and her experience of pregnancy. I come to our relationship with my knowledge of labor and birth and my experience of working with thousands of women. The two of us negotiate what is going to be the optimal outcome. Together, we define what are the right conditions for this pregnancy and birth. If I have a woman who wants no medication and no intervention, I will work with her and do try to oblige her, but I also have the obligation to communicate to her when intervention is needed for her or her baby."

Kathleen R., a thirty-nine-year-old biologist, wanted a natural birth where she and her husband could bond with their new baby undisturbed by hospital protocol and the flurry of doctors and medical staff. She hoped to avoid a high-tech birth with such medical interventions as drugs and episiotomy. After Kathleen wrote her birth plan, she found that her perinatologists disagreed with her on several key points. So Kathleen chose a nurse-midwife who practiced at the university hospital and used Kathleen's perinatologists as "backup" physicians. Thus Kathleen had access to the best of two worlds: the birth-is-natural world of the nurse-midwife and doula (childbirth support person) and the high-tech world of the perinatologists on call. This dual option situation is common, since American nurse-midwives work with obstetricians and call in the doctor if the need arises.

For additional support during labor, Kathleen hired her childbirth class instructor as a doula. The midwife and doula combination helped her feel confident and protected during childbirth and in control of her birthing environment.

Amanda, at age thirty-six, also chose a nurse-midwife. Even though Amanda developed a mild case of gestational diabetes (GD) and thus became moderately "high risk" during her last month of pregnancy, she remained under the care of the midwife (who consulted with the family practice doctor who had taken care of Amanda for years). Amanda's GD was easily managed with diet, and she felt comfortable having a nurse-midwife deliver her baby.

If you are interested in nurse-midwife support during childbirth but you want access to specialized obstetrical care, look for an obstetrics practice that includes a CNM.

Only certified CNMs can practice in hospitals. In some states, they can also do home births; however, in some states it is illegal for nurse-midwives to attend home births. For more information on CNMs, contact your local birth center, nursing school, university obstetrics department, or the American College of Nurse-Midwives (see appendix).

Non-Nurse Midwives: Certified Midwives and Certified Professional Midwives

"Direct-entry" midwives directly enter the profession of midwifery without going to nursing school. Like many nurse-midwives, direct-entry midwives specialize in normal, low-risk pregnancy and birth. Most direct-entry midwives specialize in out-of-hospital births either at home or in a birth center, although many of these midwives have agreements with doctors who accept patients who must be transferred to a hospital during childbirth. Because direct-entry midwives are not nurses, they do not use drugs such as Pitocin or painkillers. However, they do use natural interventions to move labor along such as positional changes, walking, and hot showers. Many are trained to do an episiotomy, if necessary.

Although many direct-entry midwives are experienced and very well trained, some are not. For instance, "granny" midwives who have learned their skills on the job and may—or may not—be well trained. If the midwife has not been nationally certified to practice midwifery, it may be difficult for the consumer to tell if she is well qualified. Consequently, if you are considering a direct-entry midwife as your care provider, choose a midwife who is certified by a national organization such as Midwives Alliance of North America or the American College of Nurse-Midwives (see appendix). "The certification gives the consumer some idea of the quality of midwifery practice," explains Shelly Girard, CPM/LM, a direct-entry midwife for thirty years who practices in Los Angeles. Girard attends home births, and she works closely with three Los Angeles obstetricians who care for her patients who transfer to a hospital for birth. When one of her patients goes to the hospital, Shelly stays with her patient and functions as her doula rather than her main care provider.

Shopping for a Health Care Provider

Look for someone with assurance—and humility.
—Dr. Watson Bowes Jr.

* * *

You may need to shop around for a physician whose attitude and experience meet your needs as a midlife mother and to interview several care providers before you find the one who is right for you.

These questions may help you sort through the care providers in your community to find the one or the practice that can best meet your individual medical needs and that best matches your birth philosophy (see Part 7).

Questions to ask your doctor:

1. How do you feel about women my age getting pregnant and becoming mothers?
2. How many pregnant women over ___ (plug in whatever age is relevant: thirty-five, forty, fifty) have you taken care of throughout their pregnancy? What percentage of them have complications of pregnancy? What kinds of complications?
3. Do you think that older women are automatically high risk and should be treated differently? If so, in what ways should they be treated differently?
4. Are you willing to work with me on setting up a birth plan? How many of your patients have a birth plan? What kinds of plans are acceptable or unacceptable to you?
5. If I have a problem during my pregnancy, may I call you to discuss it?

6. How often do you suggest that I see you during my pregnancy?

7. Do you find that older women labor differently from younger women?

8. Under what circumstances do you induce labor? Do you use Pitocin to augment labor?

9. What percentage of your patients require cesarean sections? Under what particular circumstances do you recommend cesarean sections? Do find that your older patients tend to need cesareans more often than your younger patients? Why?

10. What is your thinking on your patients' eating and drinking during labor, especially after they have been admitted to the hospital?

11. What is your thinking on hospital protocols such as shaving, enemas, IVs, continuous fetal monitoring? How many of your patients receive such procedures?

12. Do you give women who have had a previous cesarean the opportunity for a trial of labor and a vaginal birth after cesarean (VBAC)? If not, why not?

13. Do you routinely perform episiotomies? Under what circumstances do you perform them? How many of your patients need one? Do you think that episiotomies can be prevented? If so, how?

14. Under what circumstances do you use forceps or vacuum extraction? Which technique do you prefer? What percentage of your older patients require either forceps or vacuum deliveries?

15. Are your patients free to move around during labor? What is your thinking about the use of various birthing positions to help a woman progress in labor?

16. How do you feel about your patients getting in the shower or Jacuzzi during labor?

17. How do you feel about a doula being present at my birth? About my partner or other members of my family being present? About my other children being present?

18. What is your point of view on the "active management of labor"?

19. If I require a cesarean section, may my partner be present? May my partner be present in the recovery room afterward? May he or she bring the baby to me (if the baby is doing well) in recovery—and stay by my side—so that I do not need to be separated from my baby?

20. How do you manage breech babies? Do you use cephalic version to turn the babies? Do you consider versions dangerous? During what time is cephalic version most effective? What percentage of babies permanently turn to cephalic (head-down) presentation after a version? If the baby flips back to breech, do you try another version? Do you deliver most breech babies by cesarean section? Do you deliver breech babies vaginally? If so, how often do you perform this kind of delivery?

21. If you are expecting twins, triplets, or more ask: How do you manage twins or triplets? How often do you see women pregnant with multiples during the course of their pregnancy? Do you deliver twins or triplets vaginally or by cesarean section? Under what circumstances do you think it is safe to deliver them vaginally?

22. Will it be possible for me to be skin to skin with my baby (with a blanket put over us) for an hour to two hours after birth? How many of your patients do this?

23. What is your policy on babies being taken to the nursery after birth? May my baby stay with me instead of going to the nursery if it is healthy?

24. What do you think about breastfeeding immediately after birth? How many of your patients breastfeed in

the hospital?

25. If I have a cesarean section, will I be able to see and touch my baby directly after birth? Will my birth partner be able to hold the baby and to bring the baby to visit me while I am in the recovery room and/or after I return to my hospital room?

Doctors' answers to these questions will vary widely. What is most important is that you hear answers that make you feel comfortable and confident that you and your doctor agree on the issues that are most important to you. However, most doctors taking care of midlife mothers should have the following qualifications:

- The ability to listen and to empathically respond to your needs and concerns regarding pregnancy and delivery
- A philosophy that supports midlife pregnancy
- Experience with pregnant women your age or close to your age
- Ample experience diagnosing and managing diabetes, hypertension, and eclampsia
- Good surgical skills
- Medical partners that share these qualities (since the partner may actually deliver your baby)

Other Criteria

If you are pregnant with twins, triplets, or more, make sure your doctor is experienced in dealing with these potentially complex pregnancies. If having a vaginal delivery is very important to you, find a doctor who has the skill, experience, and inclination to perform alternatives to cesarean section such as turning breech babies before delivery (cephalic version) or forceps delivery.

Choosing a Midwife

Do not assume that all midwives have noninterventionist childbirth philosophies or that they all are enthusiastic about midlife pregnancy. Interview midwives to make sure you agree about important issues. You may wish to ask similar questions of midwives and doctors regarding their attitudes toward midlife pregnancy. Pay careful attention to their answers. For certified non-nurse midwives, questions regarding Pitocin, pain medications, IVs, continuous fetal monitoring, and hospital practice do not apply.

Questions to ask a midwife:

1. Do you think that women over forty can have a normal labor and a normal vaginal delivery?
2. What percentage of your patients have vaginal births?
3. Do you "labor sit"—will I have your continuous presence and support during my labor and birth?
4. What percentage of your patients end up needing Pitocin, pain medication, or a cesarean section?
5. Do you find that older women labor longer? How do you manage a long labor?
6. Do you consider birth a family event? Will you permit my partner, friends, or children to be present at the birth?
7. Under what circumstances do you think I should give birth in a hospital? At a birth center? At home?
8. What backup doctors do you work with, and at what hospital do you practice?
9. If I have a home or birth center birth, will I have access to a hospital if I need it? Which one are you affiliated with?
10. If I go through labor in a birth center but my baby needs to be in an intensive care nursery, what hospital would

she go to? How far away is it from the birth center? From my house?

11. What are your thoughts on breastfeeding? Do you encourage breastfeeding immediately after birth?

12. I would like skin-to-skin contact with my baby immediately after birth. Will that be possible?

13. Do you routinely use IVs, enemas, castor oil, continuous fetal monitoring, or episiotomy in the course of a normal labor?

14. Do you think episiotomies can be prevented? How? What percentage of your patients have episiotomies?

15. If I have a normal birth, how soon after the birth may I go home with my baby?

The Best Place

A woman will labor the best where she feels the safest and most secure. For some that will be the home, for some women that will be a hospital, and for some women that will be a birth center.
—Michelle Brill, M.P.H., childbirth educator

• • •

Where should you have your baby—at a hospital, a birth center, or at home? Although your choices in this area are growing as more states are offering midwifery services through free-standing birth centers and hospitals, your age, health, birth philosophy, and choice of care provider will determine where you give birth.

To choose the best birth setting for you and your baby, you first need to choose the kind of caregiver you want and to assess your health and your baby's health. If you choose a doctor, note that most doctors prefer hospital births. Very few doctors will attend home births, although some doctors will deliver babies at birth centers.

Carefully consider your risk factors before choosing a birth setting. If you are under thirty-five, you have no preexisting medical problems, your baby is healthy and well positioned, and your pelvis looks roomy enough to easily accommodate your baby during childbirth, you may be considered "low risk" enough to birth your baby at a birth center. If you are over thirty-five, your pregnancy is normal, and you have a pelvis roomy enough for your baby or you have previously had a baby, you may also be a good candidate for a birth center.

Until recently, many birth centers would not accept women over forty because of the concern that women forty and over may become high risk at some point during their pregnancy. However, this attitude is changing for healthy pregnant women (especially those who have already had a baby).

If you are over forty and have risk factors such as chronic health problems, a breech baby, or twins, you will "risk out" of most birth centers. In this case, your safest choice is a hospital. If you wish, you can recreate some of the supportive birth center atmosphere in your hospital room by bringing a doula to help you throughout your labor. You also can simulate the homey setting of a birth center by choosing a hospital that offers homelike birthing rooms.

Choose the birth setting in which you feel most secure. Some women feel most secure and relaxed in a hospital setting where high-tech medical care awaits just down the hall. Other women feel more comfortable at home. Home birth is gradually becoming popular, especially for second and third births, although it is still a controversial choice in the United States. If you wish to have your baby at home, make sure you are low risk enough to safely do so, that you are not pregnant with twins or more, that your baby is not breech, and that your midwife has excellent skills.

Also, make sure that your midwife has an arrangement with a physician who will take over your care if you are transferred to a hospital. The hospital should be a twenty to thirty minute drive from your home.

Even if you plan for a home or birth center birth—and do all the "right" things—you may end up going to a hospital. Thus, it is important to think through more than one potential birth place scenario—home, birth center, and/or hospital—in order to choose the birth environments that offer what is best for you and your baby.

The Hospital

Get up-to-date information about your local hospital. What happened in the past [regarding practices and policies in labor and delivery] may no longer apply.
—Dr. Allen Killam

• • •

Choosing a hospital is an important decision. Your choice will affect how you, your baby, and your family are treated during labor and birth and the degree to which high-tech procedures and equipment are used in the care that you and your baby receive. Your choice of hospital will make a difference if you need a cesarean section or if your baby requires an intensive care nursery with its sophisticated, life-saving technology.

Hospitals fall into one of three classifications: primary care (Level I), secondary care (Level II), and tertiary care (Level III). A primary care hospital is best equipped for low-risk births. If a baby born at a primary care hospital needs intensive care, the baby must be transported by ambulance or helicopter to a secondary or tertiary hospital with a neonatal intensive care unit.

A secondary care hospital usually is equipped to offer immediate cesarean surgery for the mother and some intensive care for the baby. The tertiary care hospital is best able to handle high-risk mothers and babies, since emergency cesarean sections can be quickly initiated, and babies can be well cared for in neonatal intensive care units (NICUs).

Your choice of hospital should be determined by your circumstances. For instance, if you are pregnant with multiples, you will require an obstetrician experienced with multiple births. You may need a hospital with an intensive care nursery (preferably a Level II or III) if your babies are very premature. Level III nurseries can provide the most complete kind of neonatal care for premature infants since they are the best equipped to help the smallest preemies breathe, take nourishment, and grow. The high-tech equipment of these nurseries is designed to deliver tiny doses of medications and nutrients. Your baby may not need to be in intensive care, but if he or she does, the unit is within the hospital and close to you.

In the event that your baby needs intensive care and your hospital does not have an NICU, your baby may be transferred to a hospital that has one. Although this may be in the best interests of your baby's health, it may separate you and the baby, especially if you are recovering from cesarean surgery and cannot be transferred to the other hospital. If it's possible, you can ask to be transferred to the same hospital so you can stay near your baby.

Ideally, your hospital should be able to provide you with the setting you want for birthing and getting acquainted with your new baby. As you shop for a hospital, inquire about policies that affect both your childbirth and your bonding experiences with your newborn:

1. What percentage of women undergo continuous fetal monitoring? What percentage are allowed some freedom of movement during labor and birth? Are women allowed to drink or eat snacks during labor (if they are not at high risk for cesarean section)?

2. Does the hospital have special birthing rooms with homey environments and showers or bathtubs? How do you arrange to be assigned such a room? Are there criteria you must meet before being allowed to use a birthing room? Is a Jacuzzi available in the labor and delivery ward for laboring mothers?

3. Are fathers or other family members allowed at the mother's side during both vaginal and cesarean births? Are they allowed in the recovery room?

4. Does the hospital separate babies from mothers at birth in order to bathe the baby, give it eye drops, and conduct a physical exam?

5. Does the hospital allow mothers to hold and nurse their babies uninterrupted for two hours after birth?

6. Does rooming-in mean that a baby is at its mother's side twenty-four hours a day if she wishes?

7. Is nursing encouraged? Is a nursing consultant available?

8. May the birth partner spend the night in the mother's room after the birth?

9. What is the hospital policy on bonding with and nursing a baby that is in the NICU? Does the NICU have a milk bank?

10. If the baby is transferred to an NICU at another hospital, is the mother transferred along with the baby?

Once you have decided upon a hospital, discuss your choice and your expectations with your caregiver. Whenever possible, double-check hospital policies with hospital administrators and labor and delivery nurses in order to prevent possible miscommunication about what is and is not allowed. If you ask permission for something that goes against usual policy (such as having your partner with you at a cesarean birth), get that permission in writing so that there is no confusion should you require a surgical birth late at night.

Touring the Hospital

Find out not only what is allowed but what is encouraged. It is far better to be in a hospital that routinely runs the way you would like it to than to have to fight the system.
—Marion McCartney, *The Midwife's Pregnancy and Childbirth Book*

• • •

As you approach your seventh month of pregnancy, it is prudent to tour the facility where you will give birth in order to orient yourself to the birthing or delivery rooms, the Jacuzzi (if one is available for women in labor), the nursery, and the cafeteria. Make note of the kind of room you would like: a private room, a room with a shower or bath, a room with a fold-out bed for family members.

Ask the staff about hospital policies such as rooming-in with your baby and using the Jacuzzi and birthing rooms. You also may wish to ask if your birth partner or doula will be allowed to accompany you during a cesarean section, and if you will be allowed several support people (such as doula, husband, mother) in your room during labor. Remember to ask your care provider how he or she works with hospital policies.

The Birth Center

If she doesn't have any medical problems, a birth center is a likely choice if a woman is otherwise healthy. I wouldn't use age as a

cut-off criteria.
—Dr. Susan Porto, obstetrician/gynecologist and clinical faculty at Mercy Hospital in Chicago, believes that problems in this healthy population of women are rare.

• • •

I have concerns with freestanding birth centers only because of the nature of obstetrics. I don't believe you can "risk out" everyone. But a birth center that's attached to a hospital—that's lovely.
—Dr. Donna Kirz argues that not every risky condition will be screened out at a birth center, and that it is safest for a woman to be in a birth center that is next to a hospital.

• • •

We studied 11,814 women admitted for labor and delivery to eighty-four free-standing birth centers in the United States and followed their course and that of their infants through delivery or transfer to a hospital and for at least four weeks thereafter . . . . We conclude that birth centers offer a safe and acceptable alternative to hospital confinement for selected pregnant women, particularly those who have previously had children, and that such care leads to relatively few cesarean sections.
—J. P. Rooks, N. L. Weatherby, E. K. Ernst, S. Stapelton, A. Rosenfield. "Outcomes of Care in Birth Centers." The National Birth Center Study. *The New England Journal of Medicine*, December 28, 1989; 321(26)

• • •

Birth centers are geared for women who are at low risk for complications such as high blood pressure, diabetes, heart disease, breech presentation, placenta previa, or pregnancy with twins or more. The centers are staffed by midwives or doctors who view birth as a family event. Therefore, birth centers are more likely than conventional hospital labor and delivery units to allow family and friends to support a laboring mother during childbirth. Most birth centers create an atmosphere conducive to mother-child bonding and breastfeeding and take into consideration the emotional needs of the mother, her child, and her extended family.

Birth centers are usually homey, low-tech environments that are designed to provide comfort and support but not to administer labor-enhancing drugs, like Pitocin, or to perform instrumental deliveries (using forceps or vacuum) or cesarean sections.

Although birth centers may have oxygen, IV supplies, and Isolettes, women having babies in birth centers receive fewer medical interventions than women giving birth in hospitals and are treated less like patients and more like women experiencing the normal and natural process of childbirth.

Some birth centers are freestanding, meaning they are not attached to a hospital; others are located on the campus of a hospital or are physically attached to a hospital. Most centers are separate from a hospital and are specifically designed for normal, uncomplicated births that are unlikely to require hospital care (see Part 7). Because most of the births are low risk, the staff is more likely to allow women to labor "naturally," to eat or drink during labor, and to relax in a Jacuzzi or birth pool.

If you qualify for a birth center, choose one that is within twenty or thirty minutes of a hospital (even at rush hour) and that has:

1. An atmosphere you like
2. Certified midwives
3. "Backup" doctors at a nearby hospital
4. Nurse-midwives with hospital privileges or midwives who can remain at your side to support you during your labor and delivery should you be transferred to a hospital

Arrange to meet the backup doctor in advance just in case he or she becomes your caregiver at the last minute. Most likely, everything will go well at the birth center. True medical emergencies during childbirth in a healthy woman are rare. However, if you are over thirty-five, having your first baby, or anxious about being too far from a hospital, look for a birth center located on—or near—the campus of a hospital. In that case, you are only a few minutes from a fully equipped hospital.

For some women, birth centers provide a happy compromise between home birth and hospital birth.

But are birth centers safe enough? When it comes to the issue of safety, doctors and midwives strongly disagree. Many midwives believe that birth is normal, not pathological, and that most low-risk women can safely birth their babies in a birth center.

Some American doctors agree with this "birth-is-normal" midwifery philosophy, arguing that emergencies requiring hospital care are so rare that most low-risk women can safely deliver in a birth center.

However, many American doctors are wary of birth centers. They feel that any additional risks for mother and baby mean too much risk, and they argue that a hospital birth is safer because emergencies that require surgery or other medical interventions can be handled immediately. Many doctors fear that if a birth becomes complicated by a prolapsed cord or a problem with the baby's placenta, the laboring mother may be too far from a hospital to get help in time to save the baby's life. For instance, a prolapsed umbilical cord that is compressed enough to jeopardize the baby's oxygen supply is a medical emergency that can only be "cured" by an immediate cesarean section. In some cases this surgery needs to be performed within ten minutes, which is impossible to do if the laboring woman is twenty or thirty minutes away from a hospital. Fortunately, cord prolapse is a rare event (see Chapter 27 for more).

Dr. David Walmer, Professor of Obstetrics and Gynecology at Duke University Medical Center, like many American physicians, argues against birth centers, because he feels any risk for the baby is not worth the gamble. "My gut feeling is that the risk you are taking is the child's life as well as yours. Have your children in as safe an environment as possible. All my children were born in the hospital. The gamble is relatively low [in a birth center or home birth]. The problem is that the penalty, if you guess wrong, is serious. The mom and baby may die. A lot of problems don't have early warning signs, like abruption where you have only five to ten minutes. You can take every degree of safety precautions you want, it depends on the circumstances. A complete abruption—you don't have time to go anywhere. You barely have time to get from the labor room to the O.R."

However, midwives and some physicians argue that such dire emergencies are rare, that it is not always possible to do a cesarean section in ten minutes in a hospital setting, and it is not wise to make decisions on worst-case scenarios when most births are normal events. Some care providers believe that a birth center birth may, in certain cases, be safer than a hospital birth—at least safer from medical interventions that may carry with them their own kinds of risks.

Numerous medical studies show that birth centers are safe for low-risk, healthy women who are properly screened. Studies of birth centers in New Zealand and Great Britain have shown that deliveries are safe for women who are well screened for risk factors. In the United States, the National Birth Center Study, published in 1989 in *The New England Journal of Medicine*, reported on birth outcomes for 11,814 women who were admitted in labor to eighty-four birth centers between 1956 and 1986 and found that women having babies at the birth centers had low cesarean section rates as well as low rates of emergencies during birth. The cesarean section rate was only 4 percent (less than one quarter of the national average for hospital births).

Because the women having babies at the birth centers were well screened, the rate of emergencies occurring during labor and delivery was only 7.9 percent. However, the National Birth Center Study revealed that women having their first baby had a higher emergency rate and a higher transfer rate to hospitals than did women who had previously had a baby. Many of the emergencies requiring transfer to a hospital included problems such as failure to progress in labor, fetal distress, and meconium aspiration.

If you are having your first baby, carefully weigh the pros and cons of having your baby in a birth center, since you may need to go to the hospital for medical assistance during labor—even if you do not have a medical emergency. Medical studies show that women over age thirty-five having their first babies may have an increased chance of difficult or prolonged labor that requires medication, usually Pitocin, to strengthen labor contractions and make them more efficient. Since birth centers do not administer Pitocin (because it is a powerful drug that strengthens labor contractions, and both mother and baby must be closely monitored), a woman with prolonged labor may be transferred to a hospital to receive the drug. A hospital also offers other interventions— continuous fetal monitoring, epidural anesthesia, forceps, and vacuum delivers—that may become necessary with difficult labors and are not available in birth centers.

Women over age thirty-five ended up having more transfers from birth centers to hospitals to have Pitocin augmentation of labor than did younger women, says Marion McCartney, CNM and Director of Professional Services for the American College of Nurse-Midwives, of her experience as a midwife attending births at a Maryland birth center. "These women were in labor, they weren't making progress, and they needed Pitocin to give birth," she explains. "Healthy women over thirty-five are more likely to be transferred from a birthing center to a hospital for Pitocin augmentation of labor than women in their twenties. But most of them [women over thirty-five] do fine," says McCartney—and they deliver at the birth center as planned.

Even if you need to be transferred to a hospital for your last stage of labor, says McCartney, a birth center may still be a good choice. That way, you may begin your labor in a supportive birth center with its birthing pools and massages and later, if you need to be transferred to the hospital, you can benefit from state-of-the-art medicine. Of course, there is a downside: the inconvenience caused by a transfer during active labor. But spending the majority of your labor in the relaxed environment of a birth center may be to your advantage and may contribute to your progress in labor and to your overall birth experience. McCartney argues that laboring in a birth center may, in fact, protect some women from the anxiety that contributes to long labors and to the need for medical interventions. Medical studies support McCartney's point of view. According to *The Cochrane Review*, women who gave birth in "home-like" institutional settings in hospital birth rooms or hospital birth centers (compared to women who gave birth in conventional hospital labor wards) used less pain medication during labor, were slightly less likely to have their labors augmented with Pitocin, and had a slightly greater chance of being very satisfied with their birth experience.

Some birth centers consider women who are pregnant with their first baby and women pregnant over age forty as having too many potential risk factors to give birth in a birth center. However, the criteria determining which women "risk out" and which women do not varies from birth center to birth center. Age restrictions, in particular, are changing as midwifery care becomes more popular, as more midwives acquire hospital privileges, and as childbirth over forty becomes more commonplace.

Should women over forty even attempt to have their babies at a birth center? The answer is a complex one, depending on the potential risks posed by the distance between the birth center and a well-equipped hospital, on the potential disruption involved in being transferred from one birth setting to another, and on the potential benefits of spending at least part of labor in a supportive birth center environment.

All of these factors are worth consideration. Before deciding to give birth in a birth center, carefully consider your individual circumstances as well as your feelings about childbirth. If you have no pre-existing medical problems, your baby is healthy and well positioned, and your pelvis appears roomy enough to easily accommodate your baby during childbirth, you may be considered a good candidate for a birth center.

If you have chronic health problems, a breech baby, twins, or a small pelvis and/or a big baby, you will "risk out" of most birth centers. In this case, your best choice is a hospital. If you wish, you can recreate some of the supportive birth center atmosphere in your hospital room by bringing a doula (childbirth support person) to help you throughout your labor. You also can simulate the atmosphere of a birth center by choosing a hospital that offers home-like birthing rooms.

If you feel uncomfortable because a birth center is too low-tech for you, yet you are concerned that a hospital is too high-tech, you may be offered a good compromise: a nurse-midwife associated with a hospital practice. With a nurse-midwife as your care provider in a hospital setting, you may find the best of both worlds: a supportive midwife with a "birth-is-normal" attitude to see you through your labor and access to a physician and high-tech medical care a few steps away—just in case you need them.

The Home Birth

I don't see a problem with home births if the women are appropriate candidates. In this day and age, you can get someone to a hospital if problems arise. I don't think age is a factor as long as a woman is healthy and has had no problems during her pregnancy.
—Dr. Susan Porto

• • •

I do not think it is wise for a woman to plan to deliver at home, because, in spite of all its faults, a modern, well-equipped, and well-staffed hospital is a safer place to deliver by far. No matter how good you are at vaginal deliveries, if you don't have the equipment and backup with such things as anesthesia and a surgical team, by the time you get to where you need to be it may be too late to prevent a bad outcome of a pregnancy.
—Dr. Allen Killam

• • •

There is no strong evidence to favour either planned hospital birth or planned home birth for low risk pregnant women.
—Olsen O. Jewell MD. "Home Versus Hospital Birth" (Cochrane Review). In: *The Cochrane Library*, 1, 2001

• • •

Women considering a home birth should be carefully screened to determine the safety of such a decision in their particular case. Home birth is for women who are considered to be "low-risk," meaning there is no reason to assume that the birth will be anything but normal. These women should have no heart disease or diabetes, and no family history of genetic disorders. Multiple births should not be handled at home. Breech and premature births should also be conducted in a hospital setting.
—Marion McCartney, *The Midwife's Birth and Pregnancy Book*

In the United States, home birth is controversial. Although a handful of doctors favor home births for low-risk women, most American doctors discourage home birth because they believe it is not safe. American midwives, on the other hand, tend to favor home births, but they disagree about under what circumstances home births are safe.

Even though true emergency situations are rare and healthy births are the norm, the majority of American obstetricians are nervous about home birth. Dr. Donna Kirz advises first-time mothers to give birth in a home-like environment in a hospital birthing room—but not at home. "When you're just getting started childbearing, there is a lot of room for mistakes. So if there's a riskier thing—like delivering at home—a first-time mother might not want to do that. I also think there are issues in terms of accessibility to a backup situation. To be at home gives you a distance and a time factor that is greater than if you are in a hospital. I would prefer a home-like situation in a hospital instead of a home, because you occasionally see somebody with an abruption, you occasionally see somebody have significant fetal distress, which isn't to say that you can't get away with it most of the time. But I'm not willing to just be lucky."

Many physicians, like Dr. Allen Killam, are adamantly opposed to home birth, even if a woman has previously had a baby. "Home birth is not as safe as hospital birth," warns Killam. "I am totally against a planned home delivery. You cannot predict many emergencies."

Midwives, on the other hand, tend to believe that birth is a normal event that can be as safe at home as it is in a hospital—if certain criteria are met. According to Leah Albers, CNM, and Professor of Nursing at the University of New Mexico. "Planned home birth is as safe as a hospital birth when three things are in place: 1) prenatal care with careful risk screening, 2) an experienced attendant for birth, and 3) a backup plan for unexpected complications. When these things are in place, home birth is as safe as hospital birth [for low-risk women]."

Dutch midwife Kathy Herschderfer, like many other Dutch and American direct-entry midwives, feels that birth at home is more intimate than hospital birth. "The added value of a home birth is the first hour after birth," says Herschderfer. "The intimacy of your own bed and own house and the contact with the baby—you can't do it anywhere else. The quiet, the calm, the bonding—and you don't have to abide by anyone's rules." Herschderfer thinks that both home birth and hospital birth involve some risks, but she concludes: "They are not the same kinds of risks. The magnitude of the risks are fairly comparable. In some cases, they are fairly small. The question becomes one of balancing risks."

However, even midwives who favor home birth often do not recommend it for women having their first baby, since labor with first babies may be longer and may require more medical assistance than labors with subsequent babies. "Home birth is not recommended for a first baby," says Pam Spry, CNM and Assistant Professor of Nursing at the University of Colorado.

Some midwives are especially cautious about women over forty having a first baby at home, because risk factors tend to increase for women in that age group. Laraine Guyette, also a CNM and Professor of Nursing at the University of Colorado, advises women over forty to think twice about home birth if they have not previously had a baby. "You're pushing the odds," says Guyette. "If I were over forty and having a first baby at home, I would really want to know that my care provider knew what he or she was talking about. Is your caregiver looking through rose-colored glasses? How many risk factors can the mother and caregiver tolerate and still feel comfortable about the chosen birth setting? The bottom line is: If something goes wrong, can you live with the consequences?"

However, Guyette supports home birth as an option for low-risk women who already have had a baby.

Louise Aucott, CNM, an advocate of home birth, believes that some low-risk women over forty are well suited to home birth, especially those who want to have control over their birth environment. "Home birth should be a legitimate and available option for every woman," argues Aucott. "There are some women for whom it is really important how they become a mother; older mothers fall into that group. They value motherhood and they want everything to be perfect: they wait until they have the right person and the right time in their career. Forty percent to fifty percent of women coming to me for home births are coming because they have so many control issues around pregnancy. These are older, well-educated, well-read women."

If you have previously had a baby and you want to give birth at home, discuss home birth with your caregivers and thoroughly go over the risks and benefits. Make sure you are familiar with your state's laws on home birth, since in some states it is not legal for midwives to attend home births; in other states, nurse-midwives or direct-entry midwives may attend home births, but only if they have a backup physician and a hospital that agrees to admit their patients. Make sure your midwife has a backup doctor and that either she or the doctor can admit you to the hospital should the need arise. Also, make sure that the midwife has a solid plan for transporting you to the hospital if you should require medical assistance during labor or birth.

Considering Home Birth

Home birth is a reasonable option for some women—but not all women. According to Leah Albers, CNM, "American women who choose home birth are swimming upstream. The women who choose home birth are women with a mission." Albers argues that home birth is as safe as hospital birth, but there is a trade-off in risks.

If you are fearful about home birth, have never had a baby, or are high risk in any way, try simulating some of the features of home birth by choosing a hospital with homey birth rooms or a birth center attached to a hospital.

To safely undertake a home birth, make sure that your midwife is certified and has good references and credentials, that she has reliable physician backup should an emergency arise, and that she has made careful plans for possible transportation to a nearby hospital. Also make sure that you:

- Are comfortable giving birth at home
- Are low risk (a healthy woman with no risk factors: no breech or transverse presentation, no multiples, no premature babies, no hypertension or significant diabetes)
- Are within twenty to thirty minutes from a hospital—even during rush hour
- Have a "proven pelvis" (in other words, you have had a previous vaginal birth) or your pelvis is clearly roomy enough to accommodate your baby

If you choose home birth, understand that home birth requires careful preparation. You need to find a birth attendant who is skilled at early management of obstetrical, fetal, and neonatal emergencies (meaning someone who can diagnose fetal distress or serious obstetrical problems in time to transfer you to a hospital; manage a baby in respiratory distress; and, if necessary, resuscitate a baby after birth).

Carefully consider how you would deal with a problem with the baby if you give birth at home. Realize that if you live in the United States and anything goes wrong at home, you may be blamed by your family, your friends, or your doctor since home birth remains controversial. Would you also blame yourself, or would you feel that your home birth was as safe as hospital birth? This is an important question to answer before you choose home birth.

For a home birth, you may hire either a certified nurse-midwife (CNM) or a certified "direct-entry" midwife (CPM or CM). Your midwife should also be licensed by your state (see Chapter 4 and Chapter 17). Research your options and look into the qualifications of the various midwives. Both CNMs and direct-entry midwives have national organizations that can help you find qualified people in your area (see ACNM and MANA in the appendix).

Your insurance company may or may not reimburse home births. Some companies reimburse CMs and CPMs as well as CNMs. Call your insurance company to see if it reimburses all certified midwives or only certified nurse-midwives. Find out if the company covers home birth as extensively as birth center or hospital birth.

Home Birth in Holland

Women in Holland frequently have babies at home, especially second or third babies, and they have one of the lowest infant mortality rates in the Western world, says Marion McCartney, author of *The Midwife's Pregnancy and Childbirth Book.* Most Dutch physicians support home births for low-risk women. The doctors care for women with problem pregnancies and leave normal pregnancies to the care of midwives who, in Holland, are considered primary caregivers and medical professionals. Thirty percent of Dutch women give birth at home. Only 10 percent of pregnant Dutch women have cesarean births, which is about half the cesarean rate of the United States.

"The Dutch are an anachronism," says Kathy Herschderfer, Dutch midwife and researcher. Not only do Dutch women prefer home birth—so do Dutch insurance companies. But are the Dutch unusual because they trust in the safety of home birth or because the makeup of their population and genetic heritage contribute to the safety of home birth in Holland? In other words: do tall Dutch men marry tall Dutch women with sufficiently roomy pelvises to safely have babies at home? While many American doctors and midwives point to this good genetic match between Dutch men and women as the reason for home birth's success in Holland, midwife Herschderfer disagrees. She argues that given extensive immigration to Holland from Asia and Africa, Dutch people (like American people) often marry small Indonesian or Asian people, and that the "genetic similarity" theory does not hold up.

Part Three

Getting
Pregnant

Chapter 5
The Good News

You probably narrow your opportunities as you grow older—but this never means that they're not there.
—Dr. Margaret Bates, obstetrician/gynecologist, Los Angeles

• • •

You may worry that you have postponed pregnancy too long and that you may be too old to conceive or raise a baby. Although there is some basis for concern about your fertility, increasing numbers of women in their thirties and forties are getting pregnant and having healthy babies. According to the final data on births in the United States in the 1999 *National Vital Statistics Report*, birth rates for women in their thirties have increased steadily since the mid-1970s and are at their highest in three decades. From the late 1970s to 1999, the birth rate for women aged thirty to thirty-four increased by 70 percent, reaching a record high, and the birth rate for women aged thirty-five to thirty-nine more than doubled. Preliminary reports from statistics for the year 2000 indicate that birth rates continue to increase for women in their thirties. (The 1999 *National Vital Statistics Reports*, published April 17, 2001, provides the "final" national statistics on births in the United States in 1999. The preliminary birth data for 2000, published July 24, 2001, provides statistics for 2000. Final data for 2001 will not be available until 2002.)

U.S. birth statistics also bring good news to women in their forties. For women aged forty to forty-four, the birth rate increased by 95 percent from 1981 to 1999, according to the 1999 *National Vital Statistics Reports*. The total number of births to women aged forty-five to forty-nine rose 15 percent from 1998 to 1999. Even though there are more births to women in this age group, there are more women in this age group than in previous years because many baby boomers are now in their mid- to late forties.

Women in their fifties have only recently figured in national birth statistics. The *National Vital Statistics Reports* for 1999 shows that the number of births to women aged fifty to fifty-four are increasing, primarily due to new reproductive technologies such as egg donation. Still, the numbers of births are relatively small, so small that the statistics for 1999 pool the women aged fifty to fifty-four with those aged forty-five to forty-nine; all together, women aged forty-five to fifty-four had about 4,174 babies that year.

If you are in your thirties or forties, it is not time to give up on your fertility, but it is time to make some decisions. The clock is ticking. You must use your time well if you hope to become pregnant. Dr. Margaret Nusbaum, an Associate Professor of Family Medicine at the University of North Carolina, counsels many of her patients who want to have babies to do so in their thirties. "Usually I think of thirty-five as the run-don't-walk time in terms of family planning," says Nusbaum.

The chapters in Part 3 of this book will give you suggestions as to how to make the best use of your reproductive years; how to seek appropriate medical care; and how to overcome obstacles to pregnancy such as fibroid tumors, endometriosis, blocked tubes, hormone imbalances, and aging eggs. The chapters will also provide explanations of the various treatments for infertility.

This chapter combines the pregnancy success stories of women with the clinical experience of their doctors and the evidence of medical studies in order to give you a broad view of the possibilities of getting pregnant in midlife.

The good news is that healthy women who enter pregnancy in midlife, whether they are thirty-five or forty-five, are likely to have healthy pregnancies and healthy babies. Even though older women may show higher rates of the complications of pregnancy and delivery, their odds of having a healthy baby are almost as high as those of younger women. Such good outcomes are the result of wise medical management, well-informed and health-conscious women, and the ingenuity of Mother Nature for constructing the uterus as a resilient organ that works admirably well most of the time.

However, a woman's eggs are not nearly as resilient as her uterus. The prime years for fertile eggs are between the ages of twenty and thirty. Generally, at about age thirty-two or thirty-three, a woman's fertility slowly begins to decrease. Some physicians believe that fertility decreases dramatically in a woman's mid- to late thirties. According to Dr. Mark Sauer, a pioneering reproductive endocrinologist who has been supportive of women seeking pregnancy in midlife, "Fertility declines in the early to mid-thirties. A lot of people assume it is forty, but nothing changes dramatically between thirty-nine and forty. Fertility starts to significantly change at around thirty-two or thirty-four. It takes a major plummet from thirty-four to forty."

Other doctors believe that the relationship between a woman's age and her fertility is more of an individual thing.

According to Dr. David Walmer, Associate Professor and former Director of the IVF Program at Duke University Medical Center, it is difficult to make general statements about when a woman's fertility will decline. "There isn't any particular age at which a woman's fertility starts to decline," says Walmer. "There is a gradual progressive decline in fertility over the years. Every woman's fertility declines at a different rate. That means that some women who are thirty-seven or thirty-eight may have no difficulty getting pregnant very quickly. Some women will have problems much younger than that."

However, even if your fertility decreases, you may still remain fertile enough to have a baby well into your forties, although pregnancy may take you longer to achieve at forty than at thirty.

Statistics on age-related fertility are averages—not absolutes. Use statistics as a guide to help you make choices about when to get pregnant, but do not assume that statistics determine your fate. Recognize the biological realities of getting pregnant in midlife without giving up before you even try. You may be one of the women who fall happily outside the bell curve of fertility statistics and remain fertile into your forties. Or you may not be so lucky.

If you are over thirty-five, carefully consider how long you will wait to let "nature take its course" before seeking medical assistance in getting pregnant. Although couples are not considered "infertile" until they have unsuccessfully tried to conceive for one year, you may not wish to let a whole year go by. "If someone is forty years old and hasn't gotten pregnant in six months, I'd start intervening. In a twenty-one-year-old, I'd wait a year," advises Dr. David Walmer. Many obstetricians and fertility specialists recommend that women over age thirty-five try to get pregnant for at least six months before seeking medical treatments for infertility.

Do not take the pregnancy success stories in this chapter of women who conceive naturally or with a little help from medical technology in their late forties or fifties to mean that you should wait that long to try to get pregnant. Joanne got pregnant without fertility drugs at age forty-nine, but she is the exception—not the rule. Jessica had a successful IVF pregnancy at forty-six, but she, too, was an exception. Some women are not so fortunate and spend thousands of dollars on fertility treatments that do not produce a baby.

Although some of the women in this chapter became pregnant without help from fertility drugs or medical technology, others became pregnant with the help of one or more of the following treatments for infertility:

- Artificial insemination (AI): the sperm are placed in a catheter and deposited near a woman's cervix.
- Intrauterine insemination (IUI): the sperm are inserted, by way of a catheter, through the woman's cervix and into her uterine cavity.
- In vitro fertilization (IVF): the sperm and eggs are placed in a petri dish, the fertilized eggs are allowed to develop for several days, and the resulting embryos are transferred to a woman's uterus.
- Gamete intrafallopian transfer (GIFT): the sperm and eggs (the gametes) are surgically inserted into the woman's fallopian tube where, it is hoped, fertilization will occur in the "natural way" within the woman's body.
- Zygote intrafallopian transfer (ZIFT): several zygotes (embryos at an early stage of development) are surgically placed in the woman's fallopian tube.
- Egg donation: the sperm and donated eggs (usually from a young donor) are placed in a petri dish, the fertilized eggs are allowed to develop for several days, and the

resulting embryos are transferred to the recipient woman's uterus.

- Intracytoplasmic sperm injection (ICSI): the sperm are injected into the egg, placed in a petri dish, allowed to develop into embryos, and transferred to the woman's uterus.
- Ovulation induction: the mother-to-be takes fertility drugs to produce one or two eggs per menstrual cycle.
- Superovulation: the mother-to-be or egg donor takes fertility drugs to produce anywhere from four to twenty eggs per menstrual cycle.

See Chapter 6 for further descriptions of each of the above treatments.

Sometimes It Just Takes a Little Longer— and Sometimes It Doesn't

The Stories of Holly, Anna, Rhonda, Jennifer, Sharon, Claudia, Cheryl, and Kathleen R.

As you move into your thirties and forties, your odds of producing a viable egg that is capable of being fertilized and growing into a baby are not as high as when you were younger, but this does not mean that your reproductive years are over. You may still ovulate viable eggs, but possibly not every month. Consequently, it may take you a little longer to get pregnant.

For some of the women whom I interviewed for this book, getting pregnant was easy. For others, getting pregnant took months or even years. The anecdotes in this section on getting pregnant are success stories, representing possibilities that may or may not resemble your own personal circumstances. They also reflect wide variations in fertility treatments received by the women I interviewed. Both the treatments and the results sometimes conflict with what may be recommended by most infertility specialists or by what is expected on the basis of current statistics from studies of infertility treatments. For instance, Claudia, at age forty-three, became pregnant via IUI (intrauterine insemination), although some doctors do not recommend this procedure for women in their forties.

The anecdotes reflect the wide variety of medical practice when it comes to medications and procedures like IVF, GIFT, and ZIFT. They also reflect great individual variation in women's responses to fertility treatments and in their ability to get pregnant with or without medical assistance. The anecdotes are not intended to promote certain fertility treatments, to disparage others, or to give you medical advice.

Holly, Thirty-six
It wasn't hard for us to get pregnant. Soren is a wedding-day baby.

Much to her surprise, Holly became pregnant the first month she tried. She had anticipated that becoming pregnant would take a while because of her age. The pregnancy went well, except for some occasional spotting that persisted through eight months of her pregnancy. Her doctors believed that the spotting was caused by expanding fibroid tumors and examined Holly each month to make sure everything was going well. Although Holly's anxiety was greatly increased by the bleeding, in other respects she had a normal pregnancy and was able to commute to her job and to continue working full-time as a lawyer until the day she gave birth to a healthy boy named Soren.

Holly felt that she had a baby at the right age for her. She was more settled and calm at thirty-six than she was at thirty, and she had accomplished many of things she had wanted to do: she had worked with troubled teens, graduated from law school, traveled abroad, and landed an excellent job. Holly was ready to be a mother.

When Holly was almost thirty-nine, she tried to have another baby. It was harder for her to get pregnant, and when she finally did, the pregnancy ended in miscarriage.

Anna, Thirty-nine

I got married. I didn't try to get pregnant. I was just under the assumption that I just wasn't going to get pregnant. I was using a diaphragm, and I also knew that women my age were needing medical intervention to get pregnant—and that seemed more common than not with my peer group. When I found out I was pregnant, I took one of those pregnancy tests and said, "oh right . . . I'd better get one of those blood tests because this can't possibly be correct."

Anna became pregnant the month she married Michael. She had wanted to become pregnant in her twenties, but both she and her first husband were in the music business, and they decided to pursue their careers before having a child. Anna couldn't imagine having a child in nightclubs and concert halls; she wanted a baby only if she could bring it up in the right environment.

The years went by. Anna divorced. She remarried when she was thirty-nine, and that month she became pregnant. She was excited but also terrified because when Anna became pregnant in the late 1980s, women over thirty-five were considered high risk. At age forty, Anna gave birth to a daughter, Julia.

Like Holly, Anna has had many experiences in life, and she feels mature and settled enough for motherhood. "I don't have issues about what I could have been if I weren't a mom. I don't feel that I missed anything."

Anna became pregnant again when she was forty-one and about to move across country. She miscarried on the trip east.

Rhonda, Thirty-seven

It took me three months of trying. Then I got pregnant. My doctor didn't think I'd be able to get pregnant because I had one tube, and it was blocked with scar tissue from the surgery from my ectopic pregnancy. The doctor said she would give me three months of trying and if that didn't work she would urge me to have her "go in" and take the scar tissue away. It took three months to get pregnant with Eric.

When Rhonda tried to conceive in her late thirties, she got pregnant with twins. One embryo implanted in her uterus, but the other one lodged in her fallopian tube. She lost both pregnancies, her fallopian tube was surgically removed, and she waited seven months to heal from the surgery before trying to get pregnant again.

The second time, Rhonda became pregnant after three months of trying to conceive, even though she had only one fallopian tube and considerable scar tissue from the emergency surgery performed to remove her ectopic pregnancy. But a woman needs only one fallopian tube to become pregnant. Luckily, Rhonda's fertility was not adversely affected, and she quickly became pregnant. She had a healthy pregnancy and gave birth to a robust baby boy, Eric, by cesarean section.

When she was forty-one, Rhonda adopted a child, a Guatemalan girl, because she believed that going through another pregnancy would be too physically difficult for her given her previous surgeries and the demands of parenting her son. She advises other women to start pregnancy earlier than she did in order to optimize their fertile years: "I've heard so many women say, 'I've got time.' But women don't factor in the likelihood of having several miscarriages. Multiple miscarriages reduces the time. You have to wait awhile after you miscarry. I advise women that if they are thirty-five, they should get on it right away. I wish that I had started earlier."

Jennifer, Thirty-four and Thirty-nine

My doctor said, "Count on a year. It's frozen sperm—not as potent as fresh." He said there was a 60 percent success rate after a year. I told myself I'd wait a year. If I didn't succeed, I'd give up. I miscarried the first time. The next month I went again [to be artificially inseminated]. That one took. That's Jamie.

Jennifer, a single mother, became pregnant at age thirty-four following her second attempt at artificial insemination with frozen donor sperm. Her doctor thought it would take her longer than that, since pregnancy rates tend to be lower with frozen sperm than with fresh sperm. Before going ahead with the insemination, Jennifer's doctor performed a hysterosalpingogram, an x-ray test where dye is injected through the cervix into the uterus and fallopian tubes to make sure there are no physical obstructions in the uterus and tubes that might prevent pregnancy. Her tubes were fine.

To prepare herself physically for pregnancy, Jennifer gave up chocolate, coffee, and alcohol in order to protect her fertility. When the day of her insemination arrived, Jennifer brought a small charm with her to the doctor's office: a purple, egg-shaped pin. "It looked like a baby in utero. It was a kind of metaphor that made me feel like I had a focus when I held it in my hand." She got pregnant the first time, miscarried, tried again, and promptly became pregnant with her son, Jamie.

When she was thirty-nine, Jennifer quickly became pregnant again with frozen donor sperm, and she gave birth to another boy.

Sharon, Forty-three

For a very long time, most birth control didn't work for me. Throughout my twenties and thirties, I got pregnant on IUDs and birth control pills. But when my husband and I started trying to get pregnant in my late thirties, it just wasn't working.

When I was forty, we started thinking about IVF. It took several tries to work. The last time, they transferred three fertilized eggs, and at first all three implanted. One of them didn't develop. Two eggs took.

When Sharon was in her late thirties and ready to have a baby, she had trouble getting pregnant. Her menstrual cycles were normal, she had no diagnosable problem, but she wasn't conceiving.

First, Sharon tried IUI, with no success. Then, she moved on to fertility drugs. "I tried Pergonal, Humegon, all the different drugs," said Sharon. She also tried Chinese medicine. "It's all a blur," says Sharon of the three years during which she took fertility drugs; she no longer remembers which drugs she took or for how long she took them.

When she still could not get pregnant, Sharon turned to IVF. Her cousin, an infertility specialist, offered her free treatment since she could not afford the expensive drugs and procedures. After several tries, Sharon became pregnant. Much to her dismay, all three embryos transferred during the IVF "took"—which meant she was pregnant with triplets. However, one of the embryos didn't develop, leaving her pregnant with twins.

Although Sharon developed a rapid heartbeat during her early pregnancy and needed to go on heart medication, she was well enough to work during her pregnancy and to go on vacation with her husband during her fifth month.

During her seventh month of pregnancy, Sharon went into premature labor and spent a week on bed rest. Eight weeks before her due date, she gave birth to her two daughters by cesarean section. The premature girls weighed three pounds at birth. After six weeks in the hospital, the babies were ready to go home. They weighed five pounds each.

The twins, Rachel and Maia, are now healthy and active two-year-olds. Sharon enjoys being the mother of twins and observing their play and their special affection for one another, but she also remembers her fear when her three-pound babies suffered many crises during their first few weeks of life.

Some infertility specialists do not recommend IVF to women who are over forty-two, because the chance of success is very low. Sharon defied medical predictions by getting pregnant on an IVF cycle and by conceiving twins, even though her doctor transferred only three embryos (a procedure not expected to produce twins in women over forty).

Claudia, Forty-three
I think I really lucked out. I was forty-two when we started. My husband had a really low sperm count, and the combination was really bad. We tried GIFT a year later. Then we tried a combination of Metrodin and CLOMID with IUI [intrauterine insemination]. It was so much less stressful [than GIFT] on my body. IUI was much less invasive. I got pregnant on my second try.

Claudia became pregnant at age forty-three by using a combination of two different fertility drugs along with IUI with her husband's sperm. She had been trying to get pregnant for a year. When Claudia and her husband didn't conceive after several months of trying to have a baby, they decided to try a GIFT cycle because Claudia's first doctors recommended the GIFT procedure.

After taking the fertility drug Pergonal, Claudia produced four eggs; the eggs, along with her husband's sperm, were inserted into her fallopian tubes. At that time, many fertility doctors believed that GIFT was the most successful of the new reproductive technologies.

The GIFT procedure began like a regular IVF cycle when Claudia's eggs were surgically removed from her ovaries. However, in the GIFT procedure, instead of the eggs being fertilized in a "test tube" and allowed to develop into embryos in vitro, the eggs and the sperm were placed back into Claudia's fallopian tubes in order to become fertilized and to develop into embryos. This technique involved surgery and anesthesia. After Claudia was put under general anesthesia, her surgeon made an abdominal incision in order to insert the sperm and eggs into her tubes.

The procedure was not successful, and Claudia was devastated and exhausted.

Because Claudia found the GIFT procedure too intense and too expensive to repeat, she sought infertility treatment at her HMO. She was offered a combination of IUI and fertility drugs, which, her doctors told her, would give her a 5 percent chance of getting pregnant. She decided to try it. She took fertility drugs (CLOMID for five days and Metrodin for three days), went in for an ultrasound to confirm ovulation, and was inseminated with her husband's sperm. The first try was not successful. However, the second time, her doctor raised the Metrodin dose. Claudia produced four healthy-looking eggs. This time, the insemination was successful, and Claudia got pregnant and later gave birth to her baby girl, Amira.

Cheryl, Thirty-one

It was very easy to get pregnant. The second time I was inseminated [at age twenty-five], I got pregnant. The second time I tried to get pregnant [at age thirty-one], I didn't have regular cycles anymore—they were anywhere from thirty to one hundred days. I probably wasn't ovulating fertile eggs. The doctor prescribed Humegon, and she recommended I get inseminated when I had five viable eggs. Looking back, that wasn't a smart choice: I'm pregnant with twins.

Cheryl, a single mother and a computer whiz, knew that she wanted children when she was relatively young. At age twenty-four, she got pregnant via artificial insemination. Cheryl had a good job, a solid support system, and was ready to have a child even though she didn't have a life partner. Her first pregnancy went well, and Cheryl adapted to single motherhood.

When she was twenty-nine, Cheryl decided to have another baby. However, pregnancy did not come easily for Cheryl the second time around, even though she was still relatively young by fertility standards. Her periods were becoming irregular, and she was having trouble getting pregnant. She tried insemination without drugs and insemination with drugs. Her doctor prescribed CLOMID to help regulate her cycles, and Cheryl took the drug on and off for several months. She said the drug made her ovulate but made her uterine lining too thin for an embryo to implant. After Cheryl didn't get pregnant, her doctor recommended a more aggressive fertility drug, Metrodin, to help her produce many eggs during her menstrual cycle, which would give her a better chance of getting pregnant. Cheryl ovulated five eggs and became pregnant with twins.

Cheryl now wishes she had more carefully weighed the aggressive versus less aggressive fertility treatments and considered whether or not she was willing to conceive twins. "I should have said, 'let's wait a few days for some eggs to die out, or let's try a lower dose of Humegon the next cycle.' I needed to balance how important it was to conceive soon and how willing I was to risk twins or high-order multiples."

Fertility drugs such as Metrodin, Humegon, and Pergonal (drugs that stimulate the development of many egg follicles during a menstrual cycle) frequently have been responsible for the conception of high-order multiples—three, four, or more babies—in women who take these drugs. CLOMID sometimes results in twins but rarely in high-order multiples.

Luckily, both Cheryl and her babies remained healthy throughout the pregnancy. She gave birth to a six-pound boy and a five-pound girl at forty weeks gestational age, had a vaginal birth, and took the babies home from the hospital after two days.

Kathleen R., Thirty-nine

All of this stuff takes a long time. The tests, the procedures, and deciding what to do next. Before you know it, six months are gone. A year is gone.

For Kathleen and her husband, having a baby was a difficult process that took them four years. When she first started tracking her menstrual cycles with basal temperature readings, Kathleen was thirty-five. When her temperature chart showed no ovulation, her obstetrician referred her to an infertility specialist. He did an x-ray test to see if her tubes were open. "He shuttled me into a hysterosalpingogram, forgetting, or not addressing, the ovulation problem," says Kathleen. The x-ray showed that both her tubes were closed, and the doctor recommended surgery to repair her tubes.

Kathleen delayed the surgery for two reasons: her insurance wouldn't pay for it, and she was scared. She lost precious time waiting for a new insurance policy to take effect. As soon as she was insured, Kathleen switched to another doctor who performed the same test and found the same tubal problem. Kathleen had the surgery, which successfully repaired one of her fallopian tubes. After surgery, she started taking fertility drugs to get pregnant.

Kathleen and her doctor had forgotten about her ovulation problem—but not for long. Not surprisingly, her ovaries showed little or no response to the drugs. Her doctor referred her to the IVF clinic where blood tests revealed the source of her ovulation problem: "The doctor called to tell me my prolactin was high. 'You have a tumor in your pituitary.' Another shock. 'Don't worry. It's benign. Two percent of the population have these. It's causing your prolactin to be high. High prolactin inhibits ovulation.'"

Kathleen had a benign pituitary tumor called a pituitary adenoma that raised the level of prolactin in her blood; the prolactin prevented her from ovulating and caused her infertility.

Luckily, pituitary adenomas and the resulting infertility are treatable with a drug called bromocriptine. Kathleen took the medication to treat her tumor. However, Kathleen's doctor had told her that the drug wouldn't cure her infertility and signed her up for the egg donor/recipiency program.

While she was waiting for the clinic to find her a donor, Kathleen went to the beach with her husband. She got pregnant that weekend, miscarried two months later, and became pregnant again after two months on fertility drugs. Kathleen was thrilled:

"On our second drug trial we got pregnant with Austin. I was a week late with my period. I knew, but I made myself wait a week. Then I took the pregnancy test. I was afraid to believe it. I took a picture of the test stick [that read positive]."

Kathleen was one month from her fortieth birthday when she gave birth to her son, Austin.

When Kathleen and her husband tried to conceive their second child, she again took fertility drugs. "My response to drugs was becoming very poor," Kathleen said. When the clinic retested her husband's sperm months later, the doctors found his sperm motility was way down; his sperm were damaged due to a varicocele—a swollen vessel in his testes. He had surgery to repair the varicocele, and the couple tried to become pregnant again when Kathleen was forty-two. Kathleen underwent fifteen cycles of fertility drugs (well beyond the recommended course of drug treatment) attempting to become pregnant with a second child, but she did not conceive.

Kathleen's story illustrates the importance of finding thorough, intelligent infertility care if you have tried to get pregnant for months or years with no success. Less-than-optimal care will cost you time, money, emotional and physical distress—and possibly the chance of having a baby.

Life Outside the Bell Curve

Success Stories of the Chronologically Privileged: Joanne, Auben, and Jessica

This section tells the stories of midlife mothers who have become pregnant as a result of perseverance, positive thinking, resourcefulness, effective coping strategies—and good luck. They are stories of the sometimes difficult paths to happy endings.

Women over forty may have trouble getting pregnant and have a higher early miscarriage rate than younger women. However, some of these women experience problem-free pregnancies and easy births.

Joanne, Forty-nine
Once the amnio came back and it was fine, I decided that anything after that I could handle—gestational diabetes, bed rest. Every day I felt great. I looked great when I was pregnant. It was one of those lucky things. As I got closer [to the due date], the doctors had me coming in three times a week. Everything was fine. I just sailed through my pregnancy. People were scratching their heads.

Joanne postponed childbearing until she married at age forty-five. She had always wanted to have lots of children but had not wanted to become a single mom. She waited until she met her husband, Reyn, and then tried getting pregnant. She tried for two years, using fertility treatments on and off. Then she gave up and stopped using the drugs. Two years later, at age forty-nine, Joanne became pregnant—much to her surprise. "My period was one day late. At first I thought I might be going through menopause. But I took a pregnancy test. It was positive. I got another test. It was positive."

Although Joanne's story turned out to be a successful one, it began with two serious obstacles that she had to overcome: numerous uterine fibroid tumors and medical bias. When she was only thirty, her gynecologist told her she needed a hysterectomy to cure heavy periods caused by her fibroid tumors and to prevent cancer in the future. He told her, "It is the cure for older women; you're probably not going to have children." Joanne refused the surgery and drove to the library to look up fibroids.

At age forty-six, Joanne found an experienced reproductive surgeon who agreed to remove her numerous fibroids—and preserve her uterus. Six months after the surgery, Joanne tried to get pregnant. She tried artificial insemination and then several months of Metrodin. She religiously did ovulation tests every month, but every month she was disappointed. Then one weekend, while on a cruise with her husband, she gave up.

"I couldn't remember what the nurse had said about when I needed to inject myself with a fertility drug. I had to count the days. I'm holding this vial and syringe and waiting to remember what the nurse said. Nothing was written down. It was Sunday. I was on a cruise boat. I couldn't get through to the doctor's office. I thought, 'What am I doing? This is too disconnected from having a baby.' I felt like I was a laboratory rat."

Joanne stopped tracking her ovulation and trying to get pregnant. She looked into adopting a baby. Then, when she was forty-nine, her period was one day late. She took a pregnancy test. It was positive.

This time, Joanne's experience with her obstetricians was uniformly positive. From her amniocentesis to her delivery, her caregivers were supportive. Even her amniocentesis doctor was optimistic, assuring her that since there were no studies on women forty-nine or over when it came to birth defects, she should simply consider no news, good news. He turned her from pessimism to optimism in five minutes.

When her amnio results came back normal, Joanne brought her doctors flowers, announced her pregnancy at work, and settled in to enjoy her pregnancy.

Joanne acknowledges that her spontaneous pregnancy at age forty-nine is unusual and that most women will not have such good fortune. "I feel that I'm so lucky. I hesitate to say very much, because I don't think I'm the norm."

However, Joanne's history of having fibroid tumors is not unusual for a woman in her forties. Some women have a few large tumors, some have numerous small ones, and some women have "symptomatic" fibroids that cause pain or bleeding or obstruct bowel or bladder function (see Part 5). Occasionally, a hysterectomy is necessary for a woman with fibroids, especially if the fibroids are cancerous; however, a cancerous fibroid is extremely rare.

If a woman wants to have children, and if the fibroid is benign, a skilled gynecological surgeon can remove the fibroid and preserve the uterus for future childbearing (see Chapter 8). Often, fibroid tumors cause no problems, do not interfere with pregnancy, and need not be removed.

Auben, Forty-five: A Menopause Baby

I went to my gynecologist and told him I was thinking about getting pregnant. I was forty-four. He said the best time for childbearing is in your twenties, and he gave me the whole lecture on how I probably wasn't ovulating. I told him I didn't want a lot of this fertility stuff, because I knew a woman who got sick from all the hormones. I told him: "if it happens, it happens. I don't want a lot of science fiction." He gave me CLOMID. A year went by and nothing happened. Then I started skipping periods. I started having night sweats. I went to see the gynecologist. He said, "You're having menopausal symptoms. Your ovaries aren't working anymore." I felt like he was sentencing me to old-lady-hood right there in his office. Later, I sat in the car, and I just cried. I was surprised at my emotional reaction. I didn't know I wanted to be a mother that badly.

Several months later, Auben thought she had come down with the flu. She was pregnant. "I made an appointment to see my doctor. He said, 'In my twenty years of practice, I can count on one hand the number of women your age that conceived naturally.' . . . For the first four or five months, I hardly showed at all. I felt great. My pregnancy went really well."

Unlike Joanne, Auben hadn't always known she wanted to be a mother. She had married at age twenty-three but had no interest at all in having children. By her mid-thirties, however, Auben felt her biological clock was ticking. "I started buying some baby books. I talked to my husband about getting off the pill," said Auben. At that point she was working on a Ph.D. thesis in psychology and working with children. When she told the professor on her Ph.D. committee that she was thinking about getting pregnant, he disapproved and told her she was "psychologically acting out" and avoiding finishing her degree. Auben didn't think about pregnancy again until she was forty-three.

When she did get pregnant, it wasn't due to monitoring her basal temperature, using ovulation kits, or taking fertility drugs. Luckily, Auben anticipated the possibility of pregnancy occurring despite menopausal symptoms such as hot flashes, and she took steps that made a healthy pregnancy possible: she didn't get back on the pill, and she didn't take Accutane, a drug prescribed by her dermatologist for acne. Auben knew that

Accutane is teratogenic (it causes birth defects in developing babies), and she didn't fill her prescription—just in case.

Auben's pregnancy was healthy and, she says, a state of amazement: "I was just totally amazed the whole nine months."

Like many women pregnant later in life, Auben found the prenatal testing a scary time. She seriously considered having the baby even if he was abnormal. He wasn't.

It turned out that Auben's hot flashes were indications that her hormones were fluctuating and although she was transitioning into menopause, she was not there yet. Before assuming you are in menopause, it is wise to get several blood tests, several months apart, measuring your blood levels of estrodial, follicle-stimulating hormone (FSH), and luteinizing hormone (LH). If you are still hoping to become pregnant, hold off on hormone replacement for a while to avoid exposing a developing fetus to the designer estrogens or progesterones present in some hormone replacement regimens. Even some women on hormone replacement therapy may become pregnant if their ovaries have not yet shut down.

Jessica, Forty-seven

I made the choice to do what I had to do to get pregnant. I decided that I would have to handle every step as it went along. I understood that if I got pregnant, there was a larger chance that the baby would have Down's. I would have to take the challenges as they'd come.

Jessica falls outside the bell curve of success rates for in vitro pregnancies. IVF is not usually recommended when a woman is over forty-two years old, because the success rate is about 5 percent to 10 percent. However, Jessica was lucky and succeeded in getting pregnant by IVF when she was forty-seven years old.

Jessica and her husband tried to conceive when she was forty-one. She immediately got pregnant, but she also had five uterine fibroids that became huge, outgrew their blood supply, and degenerated. Jessica lost the pregnancy. Then she did what she had to do to get pregnant again. She had two surgeries to remove the fibroids. She took CLOMID with no results. She tried acupuncture, Chinese herbs, and raspberry leaf tea. She did a GIFT cycle at forty-three—but still no pregnancy. A series of six miscarriages followed, usually within her second month of pregnancy.

Still, Jessica was determined to have a child. At age forty-six, she found a doctor who would do an IVF cycle with her eggs and her husband's sperm. "If you're the person who is paying, you should be able to pay for what you want," Jessica argued. At age forty-seven, her IVF cycle resulted in a pregnancy and, nine months later, in the birth of a daughter.

IVF pregnancies after age forty-five are rare.

While Jessica knew that her odds were poor, she had the tenacity, the money, and the faith in her own fertility to gamble on being one of the few, lucky women to conceive a late-in-life baby by IVF.

It's a Miracle! Getting Pregnant the Egg Donor Way

Dion, Sarah, and Sharlene

The following anecdotes show the joys of "miracle babies" conceived despite obstacles of age, fibroids, and menopause. These stories of Dion, Sarah, and Sharlene demonstrate successful journeys through the high-tech world of egg donation and the unusual and sometimes difficult paths to happy endings.

Egg donation is a process by which eggs from one woman are surgically removed, fertilized, and transferred to another woman's uterus. Often the donor is in her twenties or early thirties and capable of producing viable eggs; the recipient is usually a woman who has gone through menopause or is no longer able to produce viable eggs. Egg donation is becoming an increasingly popular way to have a baby as women push their biological clock into their late forties and fifties. "It is a myth that women are too old to do this," says Dr. Mark Sauer, an expert on egg donation.

According to the study *Assisted Reproduction Technology Success Rates* (conducted by the CDC and the American Society for Reproductive Medicine) for both 1996 and 1998, the live birth rates resulting from embryo transfers using fresh donor eggs varied only slightly with the recipient woman's age. According to 1996 statistics, the national live birth rates per donor egg transfer for women under thirty-five years old (who used fresh eggs rather than frozen embryos) were similar to the live birth rates for women over forty. For women under thirty-five, the rate of live births per transfer was 39.3 percent. For women thirty-five to thirty-nine, the rate was 39.2 percent, and for women over forty the rate was 38.9 percent. In 1998, after further improvements in egg donation technology, the live birth rates with donor eggs increased. For women between the ages of thirty-five and forty-seven, live birth rates were similar and impressively high-between 40 and 44 percent.

An important note, however, is that according to the American Society for Reproductive Medicine, "success rates shown in this report are presented in terms of cycles, as required by law, rather than in terms of women. As a result, women who had more than one ART cycle in 1998 are represented in multiple cycles." In other words, the 40–44 percent does not mean that 40 percent of all the women who tried egg donation became pregnant. It means that 40 percent of all the donor egg transfers resulted in live births (and that some of these cycles could be from the same woman attempting pregnancy several times).

The women in this chapter faced daily injections given by medically inexperienced partners; pregnancies with twins; and the genetic and emotional uncertainties that may come with donor eggs. But these women agree that the end result of their struggles—making a baby—was well worth the effort.

The egg donation procedure usually dictates that both egg donor and recipient take hormonal drugs for several weeks. The donor takes powerful fertility drugs to stimulate her ovaries to "superovulate" and produce many eggs in a menstrual cycle, and the recipient may take other hormones (such as estrogen and progesterone) to prepare her uterus to receive the fertilized embryos.

Dion, Forty-six

Bonding is just bonding. I couldn't imagine being closer to them or loving them more.

For three years, Dion's life reads like a fairy tale. She fell in love, married, had twin boys, and signed a book contract with a New York publisher.

But hers is a modern fairy tale. Both the boys and the book came to her as the result of the most successful of the high-tech fertility treatments—egg donation. After eggs were donated by an anonymous twenty-five-year-old woman, fertilized in a petri dish, and transferred to her uterus as two-day-old embryos, Dion became pregnant at age forty-five. At forty-six, after a normal pregnancy, she gave birth to twins Alex and Matthew.

Like many women, Dion got her career in order before starting a family. Dion postponed childbearing until she had finished her Ph.D. and taught college for several years. In her late thirties, she was ready to have children. She looked for the right man—but didn't find him. Finally, at age forty-two, with her childbearing years waning and no permanent relationship in view, Dion decided to have a baby on her own.

For two years, she tried fertility treatments using a combination of fertility drugs and artificial insemination with donor sperm, but she never conceived. Eventually, her doctor told her about the high success rate of egg donation, recommended a doctor, and soon Dion was boarding a plane for the two-hour flight to a university infertility clinic for an evaluation.

One month later, Dion was giving herself hormone injections to prepare her body to receive donor eggs and, at the same time, falling in love. By the time her donor was ready to donate eggs, Dion's new love was ready to marry her.

Dion married, received donor eggs, which were fertilized with donor sperm, and got pregnant with twins—all in one summer. Dion and her husband, Marsh, found romance in the high-tech procedure. As Dion and Marsh gazed at the four embryos in a petri dish, she marveled, "The embryos looked like flowers. Each cell looked like a petal." The couple consider the event a kind of birthday, and they light candles to remember it.

Dion, a woman who jogged and swam regularly, experienced a normal pregnancy. Surprisingly, she was one of the few members of her pregnant-with-twins group to carry to term (instead of delivering prematurely). Although some of the younger members of the group required bed rest, Dion did not.

Although the outcome was good, Dion's last trimester of pregnancy was not without anxiety. Since she was pregnant with twins, she was automatically considered high risk. During her last weeks of pregnancy, she hooked herself up to a fetal monitor at home several times a day and transmitted the results by phone to Stanford University Medical Center. If the babies were in distress or premature, she would go to Stanford by helicopter since Stanford had a neonatal intensive care unit. If the babies were fine, she would have the babies at a local hospital. The babies were fine, and there was no chopper ride for Dion— but there were weeks of uncertainty preceding the birth.

Dion and Marsh have been candid about the egg donation with family, friends, and doctors. "Nobody has been
appalled. . . . The bottom line is, you've got this cute kid.
That's what people see, not the abstraction of biogenetics."

Dion plans to tell her boys of their unusual mode of conception when they are older. "Marsh and I feel they have the
right to know."

Two years after the boys were born, Dion wrote a book on
assisted reproduction.

Sarah, Forty-six and Forty-eight
*I'm in love with my son. I was in love with him during
the pregnancy.*

Like Dion, Sarah had postponed childbearing while she
was building a successful career. And, like Dion, she has lived a
charmed life. At age forty-one, Sarah decided it was "time" to
start a family. In her typically efficient fashion, she gave herself
six months to meet a man. She put an ad in the personals for a
man who wanted marriage and children. Within months, Sarah
had three marriage proposals.

Sarah married at age forty-two and tried to get pregnant.
She didn't conceive. She took the fertility drug Pergonal for two
years. Still no pregnancy. Sarah also took CLOMID for a while,
with no success. Finally, at age forty-five, she turned to egg
donation. "My ob-gyn thought women in their forties need a
little help to get pregnant. I took a year of Pergonal. After seven
or eight months my doctor said, 'You might want to consider
egg donation.'"

So Sarah found an egg donor. Because she didn't want the
donor to be a stranger, she found someone she knew. The first
time Sarah's infertility specialist transferred embryos derived
from the younger woman's eggs, Sarah did not become pregnant.
She decided to try again, this time using frozen embryos left over

in "storage" from the first attempted egg donation cycle. "It was my last attempt. You have to feel like you've given it your all. It worked." Sarah became pregnant at age forty-six.

Sarah encountered some problems during her pregnancy, but nothing serious. Her uterine fibroids grew but posed no threat to the pregnancy. Her bag of waters broke one month early—at thirty-six weeks—but she took antibiotics to prevent infection. However, when her cervix wasn't dilating and her baby had a "nonreassuring" heartbeat on the monitor, she had a cesarean section. Even though Sarah had a touch of preeclampsia—with leg swelling and elevated blood pressure—both she and the baby were fine. Seven days after her cesarean, she came back to work to take care of some unfinished business. She was back at work full-time within two weeks.

Sarah maintains contact with the donor, who is a family friend. The donor now has had a baby of her own.

Two years after the birth of her first child, Sarah found another egg donor—a friend of the first donor. When Sarah was forty-eight, she gave birth to her second baby by cesarean section.

Sharlene, Forty-eight and Fifty-two

I wanted a baby so bad that a donor didn't matter. It was that or adoption. And at our age adoption was not a good option.

Sharlene married her high school sweetheart. She stopped using birth control in her late twenties, assuming pregnancy would just happen. It didn't. Meanwhile, she worked, traveled, suffered a serious work-related injury, and developed rheumatoid arthritis. She was forty-two when she and her husband decided to pursue having a baby via medical technology if they weren't able to get pregnant the natural way. Sharlene took CLOMID for several months. Then she tried AI plus CLOMID for several months. Her doctor made her take a break in between drug cycles to give her ovaries a rest. Then she went on to try Pergonal for four or five cycles, again with rests in between cycles. She experienced no adverse side effects from the drugs, despite a high dose. Sharlene did not get pregnant.

Sharlene was forty-three. She wanted to try IVF, but her doctors advised against it because they said it wasn't cost effective; she wasn't producing enough eggs. It was at this point that Sharlene and her husband decided upon egg donation.

Sharlene felt compelled to have a baby: "You're not rational once you get into the whole system. Sometimes you are really not thinking about what you're doing. It's a passion you are trying to achieve at any cost."

She and her husband decided that they did not want to know the egg donor or have her become involved in their lives. However, Sharlene would have liked a bigger role in choosing the donor. "The doctors don't give you a big file and say, 'Pick.' They ask you what your preferences are and come up with three donors. They're still ultimately picking and choosing."

The first donor didn't work out, but after six months the couple found another donor. Of the sixteen eggs that were harvested from the egg donor, fourteen made good embryos. Sharlene's doctor transferred four of the fresh embryos to her uterus and froze the remaining ten.

Sharlene did not become pregnant, so she tried again. Her doctor transferred four frozen embryos, and Sharlene got pregnant and had a healthy pregnancy and a vaginal birth.

Sharlene did not discuss the egg donation with most of her friends, although she plans to tell her daughter later on in order to give her an accurate family and medical history and prevent her from worrying about Sharlene's familial diseases. "My mother had breast cancer. Ryan doesn't have to fall into that category."

Sharlene told most of her friends and family that her daughter, Ryan, came from a frozen embryo, which was true. "I'm pretty open about it now. It's a miracle."

Sharlene became pregnant with her second egg donor baby (the genetic sister of her first baby since both children were conceived using eggs from the same donor) after two embryo transfer procedures with her remaining frozen embryos. The pregnancy went smoothly, and she experienced few problems even though Sharlene was now fifty-two. However, this time the baby's placenta implanted low in the uterus, and her doctors worried that Sharlene might have placenta previa, a condition in which the baby's placenta implants low in the uterus near the cervix and sometimes obstructs the birth canal (see Part 8). But as her uterus expanded, it brought the placenta along with it, and the placenta no longer obstructed the birth canal. Sharlene was relieved.

For this pregnancy, Sharlene hired a doula, since she had experienced a long labor with her first child. Her labor began much as it had the first time: her bag of waters suddenly broke. But when she arrived at the hospital, Sharlene started bleeding and continued to bleed. The placenta was separating from her uterine wall, a condition known as placental abruption, and she was rushed into the operating room for an emergency cesarean section.

Placental abruption can cause serious bleeding that puts both mother and baby at risk. There are some reports of increased incidence of placenta previa and placental abruption in pregnancies conceived by reproductive technologies such as IVF and egg donation, but there is no hard evidence.

Both Sharlene and her newborn daughter, Erin, did well, although Sharlene needed a blood transfusion and spent the day in a recovery room separated from her baby. Sharlene breastfed her baby (even though she was in menopause when she became pregnant with her second egg donor child). Now Sharlene enjoys motherhood and marvels at her daughters who, not surprisingly, resemble one another: "Both my babies came from frozen embryos [from the same donor]. They look like twins."

Chapter 6
Your Odds for Successful Midlife Pregnancy

From a statistical basis—if you can—plan to have a baby before forty.
—Dr. Allen Killam

* * *

I have so many patients who are kicking themselves for waiting.
—Dr. Alice Domar

* * *

U.S. pregnancy statistics tell a story that is both heartening and sobering. Increasing numbers of women over age thirty are getting pregnant and having healthy pregnancies, although pregnancy rates start to gradually decline in women over age thirty-five.

If you are thirty to thirty-four, your odds for a healthy pregnancy are good. According to the 1999 *National Vital Statistics Reports,* increasing numbers of women are having babies in their thirties and forties. However, at forty, women are not generally as fertile as they were at thirty. In 1999, the birth rate for women aged twenty-five to twenty-nine was 117.8 per 1,000 (over one million births) while the rate for women thirty to thirty-four was 89.6 per 1,000 (892,400 births). From age thirty-five to age thirty-nine, the birth rate went down 38.3 per 1,000 (434,294 births). Although women aged forty to forty-four had a birth rate of only 7.4 per 1,000, that number represents more than 80,000 births. More importantly, the national age-related birth rates do not indicate your odds for having a baby! The statistics do not take into account the number of women in the older age groups who have stopped trying to become pregnant; many women in these groups are *not* trying to get pregnant, a factor that may make your odds seem lower than they actually are.

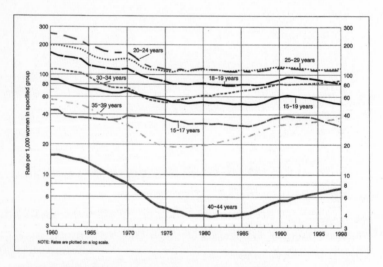

Figure 6-1: Birth rates by age of mother: United States, 1960–1999

From: Births: Final Data for 1999, *National Vital Statistics Reports,* Volume 49, Number 1, April 17, 2001 (from the Centers for Disease Control and Prevention, National Center for Health Statistics, National Vital Statistics System).

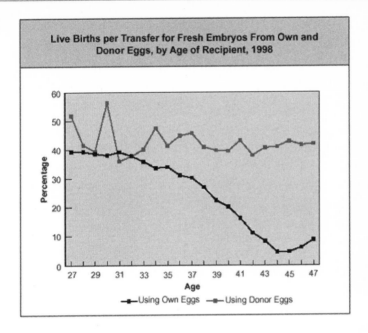

Figure 6-2: Comparison of live births from donor eggs with live births from IVF with a woman's own eggs by age of woman.

From: CDC's Reproductive Health Information Source. *1998 Assisted Reproductive Technology Success Rates. National Summary and Fertility Clinic Reports* *(www.cdc.gov/nccdphp/drh/art98/index.htm)*.

Statistics show that women aged forty-five through fifty-four are still having babies but at the reduced rate of 0.3 to .09 in 1,000, depending on ethnic background (women of Asian or Pacific Island descent have higher rates in this age group than white, black, or Hispanic women).

If you are over forty, you need not give up hope of pregnancy. Thousands of women your age continue to have babies.

The preliminary 1999 birth statistics show that among women aged forty-five to fifty-four, there were 4,330 births for that year, although many of these births may have resulted from assisted reproduction procedures such as IVF with donor eggs.

When you consider your odds for pregnancy, keep in mind that statistics reflect *average* fertility rates, which are calculated by including the rates of women who are less fertile than others in their age group with the rates of those who are more fertile than others in their age group. Despite the averages, some women will remain fertile well into their forties. You could fall anywhere along this continuum, depending on your individual biology, your family pregnancy history, your current medical condition, and your partner's fertility. Consequently, you should not take national fertility statistics as absolute prophecy about your individual reproductive future.

Use statistics as a rough guideline to help you plan the timing of your pregnancy. If you are having trouble getting pregnant, see a reproductive endocrinologist who can assess the reproductive health of both you and your partner. If you do not conceive after a reasonable period of time (a year if you are in your early through mid-thirties, six months in your early to mid-forties, and three to six months if you are over forty-five), you may wish to try assisted reproduction treatments such as IUI, IVF, GIFT, or egg donation.

Eggs and Ovulation

It's egg quality [that makes the difference in getting pregnant]. We can fix most ovulation problems. We can make most women recruit eggs. The question is the quality of the eggs you're getting.
—Dr. David Walmer

If you put off pregnancy and if you run into problems, time might be one of the problems. Time should be on your side, not against you.
—Leda, at age thirty-nine, had a baby girl after trying to have a baby for six years

⁕ ⁕ ⁕

Even if your ovaries produce eggs, you ovulate regularly, and you have regular periods, it is the *quality* of your eggs and ovulation that will determine if you can become pregnant. Healthy eggs and hormonally normal ovulation are essential ingredients for fertility.

Dr. Mark Sauer and Dr. David Walmer, both directors of university-based infertility programs, provide realistic yet sympathetic perspectives on the quality of eggs and ovulation in women over thirty. Dr. Sauer, a reproductive endocrinologist at Columbia University and one of the "fathers" of egg donation technology, advises women to consider biological time limits if they plan to postpone pregnancy, especially if they want to have a child with their own eggs rather than donor eggs.

"Age-related infertility is not a disease. It's a normal human condition and biologically determined. . . . Women should be aware that reproductive capacity is not endless," advises Sauer, who worries that women will end up disappointed if they assume they can beat the odds. He sympathizes with the plight of American women who postpone pregnancy until they develop a solid relationship and career—only to find that their fertility has waned in the meantime. "You're raised as a woman in American society geared toward childbearing. You wait for Mr. Right. You become an attorney and find yourself in your early thirties or forties and, through no fault of your own, you are reproductively challenged. It comes as a shock."

Sauer points to studies of the Amish and of Islamic villagers as proof that a decline in female fertility is natural and measurable. He maintains that the numbers from "natural population curves" derived from studies of Amish women (who do not use birth control and get pregnant from their teens into their forties) give some indication of about how long women remain fertile.

Dr. David Walmer, a reproductive endocrinologist at Duke University Medical Center, agrees that egg quality declines as a woman grows older, although he stresses that a woman's fertility is an individual thing, and you never know at what age fertility will decline in a particular woman.

Many women think that as long as their hormone levels are normal, they are fertile. While this may sometimes be true, says Walmer, sometimes it is not. Even if a woman ovulates normally and has regular menstrual cycles into her forties, her egg quality may not be normal:

"It's not hormones. It's the quality of the egg and the likelihood that each egg that a woman has left can develop into a baby. Of the three things you need to get pregnant—sperm, eggs, and a uterus—two of them are renewable resources and one is not. The lining of your uterus is thirty days old, because you make a new one every month. Men make new sperm every ninety to one hundred days. And women make all their eggs before they're born. So when a woman's forty, her eggs are forty years old."

Of course, there are always exceptions. Occasionally women in their forties have eggs that remain fertile and capable of conception, although conception may take longer or require some help from reproductive medicine.

If you are not one of these biologically lucky women, there is nothing you can do to improve the *quality* of your eggs. However, you can take hormonal fertility drugs to increase the *quantity* of eggs you ovulate each month in order to increase your odds of getting pregnant (see Chapter 7).

If your doctor suspects that you are not ovulating, that your egg quality is poor, or that hormonal imbalances are interfering with your ovulation, he or she may take blood or urine tests to help assess your hormone levels and ovulation. Unfortunately, you cannot count on these diagnostic tests to define the quality of your ovulation or your eggs, since tests for ovulatory problems do not always offer precise results. Ovulation kits can determine an LH surge, which usually indicates if you are ovulating, and ultrasound scans can actually visualize the egg follicles. But neither test determines the actual quality of your eggs.

Diagnosing female fertility problems remains a challenge, despite tests of a woman's hormone levels, says Walmer:

"We can look at hormone levels to try to get an assessment of fertility, but most of those [changes in] hormone levels are very late indications of a loss of fertility. The vast majority of the population will have normal numbers even if their fertility is diminished. We can do a CLOMID challenge test. A Day 3 FSH. A Day 3 estradiol. Abnormal numbers are bad news, but normal numbers are not necessarily good news. We need to tailor the lab test to the individual patient."

Furthermore, an individual woman's hormone levels may vary significantly from menstrual cycle to menstrual cycle. Consequently, it is difficult to diagnose ovulation problems and to clearly categorize the quality of a woman's ovulation. "Nothing in nature is that rigid. You're going to have a spectrum from good to bad. We don't have a yardstick to distinguish between primo cycles and those that are borderline," says Walmer.

One of the most controversial diagnoses in the area of hormonally related ovulatory problems in older women is *luteal phase defect*—a condition in which the corpus luteum (part of the egg follicle that remains on the ovary after ovulation and that releases progesterone during the weeks after an egg is released) does not produce as much progesterone as it should. This failure results in a progesterone deficiency that may interfere with the successful implantation of an embryo. Sometimes frequent early pregnancy loss is attributed to luteal phase defect—which is why some doctors give women additional progesterone to "support the pregnancy" during the last part of their menstrual cycle or during their first trimester of pregnancy. (See Chapter 7.)

However, some doctors argue that early pregnancy loss is more often due to genetically flawed eggs and embryos than to hormonal imbalances. Although progesterone may support some high-tech pregnancies (such as pregnancies achieved with donor eggs where the egg recipient is making none of the natural progesterone that comes with ovulation or early pregnancy), it has not been proven to prevent miscarriage in women who have become pregnant without high-tech interventions. "There is no data that supplementing pregnancy with progesterone—even if a woman has had a history of recurrent pregnancy loss—improves her likelihood of success," says Walmer.

Like many other reproductive endocrinologists, Walmer believes that low progesterone levels may result from an unhealthy pregnancy that is not meant to be and that adding progesterone isn't going to save such a pregnancy.

Whether luteal phase defect is truly a common problem among women is the subject of medical debate. According to Dr. Sauer, "Luteal phase defect is overdiagnosed. It is easier to treat it than to see if it exists, although it probably exists in a small number of women."

The debate is not easily settled, however, since the tests (endometrial biopsy and blood progesterone levels) used to diagnose the condition often yield confusing or misleading results. "We have tests that people use, but these tests are not very good at discriminating between normal and abnormal patients," says Walmer. For instance, a woman's blood progesterone levels may fluctuate during the day, making results difficult to interpret, adds Walmer. "The dilemma is that everyone knows that no progesterone early in pregnancy is bad. So there must be some sort of threshold. But nobody knows what that threshold is. The problem is that we use a single blood value [a onetime test] for a hormone that cycles up and down fairly widely. When you draw a hormone level, you don't know if you're in the peak, the trough, or in between."

If your menstrual cycles are often shorter than twenty-seven days or longer than thirty-six days, you may have an ovulation problem, says Walmer. See a reproductive endocrinologist in order to identify the cause of the menstrual irregularity. Sometimes irregularities are due to polycystic ovarian syndrome (PCOS) or other hormonal conditions that may respond to hormonal drugs.

Do not self-prescribe these drugs, and do not use them without a doctor's supervision. Hormonal drugs may have powerful side effects and should be taken only when specifically prescribed and while under the careful monitoring of a physician.

Sperm: The Male Factor

We tried to get pregnant for about a year. We thought it had to be the woman. But Jeff was sterile. His sperm count was 3. Not 3,000, but 3.
—Stacy became pregnant when she was twenty-eight and then again when she was thirty-two through ICSI—a high-tech procedure whereby her husband's sperm were mechanically inserted into her eggs.

*If the husband is thirty, age is not a problem, but if the husband
is forty, there could be problems like varicose veins or previous
infections.*
—Dr. Allen Killam

• • •

For couples with fertility problems, about 40 percent of the
time, the male partner is either "the sole cause or a contributing
cause of infertility," according to the American Society for
Reproductive Medicine (1999, Media Fact Sheet on Infertility).
About 40 percent of the time, the female partner has the fertility problem. However, sometimes the fertility problem results
from the combined effect of the structural, medical, or age-
related problems of both members of a couple.

The "male factor" in a couple's fertility involves both the
number of sperm and the quality of sperm that a man produces.
To test for fertile sperm, doctors assess the number of sperm
and their motility (how well they swim). Men with high sperm
counts are not necessarily fertile, since they may produce damaged sperm with poor motility or sperm that are unable to penetrate an egg.

Age may be a factor in male fertility, although sperm are
not affected by age in the same way that eggs are, since a man
continually produces *new* sperm. However, the quality or quantity of a man's sperm may decrease as he ages or may change
due to past or present health problems. Some men have medical problems or infections that diminish their fertility—conditions that may be medically or surgically treated, but with
varying degrees of effectiveness.

How to best test for and remedy sperm-related problems is
the subject of debate, partly because male infertility is difficult
to diagnose on the basis of the appearance and motility of
sperm. Many doctors dismiss the effectiveness of the "hamster

test" once used to assess the ability of sperm to penetrate an egg (albeit a hamster egg). Some doctors contend that expensive "swim-up" tests and other complex screening, as well as "washing sperm" and whirling them around in a centrifuge, are a waste of time and money. Others swear by such techniques. Many health experts argue that further research is needed to establish better diagnostic and treatment procedures and to assess current ones.

To date, the most effective fertility treatment for men with few or immotile sperm is intracytoplasmic sperm injection (ICSI), a high-tech micromanipulation procedure whereby a sperm is grasped with a tiny instrument and inserted into an egg. Usually, the procedure involves using several sperm to fertilize several eggs. After the eggs are fertilized in a petri dish, the resulting embryos are inserted in a woman's uterus or fallopian tubes.

ICSI has been dramatically successful in allowing men whose sperm were neither motile, plentiful, nor mature enough to fertilize an egg under natural circumstances to become fathers.

ICSI is an expensive, popular, and relatively new method, which may or may not have long-term side effects. Some recent studies indicate that the ICSI procedure may damage eggs or sperm, although other studies indicate that the babies resulting from ICSI procedures are healthy. Critics of the procedure question whether we should facilitate pregnancy with sperm that are otherwise unable to penetrate an egg, since we may be overriding a process of natural selection in which only the healthiest sperm are allowed to fertilize eggs and pass genes on to the next generation. Defenders of the procedure point to a growing number of healthy children born as a result of ICSI. Discuss the benefits and possible short- and long-term risks of the ICSI procedure with your reproductive endocrinologist and embryologist before undergoing the procedure.

Can Eggs and Sperm Find Each Other?

The issue that starts at thirty is getting pregnant. After age thirty, pregnancy becomes more and more difficult. By forty, there is a considerable infertility factor. Endometriosis can make conception more difficult, as can blockage of the tubes.
—Dr. Allen Killam

• • •

First, you need to answer the questions: Are there sperm, are there eggs, and can they find each other?
—Dr. David Walmer

• • •

If you have healthy eggs and your partner has viable sperm yet you still are not getting pregnant, your problem may reside in the passageways that sperm and eggs must traverse in order to meet, fertilize, and form an embryo.

As a woman over thirty, you are more likely than a younger woman to have developed problems such as endometriosis, infections, or fibroid tumors that can obstruct conception by preventing eggs and sperm from finding each other in your fallopian tubes. These conditions may also interfere with pregnancy by preventing an egg from implanting in your uterine lining. If your partner is over thirty, he also may have developed health problems that could interfere with his fertility.

Under normal circumstances, your fallopian tubes are mobile; they reach for an egg as the egg bursts out of its follicle in your ovary. However, if you have internal scar tissue or adhesions from abdominal surgeries, or if you have advanced endometriosis (a condition in which the endometrial lining of the uterus migrates to the tubes, ovaries, and/or abdominal cavity), your fallopian tubes may become stuck to other organs or too hampered by endometriosis or scarring to receive the egg. Infections from IUDs or from sexually transmitted diseases may also create adhesions and subsequent fertility problems.

If you have had infections or endometriosis, the interior of your fallopian tubes may be obstructed, possibly hindering the passage of eggs or sperm through the tube. Fallopian tubes may also be obstructed by uterine fibroid tumors.

Two tests that are commonly used to determine if your tubes are open or closed are hysterosalpingogram and laparoscopy. In a hysterosalpingogram, your doctor (or radiologist) inserts a catheter through your cervix and then injects a dye through the catheter. As the dye is injected, your doctor will take x-rays to see how well the dye circulates inside your uterus and fallopian tubes. If a fallopian tube is blocked, the dye will not be able to pass through the tube. If you have a blocked tube, your physician may recommend that you either have the tube repaired with micro-surgery or circumvent the tube by using IVF to become pregnant. IVF is an especially effective procedure for women who have mechanical obstacles (adhesions, scarring) that are preventing the egg and sperm from meeting in the fallopian tube. Surgical repair of the tube may or may not solve your problem, and it may create additional problems that result in an ectopic (tubal) pregnancy. However, if the tube is successfully repaired, you may be spared the additional expense and stress of IVF.

Laparoscopy is a surgical technique that helps your doctor see your fallopian tubes and ovaries in order to diagnose and sometimes correct reproductive-system problems that interfere with conception. During a laparoscopy, you are sedated or anes-thetized while very small incisions are made in your abdomen. An instrument called a laparoscope is passed through the inci-sion, so your physician can diagnose your problem. Your doctor can surgically remove pelvic adhesions, ovarian cysts, and some types of fibroid tumors during this procedure (see Chapter 8).

If You Are Still Not Pregnant

If somebody is approaching forty years old and hasn't gotten pregnant in six months, I'd start intervening.
—Dr. David Walmer

• • •

If I have angina, I go to a cardiologist, not a family doctor. If I have infertility, reproductive endocrinologists are the only people who can treat me.
—Dr. Mark Sauer

• • •

If you don't get pregnant, you always have the option of patience. Sometimes it takes more than a year or two to become pregnant, especially if you are in your late thirties or early forties. However, many reproductive endocrinologists suggest that women over thirty-five make the most of their remaining reproductive years and seek medical assistance if they have trouble getting pregnant.

At what point should you seek medical assistance? If you are between thirty and thirty-five, many doctors advise that you try to get pregnant for a year. If you are over thirty-five or forty, they say try for four to six months. For persisting fertility problems, seek the opinion of a board-certified reproductive endocrinologist (someone who has completed two years of training in infertility treatment and passed a national exam certifying competence) in order to identify and treat any reproductive problems that you and/or your partner may have.

Unfortunately, it is often difficult for potential patients to sift through all the clinics offering infertility treatments and decide which clinics have the most competent, ethical, and credentialed doctors. For instance, some doctors are listed in the phone book as infertility specialists, even when they do not have this special training. So how do you choose a doctor? Dr. Sauer advises women to choose board-certified reproductive endocrinologists, doctors who are specially trained to treat infertility. The infertility business has become a big business, warns Sauer, and the consumer must not take medical advertisements in the Yellow Pages at face value.

If you want to try treatments for fertility, make sure that:

a. Your doctor gives you adequate informed consent—that means balanced, unbiased information about the pros and cons of each procedure or drug you are being offered.

b. Your doctor tells you which procedures and drugs are experimental.

c. Your doctor explains why a particular treatment is appropriate for your particular condition.

d. You read the package inserts for all medications (ask your pharmacist for the package inserts—information that accompanies pharmaceutical drugs to explain the uses, the potential side effects, and the appropriate dosages).

e. You get a second medical opinion (from a doctor in a different clinic) if your doctor recommends tubal or uterine surgery, hysterectomy, or long-term fertility drug treatments (see Chapter 7).

f. You seek a second opinion if your doctor tells you that you are too old to have a baby.

g. You carefully consider the pros and cons of the various treatments offered to you.

Once you and your partner have found a doctor, get appropriate diagnostic tests and decide what to do next. If you are in your thirties or early forties, you may be offered treatments such as superovulation with fertility drugs, or fertility drugs in addition to such procedures as AI or IUI, IVF, GIFT, or ICSI—treatments that rely on the fertility of your own eggs. If you are in your mid- to late forties or your fifties and have a history of long-term infertility, or are menopausal, your doctor may suggest egg donation.

How do you know which is the best treatment for you? You don't necessarily know, which is why choosing a good doctor is so important. We live in a time where conflicting opinions and contradictory studies create a confusing world for both infertility specialists and their patients. There often are no hard and fast answers as to what infertility treatment may be best for you. Consequently, it is important for you to get the medical opinions of a specialist or two, ask lots of questions, investigate which treatments are supported by the strongest medical evidence, and respect your subjective reactions to doctors and the treatments they recommend. Only after carefully considering your choices can you make informed decisions about expensive, high-tech treatments for infertility.

Assisted Reproduction

All of the therapies that we have carry some risk. So you want to balance risk and benefit. If someone hasn't demonstrated that they have difficulty getting pregnant, then you don't want to expose them to the risks of the therapies.
—Dr. David Walmer

• • •

"We don't do anything magical," says Dr. David Walmer when he talks about his work as an infertility specialist. "We just give eggs and sperm the opportunity to do what they do naturally."

Some infertility treatments help eggs and sperm do what

they do naturally by increasing the number of eggs that a woman produces each month or by giving sperm a "boost" by placing them closer to the eggs, thus making their journey shorter. These low-tech, relatively noninvasive treatments include fertility drugs that push a woman's ovaries to ovulate many eggs (instead of only one) during a menstrual cycle and artificial insemination procedures that collect a man's sperm and insert them near the woman's cervix or within her uterus. To help nature just a little bit more, sometimes doctors use both drugs and insemination to increase a couple's odds of becoming pregnant. For many couples, these first-line treatments result in pregnancy.

Some couples who do not conceive move on to the high-tech infertility treatments such as IVF, ICSI, or egg donation in which conception takes place in a petri dish where the embryos incubate until they are three to six days old and ready to be placed in a woman's uterus. Walmer sees such laboratory fertilization as "an incredible gift" that works in accord with nature.

Assisted reproduction procedures such as IVF, GIFT, and ZIFT can only work with nature—not transform it. The procedures simply help eggs and sperm find each other and boost your monthly odds of conceiving, but they cannot make your eggs younger. For women in their mid- to late thirties, assisted reproduction expedites an event that's likely to occur anyway, although it may take a woman five or six years to become pregnant naturally, without medical intervention.

For women in their mid- to late forties who want to try the high-tech reproductive technologies, many doctors recommend egg donation instead of IVF, since egg donation can boost a woman's chances of having a baby to between 39 and 50 percent. For most women over age forty-five, the odds of becoming pregnant using her own eggs and IVF are much lower—only about 5 to 10 percent. Of course, doctors' opinions differ regarding how to view such statistical averages. For some physicians, a 5 to 10 percent chance of a woman becoming pregnant via IVF is so low that they may advise women against such a potentially disappointing route to pregnancy. Other physicians still consider IVF an option until age forty-five and sometimes later, arguing that a 5 percent chance for a woman in her late forties is better than no chance at all, and the procedure will give her an opportunity to conceive naturally with her own eggs.

Often your doctor will individualize your infertility treatments to fit your age, your medical profile, and your particular infertility problem. When he begins treatments, Dr. Walmer takes into consideration which therapies tend to be more successful for women in midlife and for women or couples who have particular fertility problems. "Population statistics describe 'people who look like you' in terms of age and reproductive problems," which does not always result in easy, clear-cut answers, says Walmer. "Everybody's stuck with the dilemma of figuring out how population statistics apply to individual couples. You figure out the population numbers and say, 'Here's what the therapies are that appear to have a benefit for someone with your problem.'"

Another reason why treatment success statistics do not provide you with clear-cut answers is that these statistics are not always based on the most solid kind of medical evidence—the kind that comes from large research studies—but rather on the doctor's medical opinion and clinical experience. Given the nature of infertility patients, it is difficult for doctors to gather "hard scientific evidence." The most reliable kind of medical evidence comes from very large studies that are "controlled, randomized, prospective trials."

To do these kinds of studies, doctors need patients who are willing to be randomly assigned to groups that either receive the fertility treatment or do not receive it. However, in the case of infertility studies, very few people are willing to be in the group that does not receive the treatment, since most of the patients desperately want to have a baby. Another problem with research on fertility treatments: many studies are simply not large enough to provide researchers with clear-cut answers. In order to do a study with meaningful statistics, doctors need to study many people. In the case of fertility treatments, there are often not enough people participating in the study for the researchers to arrive at clear-cut conclusions.

To make matters more confusing, success rates for procedures may vary from clinic to clinic, depending on the patient population of the clinic, its facilities, and the skills of its doctors and embryologists.

If many clinics consistently favor one procedure over another, you have an indication that the procedure probably produced good results, advises Dr. Walmer.

"All of us in the infertility business are faced with interpreting a literature that may have stronger or weaker evidence to support what we do . . . IVF for blocked tubes doesn't differ from program to program. There is minimal variance in certain things. Things that are consistently done from one program to another are things that have withstood the test of time. As things change, some programs change more rapidly than others. The more discrepant the therapies are from program to program is probably an indication of less evidence to support them."

Whether you choose to get pregnant naturally or with help from medical technology, you are making high-stakes choices that involve considerable uncertainty. Even if you are clear about where you stand in terms of your age and diagnosis, you must choose procedures based on conflicting medical opinion as well as on subjective factors such as what feels right for you.

When you are considering reproductive technologies, do

your research. Consult the American Society for Reproductive Medicine (ASRM) and CDC sites on the Internet to compare statistics from various fertility clinics (see appendix). Gather as much information as you can on fertility treatments in order to fully understand the benefits and risks of your options before you choose one.

The 1998 CDC Reproductive Health Information Source makes available the study called *1998 Reproductive Technology*

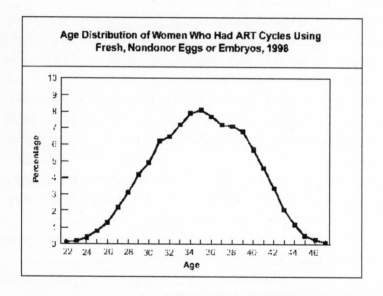

Figure 6-3: The graph shows the age distribution of women in 1998 who tried to get pregnant (using their own eggs or embryos) using assisted reproduction procedures

From: CDC's Reproductive Health Information Source. *1998 Assisted Reproductive Technology Success Rates. National Summary and Fertility Clinic Reports* (*www.cdc.gov/nccdphp/drh/art98/index.htm*).

Success Rates, which provides statistics on ART for women over thirty that may give you some of the information you need to make choices. For instance, of all the high-tech ART procedures using fresh, nondonor eggs, 30.5 percent resulted in "clinical" pregnancies. However, a clinical pregnancy rate tells you only that a certain percentage of women had pregnancies that continued long enough for an ultrasound to show the presence of a fetus—not that these women carried babies to term. More important is the "live birth rate." Of the clinical pregnancies, 82 percent resulted in live births.

For women over thirty-five, the 1998 CDC's Reproductive Health Information Source on assisted reproduction showed promising birth statistics, although pregnancy with multiples occurred much more frequently with ART procedures than with natural conceptions. With ART, women aged thirty-five to thirty-seven had a 26 percent live birth rate, and over one third of these women became pregnant with multiples. For women aged thirty-eight to forty, the live birth rate per ART cycle was 17.9 percent (27.8 percent of which were multiple births). Women over forty had only an 8 percent live birth rate with fresh, nondonor eggs; however, their live birth rates rose to 40.6 percent if they used fresh donor eggs. Thus, donor eggs almost doubled the live birth rates for women aged thirty-five to thirty-seven.

Low-Tech Treatments for Infertility

Low-tech fertility treatments include nonsurgical techniques that stimulate your ovaries to make more eggs or that give your partner's sperm a boost by placing them closer to your cervix or fallopian tubes and thus closer to their goal.

The most common low-tech procedures are AI and the use of fertility drugs such as clomiphene citrate (CLOMID or Serophene).

AI and IUI

In AI, the sperm are placed in a catheter and deposited near your cervix; they need not swim the length of the vagina. In IUI, the sperm are injected through a catheter through your cervix and placed in your uterus or fallopian tube, sparing the sperm a long journey and circumventing possible problematic interactions between the sperm and your cervical mucous.

Sometimes doctors will use a combination of IUI and fertility drugs to maximize the chance of egg and sperm finding each other and making a baby.

Fertility Drugs

If you are having trouble getting pregnant, your doctor may recommend fertility drugs either to help you ovulate one or two eggs per menstrual cycle or to stimulate your ovaries to produce many eggs. If the goal is to simply jump-start your ovulation and increase your odds for producing an egg, your doctor may prescribe one of the less aggressive fertility drugs, clomiphene citrate (also known as CLOMID or Serophene). However, your doctor may prescribe one of the more aggressive drugs if the goal is to push your ovaries to "superovulate" and "recruit" many eggs per menstrual cycle. You may produce as many as thirty-five eggs or as few as one or two, depending on the drug, the dose, your age, and the responsiveness of your ovaries. The rationale behind superovulation is that the more eggs you produce in a month, the greater your chances of becoming pregnant.

The aggressive fertility drugs, which are high tech in the sense that they are powerful and require careful monitoring, include Pergonal, Humegon, Repronex, Metrodin, and Fertinex or the recombinant drugs such as Gonal-F and Follistim. Most of these drugs use either LH (luteinizing hormone), FSH (follicle stimulating hormone), or a combination of LH and FSH.

Many doctors will start you on the least aggressive drug treatments and then move to more aggressive ones if you do not become pregnant. Says Dr. Walmer of his patients at Duke University Medical Center: "A woman tries three or four months on CLOMID. If that fails, she goes to more aggressive drugs. Of the more aggressive drugs," says Walmer, "most of our patients try three to four cycles."

A given fertility drug, such as clomiphene citrate or Pergonal, tends to work within a three- or four-month period—if it is going to work. Consequently, your doctor may first prescribe three months of clomiphene and then, if you do not become pregnant, may prescribe three months of a superovulation drug like Pergonal or Metrodin.

Some women who become pregnant during the first three months on a drug may have become pregnant without drugs, although it might have taken them longer to conceive. However, some women may be working within the limits of their last months of fertility: If they don't become pregnant soon, they may never become pregnant at all. In such cases, fertility drugs can create "miracle babies" that would never have been conceived had nature been allowed to simply take its course. Discuss your circumstances with your doctor so that you can match your drug routine with your age, your medical history, and your expectations. Given possible drug-related risks, many doctors suggest that you limit the number of your drug-stimulated ovulatory cycles.

Sometimes aggressive fertility drug treatments work "too well" and lead to pregnancies with three, four, or more babies. Doctors consider pregnancy with multiples as a *drug-related risk,* since multiple gestations can create problems for both mother and babies (see Part 6).

If you are not ovulating or are having certain problems that prevent you from ovulating, even massive doses of drugs may not help you become pregnant. Whether or not the fertility drugs are successful in promoting ovulation depends on what is causing your ovulation problem and what drug is being used (see Kathleen's story in Chapter 5).

As you grow older, your ovaries may become less responsive to fertility drugs. If the drugs recruit only one or two eggs per cycle after several months of fertility drug treatment, you may do just as well trying to conceive without drugs, since your drug-related risks may begin to outweigh your benefits.

If you take fertility drugs, make sure that your care provider monitors you each month to see if you are ovulating and how many eggs you are producing. If the drugs are not working, you will need to find out why, because you may have ovulation problems that can be corrected by other medications—and not fertility drugs.

Taking these drugs for more than six months means taking additional risks without increasing your benefits (see Chapter 7). Like any drug, more is not necessarily better. All drugs have side effects, and fertility drugs are powerful hormones whose possible side effects include: visual disturbances, growth of existing fibroid tumors, abdominal tenderness, mood swings, and breast and ovarian cysts. More serious short-term side effects include the rare but sometimes dangerous ovarian hyperstimulation syndrome (OHSS). Some studies have also raised concerns about ovarian cancer risks, although other studies have shown no risks. The issue has not been resolved. Still other scientific studies offer conflicting results as to whether fertility drugs are associated with breast or endometrial cancer (see Chapter 7).

For further information on drug side effects, ask your pharmacist about the package insert that comes with the drug, look up the drug in *The Physicians' Desk Reference*, contact the InterNational Council on Infertility Information Dissemination (*www.inciid.org*), call a university pharmacology department, or consult Reprotox or Motherisk on the Internet (see appendix).

Whatever you do, do not self-prescribe fertility drugs that you acquire on the Internet or through friends. The drugs can have systemic effects that must be carefully monitored by a physician.

High-Tech Infertility Treatments

High-tech fertility procedures include complex procedures such as IVF, GIFT, ZIFT, and ICSI as well as the powerful fertility drugs used in superovulation.

IVF (in vitro fertilization) is a procedure by which eggs are surgically retrieved from your ovaries (via a thin catheter passed through your vaginal wall or your abdomen) and then fertilized with your partner's or donor's sperm in a small petri dish (the "test tube"). Three to six days later, the fertilized eggs (embryos) are transferred to your uterus where, it is hoped, one will implant in your uterine wall and grow into a baby. Egg donation/recipiency involves the same procedure, except that the eggs come from another woman—an egg donor.

GIFT (gamete intrafallopian transfer) is a procedure in which eggs and sperm (gametes) are not combined in a petri dish. Instead, eggs and sperm are returned together to your fallopian tubes where fertilization may occur in the "natural" way: within a woman's body. Returning the gametes to your tubes involves more extensive surgery than IVF, since your doctor must make small cuts in your abdomen in order to place the gametes in your fallopian tubes. ZIFT (zygote intrafallopian transfer) is similar to GIFT, although the eggs are first fertilized in a petri dish, and the resulting embryos (zygotes) are returned to your fallopian tubes.

Among procedures using fresh, nondonor eggs, IVF accounted for 73.3 percent of babies born through assisted reproduction, according to the CDC's 1998 *Reproductive Health Information Source*. GIFT accounted for 1.8 percent and ZIFT for 1.4 percent of the babies born from high-tech procedures using fresh nondonor eggs. Although procedures using donor eggs were used less frequently than standard IVF, the procedures with fresh donor eggs offered impressively high birth statistics (see "Egg Donation and Recipients").

High-tech, assisted reproduction procedures should be performed by board-certified reproductive endocrinologists who have had training in the surgical and ultrasound techniques necessary to retrieve eggs from your ovaries and put them back (as eggs mixed with sperm or as fertilized embryos) into your uterus or fallopian tubes.

IVF

Mechanical obstacles are the clearest indication for IVF.
—Dr. David Walmer

• • •

Your doctor may recommend IVF if you have mechanical barriers, such as scar tissue or blocked tubes, that prevent your eggs from traveling from the ovary to the fallopian tubes or moving through the tubes toward the uterus, since IVF provides an effective way to bypass damaged fallopian tubes and retrieve eggs from trapped ovaries. However, if you have no mechanical barriers interfering with conception, you may not need IVF. Some reproductive endocrinologists believe that if you have no physical obstacles to conception, superovulation may sufficiently improve your fertility.

Fortunately, if you do need IVF, the success rates have greatly improved due to advances in IVF technology. Throughout the 1980s and early 1990s, the embryos transferred during an IVF procedure were often two or three days old, and doctors would transfer anywhere from two to six embryos to a woman's uterus. However, due to technological advances in the mid-1990s, the embryos can remain in a culture in the petri dish until they become *blastocysts:* six-day-old embryos. Since this technique often results in higher pregnancy rates, doctors using blastocysts may transfer only two, or sometimes three, to your uterus in order to prevent pregnancy with high-order multiples. The number of blastocysts planted in your uterus will depend, in part, on your age. If you are in your early thirties, your doctor may implant only two blastocysts. However, if you are forty, many doctors suggest implanting four or more embryos, since few women over forty end up with triplets or quadruplets, although they may end up with twins.

The successful blastocyst technology has made IVF preferable to GIFT, according to some reproductive endocrinologists, because IVF puts healthy fertilized embryos back inside a woman, whereas GIFT puts unfertilized eggs and sperm back into the woman. "I would make the argument that IVF is better [than ZIFT or GIFT]," contends Dr. Walmer. "Human reproduction is inefficient. What I mean by that is we have lots of abnormal sperm and abnormal eggs, and therefore we make lots of abnormal embryos. With standard IVF cycles, we get ten eggs. Only 50 percent or 60 percent of them will fertilize. Of the fertilized embryos, only 30 percent are capable of developing into a blastocyst—which is an embryo that can implant [in the uterine wall]. So, on average, you get ten eggs, six embryos, and two blastocysts."

The secret of IVF's recent success is that the procedure puts two to four blastocysts back into a woman's body, whereas GIFT uses a combination of eggs and sperm, which may never become blastocysts. "If you do GIFT, that means you are starting with the egg stage. You don't know which ones are going to fertilize. You have to choose how many you're going to put in the tubes. Are you going to put in ten? Most people don't. You'll put in four or five," Walmer explains.

ZIFT also uses preblastocyst-stage embryos, which creates more uncertainty than IVF. "If you do ZIFT, you're going to put in *pronuclear*, single-cell embryos in the first day or two after fertilization. Only 30 percent of those are even capable of making it to the blastocyst stage, whereas if you keep them in culture for five or six days with IVF, you only put two embryos back. Of those ten eggs, you know exactly which two to put back. This is the direction that IVF is going these days," Dr. Walmer explains.

However, the success rates for IVF decrease for women over forty. "After one month of IVF, a thirty-year-old woman has a 35 percent chance of having a baby," says Dr. Sauer, who finds the procedure especially successful in women under forty. However, Sauer argues that a forty-year-old woman will not fare as well, since her chance of getting pregnant is only 8 to 10 percent.

IVF usually involves the following basic steps, although the drugs and methods may vary somewhat from clinic to clinic and as new techniques are developed:

1. Early in your menstrual cycle, your doctor gives you injections of fertility drugs to stimulate your ovaries to mass-produce eggs. You inject yourself at home or have your partner inject you.
2. When the eggs are mature, your doctor injects you with human chorionic gonadotropin (hCG), which is used to trigger the release of eggs from your ovaries.
3. To surgically retrieve your eggs, your doctor inserts a thin needle, guided by ultrasound, through your vagina to the ovarian egg follicles. You may be sedated and sleepy, but usually you will not be totally anesthetized.
4. Your eggs and your partner's sperm will be mixed in a

culture to fertilize. The resulting embryos will be allowed to mature for three to six days.

5. The best embryos will be transferred to your uterus via a thin catheter inserted through your cervix. Usually, between two and six embryos will be transferred, depending on the procedure, your age, and the decisions you reach with your doctor about the possibility of becoming pregnant with multiple babies.

6. If you are left with extra embryos that have not been transferred, these embryos may be frozen for your future use.

7. If all goes well, one (or more) of the embryos implants in your uterine wall, develops a placenta, and grows into a baby.

IVF with "Natural Cycles"

IVF may also be performed without the use of fertility drugs. In this case, your physician carefully follows the development of your monthly egg follicles, looking for a mature egg. When a mature egg is found, it is retrieved and placed in a petri dish. Since there are far fewer eggs in a natural cycle than in a drug-stimulated one, ovulation may need to be monitored very carefully. Although pregnancy rates from natural cycles are much lower than those achieved through drug-induced superovulation, there are benefits to doing natural IVF cycles. With natural cycles you are not exposed to fertility drugs and their potential risks, and you do not have the additional expense of fertility drugs.

GIFT

GIFT is designed for women who have at least one healthy fallopian tube and a partner with healthy sperm, because GIFT allows eggs and sperm to come together and fertilize "naturally" in a woman's fallopian tubes.

Because GIFT babies are conceived within a woman's body, the procedure is approved by some religions that object to babies made in vitro—in a "test tube." At one time, it was GIFT, rather than IVF, that was recommended for women over forty, if high-tech reproduction was deemed appropriate at all. In fact, GIFT was once thought to be the most successful form of assisted reproduction next to egg donation. Therefore, it was often recommended as the most effective high-tech procedure for many women of various ages who had at least one good fallopian tube and a partner with healthy sperm.

However, IVF is now used more frequently than GIFT, since doctors believe that the blastocyst technology makes IVF more successful and reliable than GIFT.

GIFT is a more invasive procedure than IVF because it involves laparoscopic abdominal surgery and anesthesia. The procedure includes the following steps:

1. You are given fertility drugs to stimulate your ovaries to mass-produce eggs.
2. You are given an hCG injection to trigger release of eggs from your ovary.
3. When you come in to the clinic or hospital for your GIFT procedure, you are put under general anesthesia.
4. Once you are asleep, your doctor makes three very small incisions in your abdomen, inflates your abdominal cavity with gas to make it easier to distinguish and manipulate the ovaries and tubes, inserts a laparoscope so he or she can locate your fallopian tubes, and then guides a hollow needle to your ovaries in order to collect eggs.
5. You remain anesthetized while your doctors mix your eggs with healthy sperm and then inject both eggs and sperm into your fallopian tubes via a thin catheter. For

women over forty, or women who have previously been unsuccessful with IVF or GIFT procedures, a large number of eggs may be returned to the fallopian tubes.

6. Your "extra" eggs may be fertilized in vitro (as in IVF) and frozen as embryos for your later use. (Currently, laboratories are unable to freeze unfertilized eggs without damaging the delicate structure, although freezing eggs and thus repeating a GIFT procedure from the same "batch" of eggs may become possible in the future.)

7. Your doctor closes your incisions, you spend the day in a recovery room, and then you return home.

8. If all goes well, an egg is fertilized, and you become pregnant. Sometimes more than one egg is fertilized, and you become pregnant with twins or more.

ZIFT

In a ZIFT procedure, as in IVF, you are given fertility drugs to hyperstimulate your ovaries to make lots of eggs, and the eggs are retrieved via transvaginal aspiration with a thin needle and fertilized in vitro. After the fertilized eggs develop and become embryos, they are transferred to your fallopian tubes (as in the GIFT procedure). To transfer the embryos (or zygotes) to your fallopian tubes, your doctor can either (1) perform a surgical laparoscopy (see "GIFT" above) to transfer the embryos through an incision in your abdomen, or (2) transfer the embryos via a catheter inserted through your cervix and uterus and into your fallopian tubes.

An advantage of using ZIFT instead of GIFT is that your doctor is not leaving fertilization up to chance; instead of transferring eggs and sperm back into the fallopian tube to fertilize— or not to fertilize—by chance, the doctor transfers embryos: eggs that have been fertilized. ZIFT was at one time regarded as more effective than IVF. However, recently, ZIFT has become less popular than the other ART procedures. In 1998, ZIFT was responsible for only 1.4 percent of ART pregnancies.

Egg Donation and Recipients

When donor eggs are used, the age of the woman undergoing ART does not affect success as it does when a woman uses her own eggs. The likelihood of an egg fertilizing, implanting, and producing a live birth is related to the age of the woman who produces the egg.
—American Society for Reproductive Medicine, *NEWS*, February 3, 1999

• • •

Egg donation is the high-tech procedure most frequently offered to women in their forties and early fifties. In 1998, among women over age forty-six, 70 percent of all high-tech assisted reproduction procedures used donor eggs. Since egg donors are usually young women between the ages of eighteen and thirty, women who get pregnant with donor eggs have birth rates similar to young women—sometimes even better. Because the age of the eggs is the age of the young donor, the embryos tend to be healthy and are more likely to implant and become babies than are the embryos of women over forty. Consequently, the "take-home baby rates" from egg donation are the highest of all the reproductive technologies. Live birth rates for women receiving donor eggs range from 40 to 65 percent, even if the egg recipient is nearing fifty.

The egg donation/recipiency procedure resembles IVF—except that the fertility drugs are given to an egg donor, and her eggs are the ones retrieved. The donor's eggs are then fertilized with the sperm of the egg recipient's partner or the sperm of a donor. The fertilization takes place in a small petri dish, and the resulting embryos are allowed to develop (the length of time varies from clinic to clinic) and then placed in the recipient's uterus.

Since it is the age of the donor egg—not the recipient's uterus—that is responsible for high success rates, even a fifty-five-year-old recipient stands an excellent chance of having a baby via egg donation—especially if she is willing to make up to three attempts. However, the process is very expensive, because the recipient is paying for the donor's fertility drug treatments, her surgery, and her physical discomfort. An egg recipient will pay the egg donor anywhere from $2,500 to $5,000. (Some donors have received over $10,000, although such fees are currently considered excessive.) The donor is usually paid by the doctor, who collects the donor's fee plus the costs of the procedure from the egg recipient. The entire cost of the procedure amounts to anywhere from $13,000 to $18,000.

Because donor eggs are often fertile, many of the embryos may "take," thus increasing your odds of becoming pregnant with twins or triplets. Pregnancy with multiples is the most obvious and frequent risk of the egg donation procedure. Other more subtle risks include the uncertainties of an anonymous donor's genetic heritage, the unpredictability of the recipient's response to carrying a baby that is not genetically hers, the complex emotional and ethical decisions involving whether or not to tell a child of its egg donor origins, and the possible side effects of progesterone—a hormonal drug to which both mother and baby are exposed during the first ten to sixteen weeks of pregnancy.

Egg donation/recipiency programs differ as to age cutoffs; health criteria; and medication, incubation, and embryo transfer protocols for women hoping to have babies. Some programs have an age cutoff of fifty, the average age of menopause, while others offer egg donation to women up to fifty-five years old.

Although most programs require egg recipients to be in general good health, programs differ when it comes to such health issues as uterine fibroids. Some egg donation programs accept women with uterine fibroid tumors as long as the tumors do not distort or occupy the uterine cavity. Other clinics are concerned with the size of a woman's fibroids and may require that a woman with "large tumors" have a myomectomy (surgical removal of the fibroids) before an egg donor pregnancy will be attempted. Of course, different doctors have different ideas of what "large" means, and you may wish to get a second opinion if your doctor thinks you should avoid pregnancy or have surgery on the basis of tumor size alone. The rapid growth of a fibroid is another matter, since it is an indication that the fibroid may need to be removed without too much delay (see Chapter 8).

Other protocols that will differ from program to program include what kinds and doses of medications are given, how many embryos are transferred to the recipient woman's uterus, and at what stage of the development the embryos are be transferred.

Transferring many embryos increases the odds of getting pregnant, but it also increases the odds of pregnancy with multiples. Although having two or three babies at once may seem like a bonus, pregnancy with multiples will greatly increase risk factors for both the woman and her babies. Many doctors try to control the number of babies by limiting the number of embryos transferred. Dr. Walmer uses the developmental stage of the embryo and the age of the eggs to determine how many embryos he will transfer: "With donor eggs in a forty-year-old woman, if we put in three embryos on Day 2, the woman has a 40 percent chance of getting pregnant. If we put in two blastocysts [older and more developed embryos] on Day 6, she has a 65 percent chance of taking home a baby."

Some doctors prefer to transfer blastocysts because healthy blastocysts are more likely to "take" than three-day-old embryos. Other doctors prefer to transfer the three-day-old embryos. Discuss with your doctor which procedures he or she prefers. (See Part 6 and Chapter 7.)

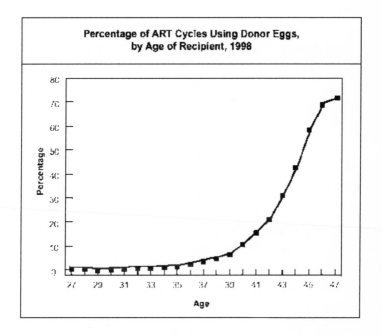

Figure 6-4: Percent of assisted reproduction cycles using donor eggs, by age of recipient, in 1998. The number of women using egg donation climbs after age forty-one

From: CDC's Reproductive Health Information Source. *1998 Assisted Reproductive Technology Success Rates. National Summary and Fertility Clinic Reports* (www.cdc.gov/nccdphp/drh/art98/index.htm).

Future Technology or Science Fiction?

In the future, the technology of assisted reproduction may offer other compelling ways of helping nature do what it does naturally, especially for women who postpone pregnancy. Some researchers have successfully frozen eggs from animals, and a few researchers have frozen eggs from humans. Although doctors imagine a time when women in their twenties can freeze their eggs and "bank them" for use in their thirties or forties, this time has not yet arrived.

In the future, infertility medicine may also be able to transfer the nucleus of your egg—the part that contains your genes—to the cytoplasm (cellular material) of a younger woman's egg, thus creating a way for you to have a child that is genetically yours. This technique, called *nuclear transfer,* was developed by Dr. Jamie Grifo, a reproductive endocrinologist at the New York University Medical Center in New York City. Dr. Grifo's interest in nuclear transfer was sparked by the question: What makes an older woman's egg different, and less viable, than a younger woman's? The difference, says Grifo, "all boils down to chromosome abnormalities." He theorizes that by taking the chromosomes out of an "old egg" and putting them in a young donor egg, scientists could solve infertility problems. The solution would be based on replacing the "old" cellular mechanisms that pair chromosomes during the early embryonic development of a baby with new cellular mechanisms that could help the fertilized egg divide its chromosomes normally and produce a healthy baby. However, the FDA is being cautious and has confined Grifo's research to mice.

Chapter 7

The "Drugs of Pregnancy": Making Informed Choices About Fertility Drugs and Progesterone

CLOMID made my periods like clockwork and regulated them. In one month, I got pregnant.
—Leda, a DES daughter, had ovulatory and conception problems. She became pregnant one month after using clomiphene citrate.

* * *

Women are so desperate to get to the end point they want [pregnancy] that they are vulnerable to exploitation. The most important thing to do is to educate women about the problems, the success rates, and the risks and to let them apply their own value systems to this information.
—Dr. David Walmer

* * *

Thousands of women take hormonal fertility drugs each year in hopes that these drugs will enhance their ovulation and increase their chances of getting pregnant. Frequently, the drugs work. They can correct a woman's ovulation problem or spur her ovaries to produce more eggs, thus increasing her odds for conception. After years of trying to get pregnant, some women conceive after one to three cycles of drug use. Of course, some of those women might have conceived eventually, but the drugs sped up the process. Other women may never have conceived without drugs.

After hearing fertility drug success stories, you may want to take fertility drugs to help you become pregnant, if you have fertility problems. If you don't conceive after six months or a year, you may be tempted to continue taking the drugs, hoping each month that you will become pregnant. Kathleen R. did fifteen ovulation cycles with injectable drugs plus CLOMID. She felt compelled to keep trying.

But before you take fertility drugs for prolonged periods of time, it is important that you carefully consider possible drug-related risks. Like all drugs, fertility drugs have potential side effects, and these side effects may increase if you take the drugs too long or at too high a dose. Even though some fertility drugs come from "natural hormones"—and many people argue that natural compounds are safe—others argue that no hormone, even a "natural" one, is safe in excess amounts. The *dose* of a compound determines its safety even when it comes to "natural" products like vitamin A.

Clomiphene citrate (CLOMID, Serophene) is often the first fertility drug that doctors prescribe if a woman has ovulatory problems, since this drug has effectively treated some ovulatory disorders. Doctors prescribe clomiphene citrate to help women who have ovulatory problems produce one to two eggs and to help normalize their menstrual cycles. According to the 1996 Hoechst Marian Roussel pharmaceutical company package information for CLOMID, studies of the drug done between 1964 and 1978 showed that "pregnancy occurred in 35 percent of 5,154 patients with ovulatory disorders."

If a woman's ovaries do not respond to clomiphene citrate after three months or if she is undergoing a high-tech procedure such as IVF or GIFT, her doctor may prescribe one of the more aggressive ovulation induction drugs such as Pergonal, Humegon, Repronex, Gonal-F, or Follistim. These drugs make a woman's ovaries mass-produce eggs—sometimes as many as ten to twenty in one menstrual cycle. This process is called *superovulation* or *controlled ovarian hyperstimulation*. The superovulation drugs consist of such hormones as FSH (follicle stimulating hormone), LH (luteinizing hormone), and human menopausal gonadotropins (hMG), the same hormones that women produce during a normal menstrual cycle. Some of these powerful drugs come from natural sources, others are made in purified form from recombinant DNA.

Although the benefits of fertility drugs are well known, some of the risks are not. This chapter discusses these risks, including some of the more controversial research hinting at a link between fertility drugs and ovarian cancer—studies that some doctors may not tell you about in much depth or detail. It provides you with information on "the drugs of pregnancy" (fertility drugs and progesterone) so that you can make informed decisions in your best interest.

Each woman who reads this section will need to arrive at her own conclusions, depending on her own medical history and her own perceptions of risk and benefit. By becoming informed about guidelines for the use of fertility drugs, side effects, and precautions, you will be able to intelligently participate with your doctor in deciding which drug you should take and for how long.

Partial List of Current Fertility Drugs Used for Ovulation and Superovulation

clomiphene citrate (synthetic antiestrogen or weak estrogen): CLOMID, Serophene

follitropin (recombinant FSH): Follistim, Gonal-F

menotropins (hMG): Humegon, Pergonal, Repronex

urofollitropin (FSH): Fertinex, Metrodin

Guidelines for Fertility Drug Use

Ovulation induction drugs, such as clomiphene citrate (designed to help you ovulate and produce one or two eggs per menstrual cycle), and *superovulation* drugs, such as Pergonal, Humegon, and Fertinex (designed to stimulate your ovaries to produce many eggs per menstrual cycle), are powerful hormonal agents that should be used according to the guidelines suggested by the FDA, the United Kingdom Committee on the Safety of Medicines, the American Society for Reproductive Medicine (ASRM), and the pharmaceutical companies. In order for you to intelligently participate in your fertility drug treatment, it is important for you to fully understand how these drugs can be used most effectively and safely.

Clomiphene Citrate (CLOMID, Serophene): A Popular Ovulation Induction Drug

Clomiphene citrate (CLOMID, Serophene) is appropriate for women who are not ovulating at all or whose ovulation is irregular. According to the Hoescht Marion Roussel package information on clomiphene citrate, the drug is usually effective within three months. The company recommends that the drug should be taken for no longer than six months and that drug dosages should begin at 50 mg for five days and should be increased to 100 mg for five days only if the smaller dose has not been effective. In 1995 the United Kingdom's Committee on the Safety of Medicines issued guidelines restricting the use of clomiphene citrate to six months, according to an article on ovarian cancer on the BBC online network, November 24, 1998.

Women taking clomiphene citrate should be monitored by their physicians. Hoescht Marion Roussel, in its 1996 drug information on CLOMID, encourages physicians to monitor women who are taking clomiphene to make sure that they are ovulating, that their ovaries have not become enlarged or developed cysts, and that they are not pregnant. Since clomiphene may interfere with the development of healthy cervical mucous or healthy uterine lining, it may interfere with conception or implantation. In an article entitled, "Clomiphene Citrate: Use and Abuse," The InterNational Council on Infertility Information Dissemination (INCIID) recommends that physicians monitor cervical mucous production and a woman's monthly response to her clomiphene treatment.

CLOMID Prescription Information as of February 1996

Treatments of the selected patient should begin with a low dose of 50 mg daily (1 tablet daily) for five days. The dose should be increased only in those patients who do not ovulate in response to cyclic 50 mg CLOMID. A low dosage or treatment course is probably recommended if unusual sensitivity to pituitary gonadotropin is suspected, such as in patients with polycystic ovary syndrome (see WARNINGS: Ovarian Hyperstimulation Syndrome: The patient should be carefully evaluated to exclude pregnancy, ovarian enlargement, or ovarian cyst formation between each cycle).

* * *

. . . When ovulation occurs at this dosage, there is no advantage in increasing the dose in subsequent cycles of treatment. If ovulation does not appear to occur after the first course of therapy, a second course of 100 mg (two 50 mg tablets recommended as

a single daily dose) for 5 days should be given. This course may be started as early as 30 days after the previous one, after precautions are taken to exclude the possibility of pregnancy. Increasing the dosage or duration of therapy beyond 100 mg/day for five days is not recommended.

* * *

The majority of patients who are going to ovulate will do so after the first course of therapy. If ovulation does not occur after three courses of therapy, further treatment with CLOMID is not recommended and the patient should be reevaluated. If three ovulatory responses occur, but pregnancy has not been achieved, further treatment is not recommended. If menses does not occur after an ovulatory response, the patient should be reevaluated. Long-term cyclic therapy is not recommended beyond a total of about six cycles (see PRECAUTIONS).

From: Hoescht Marion Roussel, the Pharmaceutical Company of Hoescht, *CLOMID Prescribing Information as of February 1996.*

Superovulation Drugs

If CLOMID is not effective, doctors may prescribe more aggressive drugs such as Metrodin, Humegon, or Fertinex to make a woman's ovaries "superovulate" and produce many eggs, thus improving her odds for getting pregnant. According to INCIID, the superovulation drug Pergonal does not interfere with the production of normal cervical mucous, thus offering an advantage over clomiphene (INCIID, "Overview of Injectable Fertility Drugs," 1999). However, gauging the correct amount of Pergonal for a given woman is a complex process that involves a risk of overstimulating the ovaries.

Superovulation drugs have been linked to ovarian hyperstimulation syndrome (OHSS), a potentially life-threatening condition that may include ovarian enlargement, abdominal swelling, fluid retention, and difficulty breathing. Superovulation can also result in the birth of high-order multiples (e.g., quadruplets or quintuplets), which carries health risks for the mother and the babies. Because of these concerns, drug companies and INCIID alike advise women taking superovulation drugs to be carefully monitored by a physician trained in fertility medicine.

Guidelines for Injectible Fertility Drugs

PERGONAL (note: The description for Humegon is similar)

Indications and Usage

"Pergonal and hCG given in a sequential manner are indicated for the induction of ovulation and pregnancy in the anovulatory infertile patient, in whom the cause of anovulation is functional and not due to primary ovarian failure.

Humegon and hCG may also be used to stimulate the development of multiple follicles in ovulatory patients participating in an in vitro fertilization program."

Contraindications

"Pergonal is contraindicated [not recommended] in women who have:

1. A high FSH level indicating primary ovarian failure.
2. Uncontrolled thyroid and adrenal dysfunction.
3. An organic intracranial lesion or a pituitary tumor.
4. The presence of any cause of infertility other than anovulation, unless they [the women] are candidates for in vitro fertilization.
5. Abnormal bleeding of undetermined origin.
6. Ovarian cysts or enlargement not due to polycystic ovary syndrome.
7. Prior hypersensitivity to menotropins.

8. Pergonal is contraindicated in women who are pregnant and may cause fetal harm when administered to a pregnant woman. There are limited human data on the effects of Pergonal when administered during pregnancy."

Warnings

"Pergonal is a drug that should only be used by physicians who are thoroughly familiar with infertility problems. It is a potent gonadotropic substance capable of causing mild to severe adverse reactions in women. Gonadotropin therapy requires a certain time commitment by physicians and supportive health professionals, and its use requires the availability of appropriate monitoring facilities . . . [It] must be used with a great deal of care.

"Multiple Births. Data from clinical trials revealed the following results regarding multiple births. Of the pregnancies following therapy with Pergonal and hCG, 80 percent resulted in single births, 15 percent in twins, and 5 percent of the total pregnancies resulted in three or more conceptions. The patient and her husband should be advised of the frequency and potential hazards of multiple gestation before starting treatment."

From: *The Physicians' Desk Reference*, p. 2,946. (Edition 54). Montvale, NJ: Medical Economics Company, Inc., 2000.

Adverse Side Effects of Fertility Drugs

The possible adverse side effects of fertility drugs range from mild to severe and from short term to long term. Adverse side effects of both clomiphene citrate and the superovulation drugs include bloating, mood swings, visual disturbances, the development of breast cysts or ovarian cysts, and an increase in size of fibroid tumors. However, OHHS, a potentially dangerous short-term side effect, is associated more with the superovulation drugs than with clomiphene. A possible long-term side effect of fertility drugs may include an increased risk of borderline or cancerous ovarian tumors, although researchers are uncertain whether it is the drugs or the underlying condition of infertility that increases the cancer risk.

Superovulation Drugs and the Risk of OHSS

Nowadays, 0.5 to 1 percent of women with hyperstimulation end up in the hospital. It depends on how you monitor them and how aggressive you are [with the drugs].
—Dr. David Walmer

* * *

When Stacy, age twenty-eight, took Humegon (hMG) preceding an in vitro fertilization attempt with ICSI, she produced twenty-eight eggs even though she had taken a relatively low dose of the drug. Her doctor implanted five of the resulting embryos. One week later, when she became pregnant with twins, her abdomen filled with two liters of fluid and distended to the size of a three-month pregnancy.

Stacy was hospitalized, and drainage shunts were poked into her taut belly to draw the fluid out. But the fluid kept accumulating. "The fluids were dumping into the extra space in my abdomen. They put tubes into my abdomen to get the fluid out. I was in the hospital for ten days. I was very uncomfortable. I looked like I was three months pregnant. My abdomen was swollen and tight. I was kind of out of it. I didn't have my wits about me. My ovaries were the size of grapefruits; they were so big they were touching each other."

It took three months for the bloating to completely disappear. Stacy's doctor had briefly told her of the risk of OHSS when she decided to take fertility drugs, but he said it was rare.

He did not tell her it was potentially life threatening. Fortunately, her twins were fine, and Stacy later gave birth to full-term girls—Katherine and Elizabeth.

Three years later, when Stacy had a "maternal need to have another child," she tried another cycle of superovulation drugs. This time, Stacy produced thirty-two eggs. Her doctor suggested that, because her risk for developing OHSS again would be increased if she got pregnant immediately, she should not transfer any of the resulting embryos. Despite these precautions, Stacy developed OHSS and ended up in the hospital for three days. Her doctor froze the embryos. On her doctor's advice, Stacy waited five months—until her ovaries had returned to normal size—before thawing and transferring the embryos. Then, after several implantation attempts, she became pregnant.

OHSS is a potentially serious problem causing an imbalance in the body's fluids and electrolytes. It is a well-established side effect of the aggressive fertility drugs when "controlled super-ovulation" gets out of control, either because of a high dose, a woman's unique response to a standard dose, or a preexisting problem with ovarian cysts. OHSS is rare with clomiphene citrate, but it can occur. Women with polycystic ovarian syndrome (PCOS) are at increased risk for OHSS. Although mild forms of OHSS are common, fortunately the severe forms are rare, and the syndrome can often be minimized with careful monitoring of a woman's response to fertility medications.

According to some health experts, *about 20 percent* of women who take aggressive drugs like hMG develop a mild form of OHSS that may cause some abdominal bloating and ovarian enlargement. A moderate form is expected in about 4 to 5 percent of the cases. Serious cases of OHSS are rare and occur between 0.6 percent and 1.9 percent of the time when superovulation drugs are administered. According to Dr.

Mark Sauer, "Ovarian hyperstimulation affects 1 in 100,000 women. In a severe case of OHSS the ovaries may swell to six times their normal size. This may be accompanied by an accumulation of fluid in the abdomen or lungs, vomiting, or difficulty breathing. The most severe form of the illness occurs in about 1 percent of the cases." Severe OHSS poses risks of liver damage, kidney or liver failure, rupture of the ovary and abdominal bleeding, compromised breathing or acute lung failure due to abdominal distention. OHSS is more likely to occur if you have high estrogen levels, PCOS, or become pregnant during a drug cycle (a menstrual cycle in which you take fertility drugs).

If you are taking fertility drugs, and you experience abdominal swelling or pain along with difficulty breathing, vomiting, or diarrhea, call your doctor immediately. Minor side effects of OHSS include hot flushes, tenderness of the breast, headache, mood changes, nervousness, dizziness, nausea and vomiting, and fatigue. Although rare, it can also cause visual disturbances. Fortunately, OHSS is usually treatable. However, the more serious cases require hospitalization for days or even weeks. It is difficult to prevent, but if detected early, action can be taken to minimize the severity of the syndrome. Again, careful monitoring of your health—which includes your reporting any symptoms to your doctor—is the key.

If you develop OHSS, you face several possible options, depending on the extent of your illness and your physician's approach to the condition. Your IVF cycle or insemination procedure may be canceled, you may be taken off the fertility drug temporarily, or you may be placed on lower doses of fertility drugs the next time around. Under some circumstances, your doctor may advise you against taking aggressive fertility drugs in the future.

Possible Side Effects of Clomiphene Citrate

Although the fertility drug clomiphene citrate rarely leads to OHSS, clomiphene may produce such side effects as abdominal distention, mood swings, vision problems, the growth of fibroid tumors, and breast and ovarian cysts.

Report all side effects to your doctor, since seemingly minor symptoms may indicate potentially serious problems. Visual disturbances (flashes of light across your visual field, difficulty focusing) may make it dangerous for you to drive. Any visual disturbances should be reported to your doctor for further evaluation to determine if you need to stop taking the drug or reduce your dose. Most short-term effects are relatively mild and usually disappear with cessation of drug therapy, although ovarian cysts may require monitoring.

Take special care to determine that you are not pregnant before taking clomiphene; in a University of San Francisco study, the drug was found to cause birth defects in both animals and humans if it is taken during early pregnancy.

Do Fertility Drugs Cause Cancer?

Research to date demonstrates conflicting results, with some investigators reporting an increased risk of ovarian cancer with fertility drugs, whereas others do not. The likely magnitude of risk, if one believes a risk exists, may be two or three times that of the general population which is at most 4–5% in a woman's lifetime. The present uncertainty makes it challenging to apply this to today's practice of medicine. With continued efforts worldwide, we hope an understanding of this will be forthcoming.
—A. N. Beltsos and R. R. Odem, "Ovulation Induction and Ovarian Malignancy." *Semin Reprod endocrinol,* 14(4): 367–374, 1996

I feel it is highly unlikely that fertility drugs are associated with an increased risk of ovarian cancer. Rather, it is likely that they actually confer benefit to the woman by providing the opportunity to become pregnant, thereby decreasing her risk of both ovarian and breast cancer.
—Dr. Mary Croughan-Minihane, Department of Family and Community Medicine at the University of California at San Francisco

❋ ❋ ❋

I think whether or not the drugs cause cancer is still an open question. There have been a couple of additional reports, but they have been small studies. We need large tudies to find an answer.
—Dr. Mary Anne Rossing, Fred Hutchinson Cancer Institute, Seattle, Washington

❋ ❋ ❋

Ovarian cancer is a rare but dangerous disease that is more difficult to detect and treat than breast cancer and more often fatal, because by the time it is detected, the disease has often spread.

Although there is no definitive proof that fertility drugs cause ovarian cancer, several studies have shown an *association* between women who take the drugs and those who develop the disease, an association that concerns some researchers.

The most frequently cited studies suggesting an association between the drugs and cancer are a 1992 study by Dr. Alice Whittemore and her twelve coresearchers from The Collaborative Ovarian Cancer Group (COCG), published in *The American Journal of Epidemiology*, and a 1994 study by Dr. Mary Anne Rossing et al., published in *The New England Journal of Medicine*.

Dr. Whittemore and the COCG researchers pooled the

data from their ovarian cancer studies and found that infertile white women who took fertility drugs had a three-fold higher chance of developing ovarian cancer than infertile women who had never taken the drugs. This represents an increase in a woman's lifetime risk from about 1.5 in 100 to 4.5 in 100.

Evidence of an association is not the same as evidence that the drugs cause ovarian cancer. But the association makes biological sense. It is consistent with two theories about the causes of ovarian cancer. The first theory holds that frequent or *incessant ovulation* irritates the ovary, causing potentially cancerous changes in the cell. The second theory states that increased amounts of hormones called gonadotropins cause ovarian cancer. Women who take fertility drugs have both incessant ovulation and increased levels of gonadotropins (since many fertility drugs either contain or stimulate gonadotropins).

Biologically plausible theories may turn out to prove nothing substantial, but they can be the first hint of a problem. Consequently, several federal agencies became concerned about a possible link between fertility drugs and ovarian cancer. The FDA asked drug companies to include a cancer warning in fertility drug package inserts, and researchers at the National Institute of Child Health and Human Development wrote an editorial on fertility drugs for the February 1993 issue of *Fertility and Sterility*.

Dr. Whittemore's study used a "case-control" design, a preliminary approach intended to find possible leads for further investigation. After the Whittemore study, the NIH funded a study by Dr. Mary Anne Rossing to pursue further the possible association of the fertility drug clomiphene and ovarian cancer. Focusing on the most widely used fertility drug, clomiphene citrate, Rossing and her colleagues examined the medical records of women who had taken this drug between 1974 and 1985 and compared them to infertile women not taking this drug.

When Dr. Rossing and her colleagues completed their study, they found that infertile women who took clomiphene citrate for twelve cycles or more had an eleven-fold greater chance of developing ovarian cancer than infertile women who did not take the drug.

Interestingly, Rossing found that women who already had children had an increased cancer risk if they had used clomiphene for a year or more. Rossing writes, " . . . our results indicate that the risk was elevated among both gravid [women who had had babies] and nulligravid women [women who had never had babies]."

In comparing the groups of infertile women who took clomiphene with those who did not, Rossing also found that the cancer risk increased in women who took clomiphene, whether or not the underlying cause of their infertility was ovarian in nature. This finding shows that the increased cancer risk was not due solely to ovarian problems. Rossing writes, "The risk of ovarian tumors [malignant and borderline] associated with long-term use of clomiphene was increased among both the women with ovulatory abnormalities and those with no known ovulatory abnormalities. These results suggest that the increased risk associated with the use of clomiphene is not merely a reflection of the presence of ovarian abnormalities that may be indications for treatment with this drug."

As a result of Rossing's study, The Committee on the Safety of Medicines in the United Kingdom recommended that women not take clomiphene citrate for more than six months.

However, the question of the association between fertility drugs and ovarian cancer is by no means fully answered. Several studies done in the 1990s found no association between the drugs and ovarian cancer. From 1996 through 2000, studies from such countries as Denmark, Italy, Israel, Australia, the United States, and Great Britain reported contradictory findings regarding the possible drug/cancer link. Currently, it is unclear whether or not fertility drugs cause cancer or, if they do cause cancer, what drugs and what doses are the most carcinogenic. It may not even be possible to do the definitive studies to completely answer this question (see below).

The Debate

To fully understand the debate about whether fertility drugs are somehow linked to ovarian cancer, it is important for you to understand what the scientific studies—and the conflicting and sometimes volatile reactions to them—mean.

Dr. Alice Whittemore and her colleagues from the Collaborative Ovarian Cancer Study Group (COCG) conducted a type of preliminary study called a "case-control" study. It compares women who have ovarian cancer ("cases") with some comparable group of women who don't have ovarian cancer ("controls") to see what might be different about them. Case-control studies are often where medical scientists start when trying to find possible risk factors.

According to Dr. Bernadine Healy, former director of the NIH, such studies should be taken seriously: "These are the kinds of observational studies that led us to our concerns about cholesterol levels. These are the kinds of studies that have led us to our concerns about tobacco. That's where you first start in terms of identifying risk."

However, scientists realize that case-control studies have limitations and do not provide final answers. Instead, they suggest possible connections that need to be followed up by further research. Whittemore's study did just that; it identified fertility drugs as a possible risk factor for ovarian cancer and suggested a new direction for future studies. It was the preliminary study that laid the groundwork for Rossing's work.

Mary Anne Rossing sees Whittemore's work as one step in the process of scientific investigation. "I think that the Whittemore study was a well-conducted study. It was solidly conducted for the kind of study it was. It did receive a lot of negative reviews in the medical community, and those reviews were widely read and formed the basis for a lot of doctors' opinions."

Rossing's 1994 study, on the other hand, was a *"retrospective cohort"* study. It was designed to more precisely investigate the association of fertility drugs with ovarian cancer and to find whether the cancer risk was associated with any particular kind of infertility or with a particular drug. This study also found an association between ovarian cancer and infertility drugs (see text).

But even a cohort study is not the optimum design for really answering the question, because women who take certain kinds of fertility drugs—or who have to take them for a longer time—may be different from other infertile women in important ways. It could be these differences, not the drugs, that are responsible for the cancer. The most reliable kind of scientific study, a "prospective, double-blinded randomized clinical trial" (RCT), has not been conducted—and may never be conducted.

Why wouldn't such an important study be done? There are both practical and ethical reasons. First of all, the most important aspect of the RCT is randomization: participants are assigned by the luck of the draw to either a group that receives the drugs or a group that receives a placebo (sugar pill). Randomization balances out the two groups in terms of their medical history, type of infertility, or any other factors that might be the real cause of cancer. If a difference in cancer risk is still found between women who take fertility drugs and those who do not, it would provide stronger evidence that the drugs are actually responsible for ovarian cancer.

But in order to have a randomized clinical trial, the participants must be willing to be randomized. Most infertile women seeking pregnancy would want the drugs, not the placebo. Second, most doctors would not want to give the drugs to patients in a clinical trial if they had serious questions about the drugs' safety. Thus, the most reliable kind of research regarding the fertility drug question is, at this time, neither practical nor ethical.

The current uncertainty means—and this is the important message to women thinking about taking fertility drugs—that each woman has to evaluate the evidence, imperfect as it is, and make a decision that she feels comfortable with. Part of that decision involves weighing the possibility of getting cancer against the benefit of getting pregnant. Even if the odds of developing cancer are very small, women must factor in the potential seriousness of the disease. As Dr. Bernadine Healy puts it: "If you talk about the risk of bleeding that you can get over, or a little bit of pain or discomfort, that is very different from a risk of ovarian cancer. . . . Even if the risk is a relatively low risk but the event is a catastrophic one like death or cancer, then that is a very different matter" (Dr. Bernadine Healy in a 1995 interview with the author for the newspaper series "The Fertility Gods" in *The Chapel Hill News*).

On the other hand, the emotional benefits of becoming a parent are many. Furthermore, a woman may physically benefit from pregnancy, since women who become pregnant and have babies have lower risks of ovarian cancer than those who do not.

What the Experts Think

Opinions vary on how to interpret the existing fertility drug findings. For Dr. Robert Spirtas, an epidemiologist and Chief of the National Institute of Child Health and Human Development at the NIH, the combined results of the Whittemore and Rossing studies were sufficient to generate concern—and to fund additional research. "The two studies [Whittemore and Rossing] show a statistically significant association between the use of fertility drugs and the development of ovarian cancer. Both studies are bolstered by their biological plausibility. . . .When you add Rossing to Whittemore, you'd have to say it leans you more toward being concerned. Now our job is to get as many studies out there as we can."

Dr. Richard Marrs, a nationally known infertility specialist who practices in California, dismissed the Whittemore study but took the ovarian cancer risk more seriously after the Rossing study. In 1999, Marrs wrote of the Rossing study:

. . . *[T]he seven women who developed benign, or borderline, tumors were patients who had taken at least 12 consecutive months of clomiphene citrate during their treatment. The authors rightfully conclude that prolonged use of clomiphene may increase the risk of ovarian tumors. Today, reproductive endocrinologists and gynecologists rarely use clomiphene for such an extended period of time. But looking at this data should make you aware, as a patient, that if clomiphene citrate has not been successful within your first six months of therapy, alternative methods of ovulation induction need to be found and utilized.* (Marrs, *Dr. Richard Marrs' Fertility Book*, p. 161)

But many infertility specialists believe that fertility drugs do not cause cancer, that it is the condition of infertility itself—not the drugs—that may predispose women to developing ovarian cancer.

Until more studies are done, there is no way to know if the cancer risk is large, small, or zero. Dr. Alice Whittemore encourages women to put the possible risk into perspective and not magnify it out of proportion since "no one knows for sure if fertility drugs cause cancer." Dr. Spirtas and Dr. Rossing still consider the matter "an open question."

In a November 2001 interview, Dr. Louise Brinton, an epidemiologist at the National Cancer Institute, said,

"There are still uncertainties regarding whether an association exists between the use of fertility drugs and ovarian cancer. A number of studies are ongoing that will provide further information regarding the association. Based on the available data, it would appear that if a drug/cancer link does exist, it would be a relatively modest one. Given the rarity of ovarian cancer, the 'absolute risk' of women who take fertility drugs of developing this cancer would be small."

Minimizing Your Ovarian Cancer Risk

If the jury is still out on whether fertility drugs cause cancer, what do infertile women do in the meantime? Dr. Whittemore has good news for women with no family history of ovarian cancer: "On the basis of the current data, women who have been exposed to fertility medications but have no family history of ovarian cancer are not at high-risk," she writes in her editorial, "The Risk of Ovarian Cancer after Treatment for Infertility" in the September 22, 1994, issue of *The New England Journal of Medicine*. In the same article Dr. Whittemore advises women starting treatment for infertility to minimize exposure to the medication, for example, by using unstimulated oocytes for IVF if appropriate and by choosing to have only a few cycles of ovarian stimulation. Dr. Asher Shusan, a researcher at Hebrew University in Jerusalem, also suggests that women limit the number of fertility drug-induced cycles.

Another suggestion comes from Dr. Bruce Stadel, a medical officer with the FDA who says that suppressing ovulation reduces the risk of ovarian cancer. If you have had children or have used birth control pills for over five years, says Stadel, you already have a decreased lifetime risk of developing ovarian cancer because both pregnancy and birth control pills suppress ovulation. Research shows that birth control pills dramatically reduce your risk of ovarian cancer. After one year of birth control pills, your risk goes down 20 to 30 percent, and after five years of pills, your risk is cut in half. (Note, though, that birth control pills present medical risks for women who smoke or have cardiovascular disease, high blood pressure, breast disease, or a family history of certain cancers. Some of these risks, such as heart and breast disease, increase with age and potentially put women over forty at increased risk. Get a complete physical and clearance from your physician before going on the pill.)

Even though the cancer risk remains an open question, you may wish to take steps to minimize your risk—just to be on the safe side. Some doctors recommend that women who have taken fertility drugs:

1. Take birth control pills to "rest" their ovaries if they don't get pregnant after they have completed their drug cycles
2. Obtain ultrasound screening of their ovaries twice a year for several years and have regular gynecological exams
3. Avoid long-term exposure to fertility drugs if they have a family history of ovarian cancer, cervical or uterine cancer, breast cancer, and possibly other cancers like colon and prostrate cancer

4. Avoid exposure to the drugs if they have had cancer
5. Limit treatments with clomiphene citrate from three to six cycles total
6. Limit drug cycles with the more powerful ovulation-induction drugs to three to four cycles.

Breast Cancer and Endometrial Cancer

If the link between fertility drugs and ovarian cancer is unclear, the situation is even more cloudy regarding breast cancer and endometrial cancer. Still, there have been some anecdotal reports that fertility drugs may stimulate the growth of preexisting breast cancer. So far, there is no hard evidence of a connection, and anecdotal evidence is, by itself, highly unreliable. For example, there may be age-related, rather than drug-related, factors contributing to increased breast cancer rates. According to epidemiologist Dr. Gertrude Berkowitz, women who give birth for the first time after age thirty are at increased risk for breast cancer—and that for a first birth over age forty a woman's risk goes up even more.

Fertility drugs may also be associated with an increased risk of endometrial cancer, according to two Israeli studies conducted by Dr. Baruch Modan, an Israeli physician and cancer researcher, and Dr. Elaine Ron, a researcher from the U.S. National Cancer Institute, although it is unclear if the cancer risk stems from the underlying condition of infertility or from the use of fertility drugs. The first study, published in 1997, found that "endometrial cancer incidence was observed to be significantly increased in infertile women." The 1998 study, on the other hand, showed only an insignificantly increased risk, although the scientists concluded that the role of fertility drugs in endometrial cancer "cannot be completely excluded."

These reports do not mean that you should *not* take fertility drugs, but that if you do, you should not take them for prolonged periods of time, and you should seek medical follow-up in the years following treatment. For optimal prevention of long-term side effects, health experts recommend that infertility patients who have taken fertility drugs be closely monitored over the long haul.

Egg Donation: The Ethical Quandary

Like an infertility patient, an egg donor takes hyperstimulation drugs and will produce five to thirty eggs to be "retrieved" and donated to the recipient. Because of this, egg donors (especially those who undergo many cycles of superovulation) may be taking on some of the health risks associated with fertility drugs.

Egg donors are a unique medical phenomenon: neither a patient nor a subject participating in research but rather a person solicited to undergo a medical procedure for the benefit of someone else. Because of their unique position, egg donors have a different risk/benefit equation to think about compared to a woman with fertility problems who is desperate to have a baby. Medical experts such as Dr. Robert Spirtas and Dr. Bernadine Healy, as well as medical ethicists such as Dr. Arthur Caplan, believe that potential egg donors should be well informed about the potential risks of side effects. While this does not directly affect the woman with fertility problems who is "receiving" the donated eggs, it is something to ponder if you are considering egg donation.

Pregnancies with Multiples

The incidence of twins with CLOMID is less than 10 percent—probably in the 5 percent range. The incidence with gonadotropin-like drugs [Pergonal, Metrodin, and many others] is probably in the 20 to 25 percent range. The incidence of high-order multiples is small with CLOMID, and it is about 3 to 5 percent in

gonadotropin use without IVF. With infertility programs shifting to blastocyst [six-day-old embryo] transfers, and if the doctors limit the embryos transferred to two, the multiple pregnancy rate becomes a negligible number.
—Dr. David Walmer

• • •

Since 1980, the twin birth rate has risen by 67 percent, according to the *National Vital Statistics Report* on births for 1999—the most recent date for which final statistics are available. Although the higher-order multiple rate (the number of triplets, quadruplets, quintuplets, and more) rose a staggering 423 percent by 1998, the rate dropped slightly by 1999.

Pregnancy with twins or triplets has become increasingly common for women in their mid-forties and fifties. In 1999, twin birth rates rose with maternal age and were highest for women aged fifty to fifty-four years.

The twin birth rates rose 80 percent among women forty to forty-four years of age—and almost 600 percent among women aged forty-five to forty-nine years. Researchers attribute many of these multiple births to the increased use of fertility-enhancing therapies such as ovulation-inducing drugs and ART, which are more likely to result in a multiple gestation.

According to a November 2000 *Practice Committee Report* of the American Society for Reproductive Medicine (ASRM), the National Center for Health Statistics has estimated that "for triplets and higher-order multiple births approximately . . . 40% were attributable to ovulation inducing drugs without high-tech procedures like IVF and 40% were attributable to such high-tech procedures as IVF, GIFT, and egg donation."

You many find the idea of twins attractive, telling yourself,

"I can have my whole family all at once—two or three babies from one cycle of superovulation, egg donation, or IVF." And you are free to make this choice. There are, however, greater risks for both you and your babies (especially with triplets and more) that you may wish to consider before you choose fertility treatments that greatly increase your odds of having multiples.

If you are already pregnant with multiples and prevention is no longer an issue, please turn to Part 5 and Part 6.

Risks to Babies

The more babies you have in your womb, the higher their risk of premature delivery. As you get into higher-order multiples, the risk goes up disproportionately compared to benefits. If you have three or more babies in the uterus, you end up with an increased risk of dead or handicapped children. It is my obligation to minimize risks.

—Dr. David Walmer

⁕   ⁕   ⁕

Multiple birth is considered a "risk" of fertility drugs, because twins, triplets, and quads are often premature and thus at higher risk for medical problems than are fully mature babies. Twins are frequently born at thirty-six weeks, triplets at thirty-two weeks, and quadruplets at thirty weeks, writes Dr. Barbara Luke in her book, *When You're Expecting Twins, Triplets, or Quads.* Such "preemies" must often remain in intensive care nurseries until they are mature enough to go home.

Some medical experts think it is "normal" for twins to be slightly premature—born at thirty-seven or thirty-eight weeks instead of forty weeks—and for triplets to be born at thirty-three to thirty-four weeks (see Part 6). Fortunately, multiples born at such young ages most often do well, although they will usually spend some time in a neonatal intensive care unit (NICU).

Quads are often born at about thirty-one to thirty-two weeks, which is quite early, and they may spend several weeks in the NICU in order to allow their lungs and gastrointestinal tracts to develop. Babies born at twenty-eight to twenty-nine weeks are very premature, and they may need to stay in an NICU for a month or so.

Although very premature babies are vulnerable to respiratory and gastrointestinal problems and developmental delays, contemporary neonatal intensive care can successfully nurture most of these tiny babies. However, some of the tiniest babies may suffer long-term neurological, respiratory, or developmental problems.

Risks to Mother

Many mothers do fine during a pregnancy with twins, but pregnancy with triplets and more can significantly increase the maternal risks of pregnancy. Maternal risks for mothers of multiples include increased rates of anemia, preeclampsia, and preterm labor (see Chapter 11). Women carrying multiple babies also have an increased rate of gestational diabetes (GD), although such pregnancy-induced diabetes can usually be managed effectively.

Preventing Multiple Pregnancy

Because of the potential risks to babies of multiple pregnancies, Dr. Louis Keith, a Chicago obstetrician who specializes in multiple births, believes doctors should try to prevent pregnancies with three or more babies by carefully monitoring fertility drug use. He recommends that women seek infertility treatment from board-certified obstetricians or reproductive endocrinologists (fertility specialists) who are familiar with fertility drugs and can prescribe reasonable doses that promote fertility yet prevent the excessive egg production that may lead to pregnancy with multiples. He cautions women against buying fertility drugs over the Internet or in a foreign country in order to self-administer the drugs, since women could give themselves dangerously high dosages.

If you are already pregnant with three or more babies, the continued existence of all the fetuses may threaten the lives of some, if not all, of the fetuses. According to the ASRM's November 2000 *Practice Committee Report,* "High order multifetal pregnancy is an adverse outcome in the care of the patient. The greater number of fetuses within the uterus, the greater the risk for adverse perinatal and maternal outcome." This grim reality may lead to a stressful and sometimes traumatic choice for both parents and physicians: (1) to maintain the status quo and risk losing some or all of the babies, or (2) to "reduce down" to twins or triplets—a process by which you abort one or more of the babies. "Reducing down" or "multifetal pregnancy reduction" may be recommended by your doctor to reduce a pregnancy with four or more babies to a pregnancy with twins or triplets. It is what some physicians refer to as a "lifeboat scenario," since the procedure is intended to help some of the babies survive.

If you would not abort your babies under any conditions, your best course of action may be to prevent pregnancy with high-order multiples from happening in the first place by using low doses of fertility drugs in order to prevent superovulation or, if you choose IVF, by implanting a modest number of embryos.

Taking Steps to Prevent Pregnancy with Multiples

If you are already taking fertility drugs, receiving eggs from a younger woman, or undergoing IVF, you may be able to prevent pregnancy with high-order multiples by making any of the following choices:

1. If you are using fertility drugs alone to superovulate but are not undergoing IVF, you can choose to take lower doses of the drugs in order to ovulate a modest number of eggs per menstrual cycle.

2. If you are undergoing an IVF procedure (or are receiving donor eggs) in which the embryos are transferred to your uterus after they become six-day-old blastocysts, these embryos have an excellent chance of "taking." Therefore, you may wish to transfer only two or three embryos to your uterus—and freeze the rest for future use. That way, if all the embryos take, you may have twins or possibly triplets—but not high-order multiples such as quadruplets or quintuplets. Discuss these options with your caregivers before you begin your assisted reproduction procedure.

Note: Talk to your physician about other strategies for preventing pregnancy with triplets or more.

Progesterone: The Drug of Pregnancy

I'd give progesterone to my daughter if she needed it—and I like my daughter! But with pregnant women, you should be extremely cautious before you give anything. Period.
—Dr. Arthur Herbst, Chairman of the Department of Obstetrics and Gynecology at the University of Chicago and coauthor of *The Developmental Effects of DES in Pregnancy,* in a 1996 interview with the author

If my daughter came to the point where she needed to take progesterone during pregnancy, I'd search the [medical/scientific] literature before I'd let her do it.
—Dr. Arthur Kohrman, Professor of Pediatrics and Public Health at Northwestern University, in a 2001 interview with the author

* * *

I wouldn't give progesterone to pregnant women.
—Dr. Howard Bern, Professor at UC Berkeley and coauthor of *The Developmental Effects of DES in Pregnancy,* in a 1995 interview with the author

* * *

Every pregnancy depends on progesterone. Progesterone is an essential hormonal ingredient in the process by which a tiny embryo attaches itself to the wall of your womb. Progesterone helps your baby-to-be develop a placenta, which will nourish it as it grows for nine months. Natural, *endogenous* [made within your body] progesterone is produced by the very spot on your ovary from which the egg first erupted—the corpus luteum, or "yellow body." Sometime after your forth week of pregnancy, there is a shift away from the ovary and corpus luteum to the placenta for the production of the progesterone necessary to maintain your pregnancy. Gradually, the baby's placenta makes considerable amounts of progesterone and takes over the job of maintaining pregnancy. Theoretically, by your eighth week of pregnancy, the baby's placenta produces enough endogenous progesterone to make your ovaries unimportant as a source of the hormone.

Historically, doctors have given women *exogenous* [that comes from a source outside your own body] progesterone for two reasons: to prevent "early pregnancy loss" and, more

recently, to maintain the pregnancies resulting from egg donation. Using progesterone to prevent pregnancy loss has fallen
out of favor. However, doctors routinely give progesterone to
egg recipients for the first eight to sixteen weeks of pregnancy
to help "maintain the pregnancy." Egg recipients depend totally
on exogenous progesterone during early pregnancy, since their
ovaries have no corpus luteum to generate this hormone. (It
was the egg donor who ovulated and who has a corpus
luteum—not the recipient.)

The benefit of exogenous progesterone for egg recipients is
clear cut, since these pregnancies require exogenous progesterone in order to succeed. But how much progesterone do
these women need—and for how long? The answer to this
second question of *how long* differs from doctor to doctor.
Some doctors prescribe progesterone for ten weeks into the
pregnancy, some for twelve, and some for sixteen.

"Twelve weeks of progesterone makes more sense [than six-
teen]. By then the placenta has taken over. A woman could stop
at eight weeks. Progesterone [as a medication] probably doesn't
do anything after eight weeks," says Dr. Allen Killam, basing his
argument on the biological fact that after the first eight weeks of
a regular pregnancy, the corpus luteum no longer produces most
of the hormones that you need to maintain pregnancy.

"By eight weeks, if you took out the ovaries, there'd be a
good chance of the baby making it," says Killam. "I don't think
it is necessary to give progesterone after twelve weeks. Maybe
not after eight." According to Killam, "Later in the pregnancy
you're making bucket loads of progesterone. The drugs are
pretty much a drop in the bucket, except for pretty early on."

Nonetheless, many doctors recommend that egg recipients
take progesterone for twelve to sixteen weeks to be on the safe
side in terms of maintaining pregnancy. Their reasons are
understandable: high-tech babies are hard to come by (as well

as expensive), and doctors want to do everything they can to ensure a successful pregnancy.

But are such practices on the safe side when it comes to possible drug side effects for the baby? This is an important question since thousands of pregnant women—infertility patients with ovulatory problems, women at high risk for miscarriage, and women with high-tech pregnancies—are treated with exogenous progesterone each year.

Because most forms of progesterone given to promote pregnancy are "natural" forms of the hormone, many physicians believe the hormonal drug is safe. Dr. Mark Sauer, who uses progesterone in his Columbia University clinic, believes the drug has very few side effects: "You supplement the first twelve to fourteen weeks of pregnancy with progesterone. Your body makes so much progesterone as to negate anything you put in it. We use micronized, vaginal gel. There are hardly any side effects. The progesterone goes right to the pelvic blood vessels: a direct hit." Dr. Gideon Koren, a Professor of Pediatrics and Medical Genetics and director of the Motherisk program, agrees that progesterone is safe, since he has not seen abnormalities in children exposed to the drug over the last twenty years.

But there are those who disagree. Some biologists and toxicologists express concern about progesterone's effects on "developing tissue"—the baby-to-be. Dr. Lovell Jones, a research scientist and Director of Experimental Gynecology-Endocrinology at the M.D. Anderson Cancer Institute, worries about exposing babies in utero to the drug. During the mid-1970s, Jones's studies of baby mice exposed to the drug found that progesterone caused reproduction system abnormalities in the baby mice whose mothers took the drug while pregnant. Consequently, Jones thinks progesterone should be studied further before being given to pregnant women.

Again the question is one of benefit and risk. The drug offers clear benefits for egg recipients, since without the drug there will be no baby. But does progesterone effectively treat the other conditions—luteal phase defect and early pregnancy loss—for which it is prescribed? Again, there is considerable disagreement.

A Treatment for Luteal Phase Defect and Early Miscarriage

Although there is solid evidence that progesterone works to foster egg donor pregnancies, it is not clear whether progesterone is effective for luteal phase defect (see Chapter 6) or early pregnancy loss. Consequently, progesterone treatments for both conditions remain controversial.

A prospective, double-blind randomized trial (the most reliable kind of clinical study) in the 1970s showed that progesterone did not prevent early miscarriage, according to Dr. Allen Killam. "In the 1960s it was believed that progesterone would prevent spontaneous abortions [miscarriages]. Study results were promising—until they used placebo studies. When a placebo double-blind randomized control study was done, it did not show this effect. By the 1970s, the use of progesterone to prevent miscarriage had been debunked."

According to Dr. Murray Enkin and his coauthors of *A Guide to Effective Care in Pregnancy and Childbirth* (third edition), the several randomized studies on the use of progestogens (progesterone) in early pregnancy showed "no evidence to suggest that they reduce the risk of miscarriage, stillbirth, or neonatal death in women with either bleeding (threatened miscarriage) or with a history of recurrent miscarriage." However, these studies "have not been large enough to exclude an important effect in either direction (increase or decrease in miscarriage)."

Some physicians continue to believe that progesterone prevents miscarriage and to prescribe the drug during pregnancy.

When it comes to progesterone treatment for luteal phase defect, says Killam, "the medical community is divided." About 50 percent of obstetricians do not even believe that the condition called luteal phase defect really exists, or if it does exist, they believe it is overdiagnosed (see Chapter 6).

Other physicians argue that progesterone should not be used to prevent miscarriage since the majority of miscarriages are nature's way of eliminating genetic defects. High miscarriage rates in women over thirty-five are most often due to genetic flaws in the egg and embryo—problems that are not solved by progesterone therapy.

Dr. Allen Killam speculates that progesterone may occasionally have a placebo effect. A placebo effect is said to occur when a patient's condition "improves" (in this case, she maintains her pregnancy) with a medication for reasons having nothing to do with that actual medication. The placebo (a "sugar pill" that has no real medication) may improve the patient's condition due to the patient's confidence in the doctor or the medical therapy. Dr. Killam speculates that progesterone therapy to prevent miscarriage may reduce a woman's stress level and increase her confidence, which may then help to prevent miscarriage.

Ironically, certain fertility drugs may create a luteal phase defect (and a decrease in your progesterone levels) that may make it difficult for an embryo to implant in your uterus, and thus decrease your chances of becoming pregnant. "You can create a corpus luteum defect by IVF drugs," says Dr. Mark Sauer, who describes the catch-22 faced by women undergoing certain treatments for infertility. "The drugs make you ovulate, but they make the corpus luteum left by the egg defective in producing progesterone, so you need to supplement the progesterone." Thus to "cure" a fertility problem caused by some fertility drugs, your doctor may give you progesterone.

Long-Term Risks for Babies? The Scientific Debate

I truly feel that more work needs to be done before I can say progesterone is safe.

—Dr. Richard Hajek, M.D. Anderson Cancer Center

• • ◆

Are the benefits worth the possible long-term risks? The majority of physicians interviewed for this book believe that the type and amounts of progesterone currently given to pregnant women are safe. They believe that giving the drug to pregnant women simply exposes the baby to benign "natural hormones" that are normally abundant during pregnancy and that the amount of progesterone given to women corresponds to "physiologic levels" of the hormone that are normally present in women during pregnancy.

Whether such prenatal exposure to natural but exogenous progesterone may cause long-term adverse effects is not yet known for certain, since it is considered unethical to conduct clinical drug trials on pregnant women. However, many doctors think that adverse side effects are unlikely, since they have not seen problems in the generations of children exposed to the drug.

On the other hand, many of the developmental biologists and cancer researchers interviewed for this book say the drug hasn't been studied extensively enough for us to know if it is safe for developing fetuses. These scientists point to animal studies showing that the natural form of progesterone can cause problems when given exogenously during pregnancy and that the hormonal drug is not necessarily benign just because it is "natural."

According to Dr. Lovell Jones, just because progesterone may be safe for adults does not mean that it is safe for the delicate, developing fetus. "We can talk about drugs and compounds having no negative effects in humans, but we have to always remember that fetuses are not small adults, and what may be safe for an adult to take is not safe in terms of exposure to developing fetuses," says Jones, who encourages women to make informed decisions about the drugs they take during pregnancy.

"What we know, should make us cautious. From the animal data, there is a potential risk that if you do become pregnant there is the possibility that the progesterone therapy you're taking may have a deleterious effect on your offspring. That's not conclusive, but there's that potential. It is your choice, but it needs to be an informed choice."

Researchers such as Drs. Howard Bern, Lovell Jones, and Richard Hajek are particularly worried about a fetus being exposed to progesterone during its first six to nine weeks of life—during the first trimester of pregnancy. The scientists base their concerns on animal studies, since no human studies have been conducted regarding the prenatal effects of progesterone. However, baby female rats and mice exposed to the drug— during stages of development comparable to a human fetus's first six to nine weeks—have developed reproductive abnor- malities. According to Dr. Hajek, the most prominent abnor- mality observed in animals is *vaginal cornification,* a migration of uterine cells to the vagina (an abnormality also observed in DES daughters). Some researchers fear that exposed babies may develop such reproductive-tract abnormalities, although the problems may not become obvious until the babies become young adults.

Many physicians, however, do not share these concerns, since they have seen no reproductive abnormalities appearing in the adolescent or adult children of women who took proges- terone during pregnancy. Others see it as an open question. Dr. Murray Enkin and his coauthors of *A Guide to Effective Care in Pregnancy and Childbirth* (third edition) argue that given the kind of research that has been done so far, nobody knows for sure whether or not the progestogen (progesterone) drugs are safe for babies: "Although the progestogen follow-up studies have been largely anecdotal and uncontrolled, there have been suggestions from some studies that fetal exposure to the drugs may increase cardiac, neurological, neural tube and other major malformations, and female masculinization or 'tom-boyishness' in girls. Other studies, however, have failed to detect these adverse effects, and so the safety of progestogens, like their postulated benefits, remains an open question."

What You Can Do

If you are considering egg donation, for which progesterone has been proven effective in maintaining pregnancy, your benefits will be obvious—a baby. If you wish for further information about the possible risks, discuss possible side effects with your doctor. If you wish further information about the effectiveness of progesterone for other conditions, ask your doctor or contact the ASRM in Atlanta, Georgia. For additional information call Motherisk or Reprotox or check medical databases such as Medline or The Cochrane Library (see appendix).

Chapter 8

Overcoming Age-Related Obstacles to Pregnancy: Fibroids, Endometriosis, Fallopian Tube Problems

A normal consequence of being female and menstruating is that a woman may develop endometriosis. The older a woman is, the more likely she is to have it. We believe that it is due to menstruating into the abdominal cavity. Menstrual debris goes through the tubes and into the cavity. If the living cells in the debris attach and grow in the abdominal cavity, it leads to a disease process.
—Dr. David Walmer

＊　＊　＊

Fibroids are more common in older women. They are not a major problem, but they can degenerate in pregnancy and cause pain or premature labor contractions. If they are very large, they can interfere with the presentation of the baby or obstruct labor and get in the way of the baby in the pelvis.
—Dr. Watson Bowes Jr.

＊　＊　＊

Some female reproductive tract problems become more prevalent with age. After age thirty, *endometriosis* (a migration of the hormonally reactive uterine lining to the fallopian tubes and abdominal cavity) and *uterine fibroid tumors* (benign muscle tumors of the uterus) may create difficulty in conceiving or in carrying a baby to term. For some women, fibroids and migrating endometrial tissue may create significant obstacles to conception, pregnancy, or delivery. Women over thirty are also more likely than younger women to have had tubal infections that block the fallopian tubes and interfere with conception. Such tubal obstacles to conception may be circumvented by IVF procedures (see the section on IVF in Chapter 6) or may be surgically repaired.

Fortunately, endometriosis and fibroids often do not create problems for conception or pregnancy and often require no treatment for infertility. In fact, pregnancy may serve as a temporary treatment for women with endometriosis. Although the hormones of pregnancy may make fibroid tumors grow larger, these growing tumors do not necessarily cause pain or interfere with the pregnancy or birth process. Many women with large or numerous fibroids have had healthy babies and normal deliveries.

If you already have endometriosis or fibroid tumors that are either symptomatic or creating fertility problems, your options consist of surgery; drug treatment; or simply trusting your body, forging ahead, and "letting nature take its course." This chapter will discuss the pros and cons of all of these options.

Endometriosis

With endometriosis you do surgery through a scope [laparoscope]; it's very challenging to suture through a scope, so your doctor should have experience. Endometriosis also may be treated with Lupron or progesterone or by getting pregnant.
—Dr. Margaret Bates

* * *

Endometriosis is a condition in which the lining of the uterus, the endometrium, flows backward through the fallopian tubes and into the abdominal cavity during menstruation. Consequently, little pieces of endometrial tissue may latch on to your tubes, ovaries, or other internal organs. Like the lining of your uterus, this tissue is sensitive to hormones and may proliferate over time. Eventually, endometriosis may cause adhesions that obstruct your ovaries, inhibit the normal movements of your fallopian tubes, or create ovarian cysts called endometriomas. Endometriosis may impair your fertility—or it may not. Just the fact of having endometriosis does not mean you need high-tech interventions in order to become pregnant. You may not require any treatment for your condition, unless the endometriosis is causing you pain.

Since endometriosis tends to worsen with time, extensive endometrial adhesions may be more common in women over thirty than in younger women. Some physicians, like David Walmer, believe that having a child at an early age may be somewhat protective against endometriosis. Since endometriosis is less likely to cause reproductive problems for women who have their children relatively early, you may want to consider getting pregnant sooner rather than later if you have this condition.

Drug Treatments

We believe that there is an association between endometriosis and fertility and when you have endometriosis . . . something may go awry between ovulation and egg pick-up by the fallopian tubes. You can get a partial correcting of infertility by treating women with superovulation and recruiting lots of eggs. We can more effectively treat infertility of women with endometriosis by in vitro fertilization. Danazol and surgery can shrink the [endometrial] implants, but there is not good evidence they improve fertility.
—Dr. David Walmer

* * *

Drug treatment for endometriosis often aims at relieving pain. The three drugs most frequently used at this time are birth control pills; danazol (Danocrine), a synthetic hormonal drug that is similar to testosterone; and leuprolide (Lupron), a drug that suppresses your production of female hormones. Danazol stops ovulation and the production of estrogen and progesterone and thus stops the monthly pain caused by proliferating endometrial tissues.

Sometimes you will respond to one drug at a certain time of your life and another drug at a different time. The only way to find out is by trial and error to discover which drug works best for you at a particular time. Lupron stops ovulation and creates a pseudo-menopausal state in which your periods stop temporarily (until a month or so after you stop taking the drug). Consequently, the endometrial tissues outside your uterus no longer proliferate and cause pain.

Both drugs may have side effects, and once again you must evaluate the pros and cons. Lupron sometimes creates memory problems along with hot flashes, vaginal dryness, and bone loss—symptoms of the menopauselike condition the drug induces. The package insert for Lupron recommends that the drug should not be used for more than six months.

Danazol may lead to weight gain and acne. Because Danazol suppresses female hormones, it also may create masculinizing side effects such as the growth of additional facial hair and the deepening of your voice as well as menopausal symptoms such as flushing, sweating, and vaginal dryness. However, if your pain is severe, the benefits of the drugs may be worth the possible side effects.

Surgical Treatments

Whether or not surgery is the best way to treat endometriosis is the subject of debate. If you are experiencing pain, many doctors will try to minimize your pain through drug treatment alone, especially as a first step.

If you are experiencing infertility, many doctors will recommend that you try IVF instead of tubal surgery. However, if surgery becomes necessary for you, there are two kinds of surgery commonly used to remove adhesions and endometrial tissue: *laparoscopy* or *laparotomy*. In either case, you will need a surgeon who is skilled in reproductive surgeries that preserve fertility.

With a laparoscopy, the operation will be performed with a small instrument called a *laparoscope,* and the surgeon will make several small incisions in your abdomen. This technique, combined with laser surgery, is often a first choice because it causes less damage to tissues and requires less anesthesia than a laparotomy.

A laparotomy is often a second choice, because it involves a much larger incision across your abdomen. However, there are times when a laparotomy is preferable, especially if the endometrial adhesions extend beyond the scope of the laparoscope.

Uterine Fibroid Tumors

Fibroid tumors are really not a fertility issue as such. Most fibroid surgeries are done needlessly. Fibroids are normal. 80 percent of women eventually will have them. The vast majority of these tumors need not be removed.
—Dr. Robert Israel, Professor of Obstetrics and Gynecology, University of Southern California Medical School

* * *

"Fibroids are not a big problem for pregnancy unless they are large or they distort or elongate the uterine cavity," says Dr. Mark Sauer, who sees many women with fibroids in his New

York City medical practice.

Uterine fibroids are common muscle tumors of the uterus, and much of the time, fibroids will not cause problems in terms of your getting pregnant or staying pregnant. However, because the tumors often are sensitive to estrogen, they can grow rapidly during pregnancy, causing you pain or even miscarriage. Fibroids also may create obstructions in the birth canal, which may lead to a cesarean instead of a vaginal birth—it depends on where your fibroids are located and how big they are.

There are three types of fibroids: *submucosal*, *intramural*, and *subserosal*. The submucosal fibroids, located inside the uterine cavity, are the ones most likely to cause problems for pregnancy, because they can prevent successful implantation of the embryo, take crucial uterine space away from a developing baby, or cause uterine bleeding.

Intramural fibroids grow within the muscular wall of the uterus and can become quite large. If they are large and close to the uterine cavity, they can distort the shape of the cavity—a circumstance that may affect your ability to get pregnant or carry to term. A large fibroid located near or in the uterine cavity may compete with the baby for blood supply or make a large uterus start to contract, resulting in third trimester miscarriage or premature labor.

Subserosal fibroids, located on the outside of the uterus, tend to be the least troublesome in terms of pregnancy, unless they interfere with the functioning of your fallopian tubes.

Drug Treatments

Drug treatments do not "cure" fibroids. There is as yet no real cure for fibroids except surgery. However, if your fibroid causes bleeding or if its size creates discomfort or other problems, your doctor may recommend that you take Lupron—a drug that shrinks the fibroid, at least temporarily. Lupron is a hormonal drug that brings your body into a temporary and drug-induced menopauselike condition that reduces your estrogen production. Since fibroids are estrogen-dependent, they will shrink as long as you are on the drug. However, the drug is not designed for long-term use but merely to stop bleeding or reduce growth so that your fibroid can be more easily removed surgically.

The benefits of Lupron are controversial, since some doctors believe Lupron makes fibroid surgery easier, while others think it makes surgery more difficult. Furthermore, Lupron has potential side effects such as hot flashes, memory loss, and other menopauselike symptoms. Discuss the drug treatment approach with your doctors, and expect some differences in opinion.

Surgical Treatments

For most women, fibroids have very little bearing on fertility. Regardless of age, the need to operate should be based on their size, the rate at which they grow, symptoms such as bleeding, and positions on the uterine wall.
—Dr. Margaret Bates, OB/GYN, Hospital of the Good Samaritan, Los Angeles

* * *

Troublesome fibroids that cause bleeding or impede conception may be surgically removed. If the fibroids are in the cavity of your uterus, they sometimes can be removed through a *hysteroscope,* a small instrument that is inserted through your cervix. The benefits of this hysteroscopic technique are that it does not require major abdominal surgery, it does not require prolonged use of anesthesia, and it can be done as an outpatient procedure. However, not all doctors are proficient at this kind of surgery, and only some submucosal fibroids can be removed this way.

If your fibroids are intramural or subserosal, your surgeon may need to use the laparotomy procedure, which is considered major abdominal surgery and requires prolonged anesthesia. Some doctors will use a laser instrument for part of the surgery, although this technique does not mean that you will be spared the surgical knife. "With 'laser' surgery, you still need an incision; the laser merely cleans up some of the bleeding," says Dr. Margaret Bates, an experienced gynecological surgeon.

The benefits of surgery are removal of fibroids and relief of symptoms. The risks of fibroid surgery include the risks of any abdominal surgery: bleeding, infection, and complications caused by anesthesia. In addition to the usual risks, laparotomy can itself cause scarring, which impedes fertility. Again, you must weigh benefits and risks with some guidance from your physician. By having surgery only when the indications are clear and by finding a reproductive surgeon committed to preserving your fertility, you will minimize your risks and maximize your odds of a favorable outcome. Very rarely the surgery may result in hemorrhage that requires the removal of your uterus in order to stop the bleeding.

About 20 to 25 percent of the time, fibroid tumors will recur, but even if they do, they may not require any medical treatment.

How do you know when to have fibroid surgery, and how do you find an experienced surgeon able and willing to preserve your fertility? Your doctor may recommend surgery if you have had repeated miscarriages, bleeding and anemia, rapid growth of the tumors, pain, or problems urinating. If your doctor suspects that your fibroid may be cancerous—a very rare but potentially dangerous situation—he or she may suggest that you have the fibroid removed immediately. Although hysterectomy is the first line of treatment for malignant fibroids, a myomectomy may be done first and the hysterectomy may be postponed until the cancer diagnosis is confirmed.

Medical opinion differs regarding whether or not large fibroids should be removed before you try to become pregnant. Some doctors recommend the removal of fibroids over a certain size—anywhere from five to twelve centimeters—while other doctors believe that even large fibroids do not necessarily need to come out, since any abdominal surgery can itself cause adhesions that interfere with pregnancy. Dr Walmer supports this conservative approach: "[I remove] fibroids only if there are problems with repetitive pregnancy loss. There is some risk of pelvic adhesions from the surgery."

Unfortunately, some women encounter doctors who advise them to have hysterectomies as a "cure" for fibroids, especially if the doctor believes that the fibroids are huge or that the woman is too old for childbearing and thus no longer "needs" her uterus. Joanne encountered this when she was still in her thirties, and her doctor told her "the cure for older women" was hysterectomy. Joanne eventually found a different doctor. When she was forty-six, Joanne had numerous fibroids removed. "My uterus was completely distended. Later I saw the surgery report and found that my uterus had been totally reconstructed." Joanne went on to have a normal pregnancy three years later.

"Any woman who is going to get a hysterectomy should have a second opinion—but not from the guy down the hallway," advises Dr. Mark Sauer, who thinks that a truly objective second opinion can not come from one of your doctor's associates or friends. Of course, if you want a hysterectomy, that is another story, but make sure you are well informed about the pros and cons of hysterectomy before having one.

Blocked Fallopian Tubes

The doctor said, "You have two blocked tubes. You need surgery." We were in shock. I was angry at my body. I felt like I had really taken good care of it all these years, and it wasn't functioning right.

—Kathleen R. had her tubes surgically repaired. The repair was successful in only one tube, yet Kathleen went on to get pregnant three times. The first time she miscarried, and the second time she gave birth to a baby boy. The third time, Kathleen developed a tubal pregnancy, which required the surgical removal of her remaining fallopian tube.

◆ ◆ ◆

Fallopian tubes can become blocked or damaged from infection, endometriosis, abdominal surgery, or tubal pregnancy. If your doctor suspects that your tubes may be blocked, he or she will most likely do a hysterosalpingogram, an x-ray test involving the injection of dye into your uterus and tubes. The dye is injected through a catheter that goes through your cervix. This test can be quite uncomfortable, depending on several factors: the skill of the person doing the exam, your level of anxiety, and the degree of obstruction in your uterus or tubes. Since some of the discomfort may be due to abdominal cramping, discuss with your doctor what kind of medications you can take before the procedure to prevent cramping. Some doctors recommend ibuprofen several hours before the test.

The benefit of having a hysterosalpingogram is that your doctor can see your uterine cavity and fallopian tubes and determine whether or not the cavity is normal and the tubes are open. A possible risk of the test is infection, although this seldom occurs. Some doctors may put you on antibiotics for a few days to prevent infection.

If your test shows that your tubes are closed, your doctor may offer you surgery to open the fallopian tube. This is very delicate surgery and should be attempted only by skillful surgeons who are experienced in tubal microsurgery. Often the surgery can be done through a laparoscope, which can minimize the risks of major abdominal surgery.

Some physicians may suggest that you try IVF instead of tubal surgery. Weighing the pros and cons of these procedures may require careful consideration and several discussions with your doctor. Although the success rates of tubal surgery are not high, if the surgery is successful, you may be able to conceive naturally—without the assistance of expensive fertility drugs and high-tech interventions. On the other hand, if the surgery is not successful, you will have subjected your abdomen and reproductive tract to an invasive procedure with some risks of infection, but you may still have the option of IVF.

Finding a Surgeon

It's a bad sign if a doctor tells you you're too old to have a baby or you don't need your uterus—that's agism and sexism. Any doctor that doesn't give you your choice—you need to question his or her approach. Question, question, question.
—Dr. Mark Sauer

◆ ◈ ◉

If you wish to have your fibroids removed, you may need to shop for a surgeon. Call nearby medical schools, hospitals, or various branches of your HMO for names of surgeons who specialize in the kind of surgery you need. Sometimes you will be referred to reproductive endocrinologists and sometimes to gynecologists who specialize in reproductive surgeries.

Compile a list of questions to ask your prospective doctors, since asking questions will give you an opportunity to learn about your problem, to compare the doctors' responses, and to choose the doctor whose answers and manner you like best.

Keep in mind that in addition to his or her answers, an important quality in a surgeon is *good judgment.*

Schedule an interview with a doctor, or interview the doctor at your first consultation. Your doctor should be willing to spend at least fifteen minutes with you discussing your particular case, your desire for pregnancy or for keeping your uterus, and your treatment options. It is best to find a skilled but conservative surgeon who is capable of performing challenging surgery but unlikely to perform unnecessary surgery.

Questions to Ask a Prospective Surgeon

1. *When you have set out to do a myomectomy, how often did you end up needing to do a hysterectomy?* A skilled doctor committed to preserving a woman's fertility should have a very low number of such hysterectomies. However, all doctors will ask your consent to do a hysterectomy as a life-saving measure to stop bleeding if this becomes necessary.

2. *How many fibroids have you taken out of a woman's uterus while still leaving the uterus intact?* Experienced surgeons may have removed as many as twenty-five to forty fibroids from a woman's uterus. Such doctors should also be experienced in removing large fibroids—sometimes the size of a twenty-five-week pregnancy or even larger. If your surgeon tells you that you have too many fibroids to preserve your uterus and you need a hysterectomy, seek a second opinion. Also seek a second opinion if the doctor tells you the fibroids can't be removed due to their size. You have the right to a second opinion. Getting another opinion is a reasonable thing to do when surgery is a possibility.

"No doctor should be flustered by a second opinion," says Dr. Sauer.

Occasionally, you may have a fibroid in a disadvantageous spot for surgery. Some doctors may feel it best to remove other fibroids but leave one or two behind if removing them could risk losing your uterus. However, if a fibroid is rapidly growing or causing serious bleeding, your doctor will probably not want to leave it behind. Discuss your situation with your surgeon, and reach an agreement that is comfortable for both of you.

3. *How bloody an operation is a myomectomy, and how many pints of blood will I need?* Find a surgeon who seems confident about his or her methods of controlling bleeding. You may need one to two pints of blood for the procedure, but a surgeon who frequently needs to replace four pints of blood is not the best surgeon for you.

4. *May I use autologous blood (blood that you donate in advance to yourself) rather than blood from a blood bank during the surgery?* Using your own blood is always better than using someone else's. Even though most American blood banks conscientiously screen for blood-borne diseases, you still are safer from AIDS or Hepatitis A, B, and C if you use your own blood.

If you have anesthesia preferences, discuss your preferences with your surgeon. Some women prefer to be "asleep" with a general anesthesia. Others prefer to be awake and to choose an epidural or spinal.

To make sure that you are in the hands of a skilled surgeon, call the obstetrics unit of a hospital with a good reputation and ask the nurses whom they recommend. Call the operating

room, and ask the nurses who is good at performing myomec-
tomies or endometriosis surgery. If you know an anesthesiologist
or operating room nurse, ask him or her to suggest a surgeon.

Recovering from Abdominal Surgery

*For the first two weeks, do nothing. You need to devote a lot of
energy to healing. Rest. Take very short walks. Don't go further
than half a block, and see how that feels. Walk around the house.
Don't sit a lot. Lie down with heat on your tummy. Do not take
on responsibilities around the house: no cooking, no ironing, no
washing. Lifting can be endangering. Do not even lift your cats.
Sex can be very endangering; it can disrupt your suture lines or
introduce infection. Recovery takes four to six weeks, maybe
more. It takes more if there's a lot of disruption to the endometrial cavity. Let your body heal. Engage your mind and spirit in
active healing.*
—Dr. Margaret Bates

◆ ◆ ◆

Recovering from a laparotomy is much like recovering from a
cesarean section (see Part 8). However, recovery may be even
more difficult, especially if you had many fibroids removed
resulting in numerous incisions in your uterus. In addition,
being under general anesthesia for a couple of hours (as is sometimes necessary) can add to postsurgical malaise. Recovery from
a myomectomy may take from four to six weeks, depending on
your physical condition, your healing ability, your support
system, and the extent of your surgery.

During the first week or two after surgery, you will need
help at home, since you will not be allowed to shop, cook,
clean, or change the kitty litter (see Chapter 28). If your partner
can take time off work, this would be a good time to do so.

Otherwise, you will need friends, family, or a hired aide to help since you may find making dinner an ordeal. Do not plan on trips, since jostling around in a car or train can hurt.

Even three to four weeks following surgery, you may find it difficult to sit at a desk; consequently, your recovery period is a poor time for work deadlines or home improvements. You may be advised to avoid driving for several weeks—don't jeopardize your healing by commuting to work or driving children to that soccer game across town.

Some women have quicker and easier recoveries than others, but you never know how you will respond to surgery until afterward, and by then, you will need a support system in place.

Part Four

You're Pregnant!: Nutrition, Exercise, and Environmental Health

Chapter 9
Fitness for the Long Haul

During your pregnancy you will "grow a baby," and the foods you eat will become essential building materials for the baby's bones, blood, muscles, and organs. Your prepregnancy diet will not be enough for the nutrition, fluid, and energy requirements of both you and your baby, and you must add sufficient nutrients and vitamins to keep up with the new demands on your body.

Usually, moderate exercise contributes to your health and the health of your growing baby by increasing your blood circulation, bringing oxygen and nutrients to your tissues, and by increasing your stamina during childbirth. However, it is important to use good judgment and not push your body too hard or begin new activities that are too rigorous.

Since your developing baby is more vulnerable than you are to environmental toxins, it is important for you to minimize your exposure to environmental pollutants and potentially dangerous food additives during your pregnancy. Try to avoid foods that are heavily sprayed with pesticides or that contain mercury or added hormones.

In this chapter, we will look at the components of a healthy nutrition and exercise program and identify environmental contaminants to avoid during pregnancy.

A Varied and Pure Diet

Many physicians and midwives agree that the most reliable diet is a varied diet that includes the basic food groups, vitamins, and minerals. How much pregnant women should eat has been the subject of debate, although most care providers agree that women should gain between twenty-five and thirty-five pounds with one baby and about forty pounds with twins.

"The baby steals from the mother what it needs," explains Dr. Donna Kirz when she encourages her pregnant patients to eat nutritious foods to "feed" their unborn baby and also care for their own nutritional needs.

For instance, if you don't eat enough calcium-rich foods for your baby, the baby will take the calcium it needs from your bones—a situation that becomes more problematic the closer you are to menopause when you need to avoid bone loss and supplement your diet with absorbable forms of calcium.

During pregnancy, you need extra calcium and other nutrients to literally *grow a baby,* which means you need all the nutrients crucial for building bone, blood, nerves, and placenta. You are making new tissue every day. To do this, you need energy (calories) and nutrients gained from a varied diet of fruits and green and yellow vegetables, grains, fats and oils, and liquids. This diet should contain daily sources of protein, calcium, iron, and folic acid. Folic acid is important even during the first weeks of pregnancy.

However, foods alone may not provide you with enough absorbable folic acid, iron, and calcium for your pregnancy needs. During pregnancy and breastfeeding, your daily needs for iron and vitamin D double; your need also increases for protein, zinc, riboflavin, and a variety of other vitamins and minerals. If you are a strict vegetarian, you should take special care to get enough protein, and you may need supplemental vitamin B_{12} while you are pregnant or nursing.

Pregnant women need about 2,300 calories a day in order to grow a healthy baby and still have energy left over for daily life. However, caloric requirements may vary according to individual differences in body weight and level of activity. For instance, athletic women will require more calories than women who are not as physically active. Women who breastfeed tend to use more calories than women who don't. Consult your doctor and a nutritionist about your individual nutritional needs.

When you can, choose fresh and relatively chemical-free foods and "whole foods" such as whole grains that are not processed. This may mean doing some research as to where and how foods are grown or prepared. When in doubt and pressed for time, buy organic produce, farm-raised fish, and hormone-free meat.

According to the March of Dimes, American adults should eat six to eleven servings per day of bread, or other whole grains; three to five servings of vegetables; two to four servings of fruit; and three to four servings of protein foods such as meat, poultry, fish, eggs, beans, or nuts. Fats and oils should be included in moderation. Pregnant women need sources of calcium: about three servings per day of dairy products or calcium-rich foods such as almonds, broccoli, and kale. Although this may seem like an excessive amount of food, keep in mind that "one serving" may be relatively small. For instance, one serving of fruit equals ½ cup of fruit or one medium piece of fruit. One serving of vegetables equals ½ cup of cooked or raw vegetables, and one serving of bread or whole grains equals one slice of bread, ½ cup of cooked rice or pasta, or ½ of a bagel. Because dietary recommendations change from time to time, discuss your dietary requirements with your doctor and nutritionist. The suggestions below are generalizations that may or may not apply to your individual circumstances.

The Ideal Diet for Pregnancy

- Dairy products or calcium-rich foods
- Protein (meat, fish, beans, peas)
- Fruits (including citrus fruits)
- Vegetables (including green and yellow vegetables that are rich in vitamin A)
- Grains
- Fats and oils in moderation (fish and vegetable oils are best)

Sugar is not essential to a healthy diet. If you are over thirty-five or forty, you may want to minimize additional sugar intake. If you have diabetes or gestational diabetes, discuss your sugar and fructose (the sugar found in fruit) intake with your health care provider and nutritionist.

Protein—Three to Four Servings per Day (74–100 g)

Cells come from protein, and your protein requirements will be high since you are "building" your baby cell by cell. Meat, poultry, fish, eggs, dairy products, beans, and lentils are good sources of high-quality protein. Average requirements for pregnant women are about three ounces of fish or meat, one cup of beans or lentils, or four tablespoons of peanut butter three to four times a day.

If you're vegetarian, you may need to eat more beans, tofu, or soy products than usual. If you are on a special diet, such as a rice or macrobiotic diet, you may need to modify that diet during your pregnancy in order to "eat for two" and to provide your developing child with the necessary components for its growth.

Calcium—Three to Four Servings per Day (1,200–1,300 mg)

Calcium builds—and rebuilds—bone. If you are over forty and beginning to lose bone, you need to be especially careful that you get adequate calcium through diet and vitamin supplements (so that you do not enter your perimenopausal years with pregnancy-induced bone loss).

Dairy products are, of course, a good source of calcium. One serving equals about one cup of milk or yogurt, one-third cup nonfat dry milk, one and a half cups of cottage cheese, two to three cups of ice cream, or one and one half to two ounces of cheese.

Supplement dairy products with some of the following:

- Almonds (¾ cup)
- Broccoli (1¾ cups)
- Collard greens (1 cup cooked)
- Kale (1½ cups cooked)
- Turnip greens (1¼ cups cooked)
- Tofu, prepared with calcium, 9 ounces
- Soy milk (see calcium contents on individual products) or soy yogurt
- Salmon (4 ounces, with bones)
- Canned sardines (3 ounces, with bones)

For calcium-rich snacks try figs, olives, and dried apricots.

Iron—(48–78 mg per day)

The human body has difficulty absorbing some forms of iron, especially when they are not combined with vitamin C. Of the supplements, chelated iron is the most absorbable. For the best absorption, take iron with vitamin C. You probably will not get all the iron you need from dietary sources, but try the following foods for some of your iron needs:

- Beef
- Carob powder
- Dried beans and peas
- Dried fruits
- Spinach (cooked—this is the most absorbable form)
- Soy products
- Dried spirulina

Supplemental iron may sometimes cause constipation. To prevent constipation some doctors suggest that you increase your bulk intake by eating more fruits and vegetables and drinking more water.

Fluids

Drink plenty of water—at least eight glasses a day. You need to stay hydrated to keep your blood volume and amniotic fluid levels normal. Adequate fluid intake is also needed to build cells, deliver nutrients via the bloodstream, and flush out toxins and waste products. Along with water, you can drink decaffeinated tea (check with your caregiver regarding safe herbal teas), fruit juice, milk, or smoothies (with ice cream, fruit juice, and/or yogurt). To avoid too much sugar or artificial sweeteners, try fresh fruit and vegetable juices, seltzer water (or sodium-free seltzer or mineral water if you have high blood pressure), and seltzer mixtures with fruit juice or a squeeze of lemon or lime.

Drink more fluids in hot weather or when you are exercising vigorously, since dehydration can lead to premature labor.

Dietary Precautions

What kinds of foods or vitamins should be avoided during pregnancy? Perhaps more than you realize, since several vitamins are toxic when taken in large amounts, and some foods contain potentially harmful amounts of chemicals. That does not mean you need to transform your diet, although you may wish to carefully choose where your food and vitamins come from.

Vitamins

Avoid overdoing vitamin A. Your total intake should not exceed 5,000 IUs a day. Do not take excessive doses of any vitamin. Some nutritionists believe that you should not supplement your diet with lecithin, since lecithin can cause brain abnormalities in rats.

You may need to supplement your diet with calcium, but avoid sources from bone meal and oyster shells since the bone and shell used may be contaminated with toxic metals such as mercury and lead. Ask your doctor and pharmacist about other absorbable forms of calcium.

Fruits and Vegetables

When you can, avoid fruits and vegetables that are sprayed with substantial quantities of pesticides. When in doubt, buy organic, at either your local supermarket, co-op, or farmer's market. When possible, buy organic grapes, apples, tomatoes, and potatoes since the regular brands may have pesticide residues. If you don't wish to buy organic produce, wash your fruits and vegetables carefully with a mild or biodegradable dish detergent (do not use dishwasher detergent or strong soaps). Avoid fruits and vegetables from countries, like Mexico, that use pesticides banned in the United States. To limit your pesticide exposure, peel produce that seems filmy, waxy, or powdery.

Fish

Farmed fish may be the safest, since it is raised in a controlled environment. Avoid fish exposed to mercury or other environmental chemicals. Tuna, bluefish, and swordfish tend to be higher in chemical pollutants than other ocean fish. Some fish from the Great Lakes as well as other freshwater fish (trout, perch, whitefish, salmon, walleye pike) tend to store environmental pollutants in their body fat. Dioxins and PCBs are found in some fish like lake trout. Call local environmental organizations to inquire about the quality and source of locally sold fish.

Meat and Poultry

When you can, buy hormone-free poultry, meat, and milk. Although many of us in the United States have come to accept hormone-fed livestock because such practices have become commonplace, Europeans are far less accepting of hormones in their food. Call your local supermarket chains and small health food markets to see if they sell hormone-free chicken and hormone- and antibiotic-free meat.

Some environmental health advocates recommend that pregnant women avoid eating animal fat, since meat and cheese may be a source of dioxin exposure.

Water

If your tap water has been found to have chemical or bacterial contaminants at levels of questionable safety, you can use distilled, filtered, and deionized spring water. You also may benefit from using a water purifier during your pregnancy.

Nitrates and Nitrites

Studies show that nitrates and nitrites do not appear to cause fetal abnormalities in animals, but some health experts have long been wary of these chemicals' potentially carcinogenic effects in adults. Consequently, during your pregnancy, you may wish to limit your intake of foods containing sodium nitrate and nitrite such as bacon, ham, hot dogs, knockwurst, liver sausage, salami, and bologna.

Herbs

Herbs may seem innocuous because they are associated with healing teas and remedies, but some herbal teas contain powerful chemicals—which is why they are effectively used as drugs in many cultures. Some herbs may cause damage to a growing baby or may stimulate your body to go into labor. Herbs that have been linked to miscarriage (intentional or otherwise) are slippery elm, cohosh, pennyroyal, mugwort, and tansy (see "Medications, Alternative Home Remedies, Vitamins, and Herbal Remedies" section in Chapter 2). Since herbs are becoming available to the American public more quickly than Western medicine can study them, be particularly cautious about drinking herbal teas. Consult with your caregiver about herbs to avoid during pregnancy.

Monosodium Glutamate (MSG)

MSG causes damage to infant animals, and it has been taken out of baby foods. You may want to limit the MSG in your diet. Check food labels for MSG, and ask your favorite Chinese restaurants if they use MSG or if they serve sauces without it.

Soft Cheeses

Some soft cheeses may become contaminated with a bacteria called Listeria, and Listeria can make you sick from two to thirty days after you eat the contaminated food. Because this infection can pose a serious threat to your baby, call your doctor immediately if you develop fever, chills, nausea, vomiting, and/or a headache.

To prevent Listeria infection, avoid soft cheeses such as feta (goat or sheep cheese), brie, Camembert, blue-veined cheeses, queso blanco, queso fresco, queso dehoja, queso de cnema, and asa dero. Use only pasteurized or hard cheeses, such as cheddar.

Sugar and Salt

If you are diabetic or have high blood pressure, high cholesterol, blood-clotting disorders, or other medical problems, discuss your diet with your physician and, if possible, with a dietician. Go over your salt, sugar, and fluid intake to determine what is appropriate for you. Salt is no longer considered harmful in pregnancy unless you have a medical condition that requires no added salt. Don't make assumptions one way or another: Ask your health care provider.

Raw Meat and Seafood

When you are pregnant, avoid all raw meat, eggs, and fish since they may carry parasites, salmonella, or hepatitis. Postpone that raw oyster appetizer or sushi dinner until after pregnancy.

Exercise

Pregnancy is a very demanding experience. One has to prepare for pregnancy like you prepare for a marathon run.
—Dr. Raul Artal Mittelmark

∗ ∗ ∗

Exercise moderately during pregnancy, but do not overdo it—even if you are very athletic. Listen to your body if it tells you to slow down. Amanda, pregnant at thirty-four and then again at thirty-eight, expected to maintain her activity level during her first pregnancy, but during her second pregnancy, she adopted a less strenuous routine:

"I think I was in a kind of denial about the change that was taking place in my body, and I wanted to stretch out the 'prechild me' as long as possible. I was playing a lot of tennis when I was pregnant with Ben [Amanda's second child] . . . I wanted to hold on to who I was—a tennis player and someone who was active. I started getting very winded. I felt I couldn't perform at the level I was used to. It was a matter of stamina and keeping up the pace. I think I gave it up in my fifth month. With Maia [Amanda's first child], however, I was swimming up to the very end. Swimming was wonderful because I didn't feel the weight on my legs. Just the feeling of being on my belly or back was liberating, since when out of the water, I could only lie on my side."

Once you are pregnant it is best to stick to a toned-down version of your familiar exercise routine. If you are beginning an exercise routine for the first time, try gentle, low-impact sports like swimming, water aerobics, walking, or bicycling. Such moderate exercise will improve your stamina and contribute to your sense of well-being without jeopardizing your muscles and joints, which must bear additional weight during pregnancy.

Your pregnant body is going through—or about to go through—changes. Your ligaments will loosen, your center of gravity will shift as your baby grows and your belly expands, and your heart will bef pumping more blood throughout your body. Furthermore, your body will require more calories in order for you to exercise and to nourish your baby at the same time.

If you already are exercising regularly, you may continue exercising—but with a few modifications:

1. Stop when you're tired.
2. Drink plenty of fluids.
3. Avoid extremes of altitude and temperature (hot saunas included).
4. Tone down your cardiovascular exertion.

Pregnant women should not push their cardiovascular system and should avoid activities that bring their heart rate over 140 beats per minute. When your heart rate increases for sustained periods of time, so does your baby's, and during pregnancy neither you nor your baby should be subjected to excessive physical strain. Sustained athletic activity such as long-distance running may pose problems since you can divert blood and oxygen away from the baby, says Dr. Watson Bowes Jr. "The fetus in the uterus has one quarter of your blood supply. When you exercise, you shift blood away from your viscera [belly] to pump it into your muscles."

Continue your familiar athletic activities such as swimming or bicycling. If you're a very good skier, then skiing is fine—if you are acclimated to the altitude and able to maintain your balance. "But if you are going from sea level to Aspen and you're twelve weeks pregnant, you should not be up on the slopes unless you are acclimated to both the altitude and the sport," says Dr. Bowes. Avoid sports like scuba diving, surfing, skydiving, rock climbing, and hiking on narrow, steep paths. Ask your caregiver about whether or not to continue with horseback riding, downhill skiing, baseball, basketball, or soccer.

It is better to modify your athletic aspirations than to injure yourself because your pregnant body is asked to take on too much of a challenge. Your balance, endurance, and agility simply are not what they were before you were pregnant. Because of the relaxation of your ligaments, you are more vulnerable to injury.

When you exercise, respect the fact that your body is changing, and do not expect your body to behave as though it were not pregnant.

Miriam, a marathon runner and overall athlete, found that during her pregnancy she had enough energy for running at least three miles a day in addition to lifting weights and playing sports but that her back didn't tolerate the strain of such activity. Due to the combination of running, hiking at 5,000 feet, and playing an energetic game of baseball, Miriam injured her back during her last month of pregnancy. Her labor was easy, but she spent her last few weeks in bed with sciatic nerve pain searing through her thigh. Miriam had an easy, quick delivery, which her doctor attributed to her athletic lifestyle. However, she required back surgery within one week of the birth.

Many care providers believe that exercise may prepare a woman for childbirth by increasing the stamina needed for labor, strengthening her muscles, and creating feelings of self-confidence and emotional well-being. However, doctors disagree as to whether or not exercise actually shortens labor. Some believe that women who exercise regularly have shorter labors; others argue that although exercise may not shorten labor or eliminate pain, it increases stamina—and that in itself helps a woman through labor. Exercise may also lessen fear and anxiety about labor, which, in turn, improves pain tolerance.

Exercise Safety

For safe exercise during pregnancy, remember to stretch before and after you exercise, wear shoes that provide adequate support for your feet and ankles (since you are carrying extra weight), monitor your pulse rate, rest if you get out of breath (you should be able to exercise and talk at the same time), avoid strenuous exercise in hot weather or during smog or ozone alerts, and drink liquids to replace the fluid you lose through vigorous exercise. Carry a water bottle or canteen with you so you can drink whenever you need to. Remember that exercise uses calories and that you need to replace these calories for both you and your baby.

Environmental Health

The higher up the food chain, the more environmental toxicants seem to be concentrated. Fish such as tuna, salmon, and trout eat other fish and are at the top of the food chain.

Good evidence that PCBs and dioxins in fish are having effects on humans have yet to be demonstrated. But I would advise pregnant women not to swim or eat the fish at any place that has been posted with a warning about potential pollution.
—John Rogers, Ph.D., reproductive toxicologist

＊ ＊ ＊

I dyed my hair for years. I didn't want to dye my hair and have all those chemicals go through my body.
—Joanne stopped dying her hair during pregnancy to protect her baby from exposure to chemicals

＊ ＊ ＊

Environmental pollution is a reality, not a fad. You are not paranoid if you worry about chemicals in the environment whether they come in the form of beauty products, weed killers, anesthetic gases, or fish. To be concerned about pollution in the environment or toxic chemicals in your workplace or your food is reasonable, and it is useful to identify potential problems and avoid them. When you are pregnant, you especially need to avoid substances known as teratogens, which can cause miscarriage or abnormalities in developing babies. But to avoid toxins—or at least minimize your exposure—you need to know what and where they are.

Pesticides

Pesticides may contain toxins that pose a danger to your pregnancy or your baby, depending on the chemical compounds of which the pesticides are composed. The safest course is to avoid pesticide use at home or in the workplace during the course of your pregnancy. If you suspect that some of your fruits and vegetables have been exposed to pesticides, wash the produce carefully with mild soap and water and rinse thoroughly (some pesticides will not break down if only water is used).

Organic Mercury

Organic mercury—or methyl mercury—can pose dangers to the developing baby in your womb by crossing the placenta and accumulating in embryonic tissues, especially the brain. Mercury is a known teratogen and neurotoxin that may cause neurological problems in children that are not apparent when they are born. To avoid mercury, do not eat freshwater fish from contaminated lakes and streams and limit your intake of ocean fish such as tuna and swordfish.

Endocrine Disrupters

Recent scientific studies have shown that dioxins and some other chemicals that pollute lakes, rivers, and oceans lead to infertility and reproductive abnormalities in just about everything—from alligators in Florida to birds in Michigan. These pollutants enter the food chain, residing in the fat of red meat, fowl, and fish. There is concern that such pollutants may impair sperm and may affect a woman's ability to conceive or to carry a pregnancy to term.

Lead

Lead may increase your chance of miscarriage. You can be exposed to lead from drinking water from lead pipes or ingesting lead-based paint or dye (a common source of exposure in small children). You may also be exposed to lead via leaded gasoline or storage batteries; if you cannot avoid contact altogether, wash your hands with soap immediately after contact with paint or batteries.

Polybrominated Biphenyls (PBBs)

These are found in industrial work settings in such forms as fire retardants. You may need to wear protective clothing or avoid contact altogether.

Polychlorinated Biphenyls (PCBs)

These are very toxic substances that can cause miscarriage or fetal growth retardation. PCBs are found in contaminated water and fish. If you swim in PCB-contaminated lakes, you can absorb the chemical through your skin.

Radiation

Radiation is also teratogenic, as was demonstrated in the birth abnormalities in babies exposed to the atomic bomb.

Household Cleansers and Polishing Agents

These chemicals may pose a risk to your baby. Switch to less toxic compounds from the local health food store or use gloves. Avoid exposure to your skin, and avoid inhaling fumes.

Solvents

Solvents can be found in industrial settings, paints, and some work environments and include such chemicals as benzene and turpentine. Avoid contact with skin and avoid inhaling fumes.

Electromagnetic Fields

The controversy regarding potential electronic source environmental hazards such as video display terminals (VDTs) and electromagnetic fields (EMFs) has not yet been resolved. Some doctors believe that study results have shown that VDTs are not a source of danger and do not increase risks to the baby. Others believe that women should sit as far away as possible from the back of other peoples' computers, since it is at that end of the machine where potential danger may lie.

Some health experts think that EMFs do not pose a hazard to babies and adults; others disagree. (See Chapter 10 for more information on toxins in your work environment. See appendix for more information.)

For more information on environmental toxins, contact:

- Motherisk *(www.motherisk.org)*
- OTIS *(www.otispregnancy.org)*
- The National Institute of Occupational Safety and Health *(www.edc.gov/niosh)*

Chapter 10

Pregnant at Work

Many women continue working throughout most, if not all, of their pregnancy. How much you work during your pregnancy will be determined by your individual circumstances, your health, and the nature of your work. If you work during pregnancy, you should definitely avoid heavy lifting, exposure to dangerous chemicals, extremes of temperature or pressure, and exposure to infectious diseases.

This chapter will focus on strategies you can use in the workplace to make your job safer and more comfortable during your pregnancy. To ensure the safety of your baby, you may need to modify your activity level or job duties while you are pregnant.

Strategies for the Workplace

I was terribly tired. I would have to pull off the road for fifteen minutes to rest. I would have to take breaks in the office and literally sleep on the floor. I'd lie on the floor and meditate for twenty minutes.
—Holly

Many women work full-time during pregnancy until the day or hour that they go into labor. Some women stop working during their last trimester. Others work part-time. Whatever you decide, keep in mind that you are pregnant. You may be a lawyer, a teacher, or an editor—but you are a pregnant one. Fortunately, most of the time you will not have to choose between career and pregnancy. You may, however, have to adjust the way you do your career. Although working while pregnant is manageable, you will need to take care of yourself in some of the following ways.

Respect Your Fatigue

If the first trimester of pregnancy leaves you feeling tired and in need of a nap, accommodate your body's need to rest. It is doing a lot of work making a placenta and a baby, and rearranging its blood volume, hormones, and chemistry. Close your office door, unroll your sleeping bag or foam pad, and lie down behind the desk or on top of the desk. If you don't have an office, try the teacher's lounge, the restroom, someone else's office, or a nice piece of grass. Amanda slept on picnic benches outside her office building and on a towel spread out on her office floor.

"I was starting to get really wiped. It was either go home and fall on a bed or rest at work. I put a DO NOT DISTURB sign on my office door and closed the door. I put a towel on the floor (the carpet was new, and I didn't want to inhale the fumes from it). I brought my phone down on the floor. I would lie down—sometimes for more than an hour. On a nice day I'd lie down and sleep on a picnic bench outside. It got me over a critical period.

If you don't have the luxury of a nap, meditate or simply slow down and take a relaxing break. If you are unable to rest at work, nap en route on the commuter train.

Tend to Your Morning Sickness

Avoid an empty stomach—it can increase nausea. Bring five to six small meals and eat every one to two hours. Concoct your own morning sickness prevention and treatment kit. Bring crackers, toast, decaffeinated tea, ginger tea, or whatever else works to diminish your feelings of nausea. Try snacks of whole grain cereals, nuts, seeds, toast, bagels, and other bland, comforting foods. Avoid spicy, greasy, and junk foods.

Eat Well and Stay Hydrated

Drink enough water—about eight glasses a day—even if this means many trips to the bathroom. Avoid the coffee and candy machines and frequent fast-food lunches. Eat well-balanced meals necessary for making a healthy baby and for giving you the mental and physical energy to do your job well. Adequate calories, protein, fresh fruits and vegetables, and calcium-rich foods are a must.

Bring Your Humor to Work

You can sometimes dispel tension, handle others' discomfort with your pregnancy, or gain control of potentially awkward situations with humor.

Your Self Image

My first executive committee meeting was the day I went into labor. It was imperative I be at that meeting. It was a four-hour meeting; by the end you could see my fingernail marks on the table. I couldn't stand. I was seven centimeters dilated and in transition. Dick almost had to carry me. You can do anything if you have to.
—Holly

I had a preterm delivery. I was trying to be super-doc.
—Dr. Susan Porto

* * *

If you work in a traditionally male-dominated field like law or medicine or if you are a paramedic or carpenter, you may feel compelled to show your male counterparts that you can do the job well—even if you are pregnant. You want to get the message across that you can do anything they can do. There is nothing wrong with rising to the occasion and doing your job well—unless it compromises you, your pregnancy, or your baby.

When you are pregnant, you can still do your job well—but *differently*. You may assume that modifying your job is not an option, or you may think that "giving in" to pregnancy is "weak." Unfortunately, such assumptions are frequently reinforced by employers who see pregnancy as an illness. However, a growing number of employers are developing more flexible attitudes due, in part, to women who have had the resourcefulness and strength to adapt their professional lives to the needs of their pregnancy. As a result, these women are better able to enjoy and protect their pregnancies.

Holly felt like she had to prove herself to the men in her new office. They'd hired her, amidst some controversy, when she was eight months pregnant, and she felt she had to show them that she was one of the boys. "They don't think I can do this job. I need to show them I can," Holly told herself as she decided to attend an executive meeting—even though she was going into labor. Her husband drove her to work, and Holly, in active labor, sat through a four-hour meeting. By the time the meeting was over, Holly was in transition.

Holly accomplished what she set out to do at work, but at the price of her labor plan: a quiet walk in the woods with her husband. By the time she arrived at the hospital, she felt stressed and deprived of an important part of her birth experience.

Sarah came back to work "to get a few things done" the week after her cesarean section (a surgery with a four- to six-week recovery period). Looking back, she thinks she was "a little macho." Cindy, a paramedic, continued lifting heavy gurneys long after her pregnancy pooched out the front of her baggy blue fire department jumpsuit. She did the job much to the amazement—and fear—of her male counterparts. Meg, an obstetrician, was doing surgeries two weeks after her cesarean section. Not surprisingly, she had a difficult recovery.

Of course, there is something rewarding in pushing yourself to the limit and accomplishing difficult tasks. The questions are: How hard do you want to push yourself, and at what cost in terms of health risks to you and your baby and your enjoyment of pregnancy, birth, and your first weeks of motherhood?

Normalizing Pregnancy: Rising above Bias

Sometimes the best strategy at work is to teach your coworkers to see your pregnancy as normal by showing them that you are neither ill nor incapacitated: You are simply pregnant in addition to everything else that you are.

How you choose to normalize your pregnancy and reeducate those in your workplace will depend on your circumstances and your personality. Humor may work for you, or it may not. Your best strategy may be "your example." To be direct and open about your pregnancy, as Holly was, may project a stronger, more assured image than hiding it or pretending it doesn't exist. Holly, a lawyer on her way up the career ladder, started a new job when she was eight months pregnant. She told the members of the law firm: "I am very pregnant, and I don't think it has affected my brain yet."

However, there are certain aspects of pregnancy that you may wish to play down, if possible, since male colleagues may not relate to morning sickness, obstetricians, and ultrasound scans.

Work settings that are traditionally male—law firms, fire departments, construction sites, taxi companies—may challenge your imagination and patience (and possibly your fortitude), but some of those who hold prejudices about age or gender might be teachable and may be more receptive to your example than to your words. Then again, they may not, in which case your challenge will be to detach and to "rise above" their biases.

Potential Hazards at Work

Hazards in the workplace may range from toxic chemicals to stress. Avoiding these hazards may be tricky, especially if they are part of your daily routine. If you have questions about the safety of your workplace, contact the U.S. Labor Occupational Safety and Health Administration (OSHA) at (202) 693-1999 or *www.osha.gov*; or contact Motherisk at *www.motherisk.org*.

Any of the activities that follow may pose potential risks to you, your pregnancy, and/or your baby.

Working with Chemicals

Some chemicals may cause miscarriage, birth defects, and preterm birth. If you work with mercury, avoid it at all costs during your pregnancy since mercury is a known teratogen that may cause abnormalities in the baby. Lead, organic solvents, PCBs, and PBBs should all be avoided. Prenatal exposure to herbicides and pesticides should also be extremely limited, since some of the chemicals may cause miscarriage, preterm birth, or birth defects. If you don't know what chemicals are potentially dangerous in your workplace, call the Teratology Information

Service at (888) 285-3410, the EPA, or OSHA.

Sometimes protective clothing and gloves will offer you sufficient protection, but always wash contaminated clothing separately from the daily clothing and linens used by you and your family. Asbestos should be avoided, and any clothing contaminated with asbestos should not be brought into your home or your washing machine.

Physical Strain

Pregnant women should avoid lifting heavy people or objects. If you are a nurse, arrange for some backup for lifting heavy patients. If you are a paramedic and accustomed to daily heavy lifting, consult with your doctor or midwife about how to manage your job and your pregnancy. You may need to modify your work tasks or to take an early pregnancy leave. Lifting heavy packages or equipment, standing for long hours on an assembly line or in a classroom, and working under very hot or cold conditions may pose risks to you and your baby. Consult your health care provider about how to make your job safe for you and your baby.

Contagious Diseases

During the course of your pregnancy, avoid direct contact with contagious diseases such as measles, mumps, chicken pox, hepatitis, HIV/AIDS, CMV (cytomegalovirus), and tuberculosis. Pregnancy is not a good time to volunteer in day care centers or pediatric clinics, since young children are frequently a source of contagious diseases that may harm your unborn baby. If you work in a hospital or clinic, talk to your supervisor and your doctor about ways to protect yourself and your baby from disease. In some cases, wearing a mask, gown, and gloves will give you adequate protection. In some cases it won't; you may need to temporarily work on a ward or in a clinic where contagion is less of a problem. Health care staff exposed to blood products should either transfer to a different position during pregnancy or take special precautions to avoid direct contact with sources of contagion.

Wash your hands and face frequently to protect yourself from common diseases such as colds, flu, and streptococcal infections, especially if you have contact with a sick coworker.

Hazards at Work

Pregnant women should avoid:

- Heavy lifting
- Insecure footing (at construction sites)
- Standing for extended periods
- Vibrating machinery
- Extremes of heat or cold
- Long hours driving a car or truck
- Exposure to contagious diseases
- Exposure to toxic chemicals—photographic chemicals, cleaning fluids, laboratory chemicals, and radioactive materials
- Exposure to frequent, excessive stress
- Physical activities such as pulling, pushing, or balancing
- Exposure to anesthesia

Work-Related Stress

Women who stand on their feet all day—whether they are stewardesses or mill workers—are put at higher risk for premature labor and preeclampsia and for poor pregnancy outcomes.

Women in high-stress jobs are at increased risk during pregnancy. It is critical that they think about modifying their work environment or taking time off. A nurse with ten- to twelve-hour

shifts on an intensive care unit is working in a high-stress environment, and it may be hard to modify that environment.
—Dr. Watson Bowes Jr.

✳ ✳ ✳

One of the most important things for pregnancy—and this is being well documented—is stress. Stress kills. Different kinds of stressors are deleterious to pregnancy. Peace of mind is healthy.
—John Rogers, Ph.D., reproductive toxicologist

✳ ✳ ✳

Whether or not reducing your stress levels will actually help you conceive, reducing stress will enhance your emotional and physiological experience of pregnancy and birth. Stress produces epinephrine, a hormone that is part of the "fight or flight" response that shunts blood away from your uterus and into your heart and limbs—your uterus is low on the body's priority list when it senses danger. If your body goes into a fight-or-flight reaction during a particularly stressful encounter at work, the blood flow to your uterus (and your baby) will be diverted to the parts of your body necessary for running or fighting. If this occurs on a chronic basis, your baby could be deprived of oxygen and nutrients.

Exposure to chronic stress may also contribute to premature labor and birth. A study of pregnant women who were doing their medical residencies (a stressful training period after medical school) showed a tendency toward preterm delivery.

Locating sources of potential stress at work, at home, or within your psyche, may help you better prevent or manage future stress. If you are not able to modify stressors such as physically dangerous or exhausting work, you may need to take a leave of absence from work, job share, or work part-time until after the baby is born.

Most of the time some simple lifestyle changes may help minimize stress. Make relaxing activities a habit instead of a rare event—walk in the woods, listen to music, get a massage, take a long weekend, meditate, swim, take a yoga-for-pregnancy class.

Business Travel

The good news is that you can safely travel by airplane, car, and train during most of a healthy pregnancy. The second trimester may be the best time to travel, since you are usually over the morning sickness of your first trimester, and you do not yet have the physical discomfort and the anxiety about delivery dates that comes with your eighth or ninth month of pregnancy.

During your last trimester of pregnancy, always consult your care provider before traveling. Avoid travel in your last month of pregnancy (you never know when labor will begin) or if you are experiencing any pregnancy-related problems such as bleeding, cramping, severe headaches, dizziness, or back pain.

For a long trip, avoid sitting or standing for more than two hours at a time. If you are sitting on a train or plane, get up and walk around every hour or two to stimulate circulation and to prevent the blood from pooling in your legs; this exercise prevents edema and blood clots. When you are seated, try putting your legs up or making circles with your feet. Aisle seats may be more comfortable and convenient than other seats, especially if you need to get up frequently to go to the bathroom. Since airplane air is very dry, you will need to drink a lot of fluid on a plane, although you should make sure to stay hydrated whatever your mode of transportation. If you are driving, take frequent breaks to get out and walk. Stop at least every two hours for ten minutes. Fasten the seatbelt under your abdomen—not on top of it or above it. Avoid long trips, especially toward the end of pregnancy; they are exhausting and hard on your back and your circulation.

If your back is bothering you, take a small pillow to prop behind it. Carry a copy of your medical records just in case you need to see a doctor during your trip. If you are traveling during your first trimester or if you have been prone to heartburn during your pregnancy, bring crackers, cereals, and bland snacks to have on hand throughout your trip.

Avoid traveling to places where you will not have immediate access to good medical care, where sanitation is poor, where you will be subjected to extreme changes of altitude, or where contagious diseases are prevalent.

Posture and Body Mechanics at Work

Many pregnant women experience backaches and muscle strains during pregnancy. Your body is changing in ways that affect your posture and your center of gravity. As your body tries to adjust to the weight and size of your pregnant abdomen, you may experience back pain or difficulty sitting or standing for long periods of time.

To prevent or relieve backaches, use an ergonomically correct chair that lends adequate support to your back and hips. If you sit at a desk, place the telephone and other necessary objects near you, since reaching across a table for something you need may strain your back. If you stand while working, put a small footstool under one foot and alternate at least every hour, shifting your weight from one foot to another.

Exercises that gently strengthen the back and stomach muscles—even isometric exercises that you can do while sitting—may help prevent or minimize back pain. If back pain becomes a problem, consult a physical therapist and physician who have experience working with pregnant women.

Part Five

Preventing and Managing Potential Problems

Chapter 11
Who Is High Risk?

At thirty-five, women are not high risk. Their pregnancies can be managed by a general obstetrician [rather than a doctor specializing in high-risk pregnancy].
—Dr. Katherine Shaw, perinatologist, White Memorial Hospital, Los Angeles

• • •

The older moms are more likely to have large or small for gestational age babies, hypertension, preeclampsia, and a higher incidence of c-section and gestational diabetes. But those are manageable problems. At the end, you'll end up with a healthy baby and mom.
—Dr. Susan Porto, obstetrician, Mercy Hospital, Chicago

• • •

Ten percent of pregnant patients will have a complicated pregnancy.
—Dr. Watson Bowes Jr.

• • •

If you are thirty-five years old or older, in good health, and you do not have preexisting diabetes, heart disease, high blood pressure, or other potentially serious medical conditions, health risks to you during pregnancy are not great enough to put you in a high-risk category—at least not by the standards of many caregivers practicing today. Women at highest risk for complications of pregnancy and birth and whose babies are also at risk are those women who, regardless of age, have preexisting illnesses. "There is a low-risk forty-year-old and a high-risk one. A low-risk forty-year-old has no pre-existing medical conditions," says Dr. Watson Bowes Jr.

These days, a woman is said to have a high-risk pregnancy if she has pre-existing conditions such as high blood pressure, diabetes, or heart disease. Her pregnancy may also be considered high risk if she develops certain conditions during pregnancy, such as pregnancy-induced high blood pressure (preeclampsia) or pregnancy-induced diabetes (GD). In this chapter, women and their doctors will talk about a variety of possible pregnancy complications and how the majority of these problems can be successfully managed.

I wanted to write a chapter on pregnancy risks that educated women without frightening them and told them the good news: that most midlife pregnancies have healthy outcomes, even if they are labeled high risk. "The bottom line is a healthy mother and baby," says Dr. Donna Kirz when she talks about risks for older mothers. "The medical literature is reassuring. Outcomes aren't much different for older women." You will find this optimistic perspective on midlife pregnancy—and some of the risks commonly associated with older mothers—voiced by many of the physicians I interviewed for this chapter, many of whom are prominent perinatologists and obstetricians.

High Risk: A Brief Historical Perspective

When I was born, in 1933, the maternal mortality rate was 1 in

200. Now it is less than 1 in 10,000. Compared with their grandmothers or parents, it is safer for a woman to have a baby at age 45 today than it was at age 20 forty years ago.
—Dr. Allen Killam

* * *

When Dr. Donna Kirz was training to become an obstetrician in the late 1970s, doctors commonly categorized a woman over age thirty-five and pregnant with her first baby as an "elderly primigravida." Some doctors didn't view a woman as "elderly" until she was forty, but whether doctors found a woman old at thirty or forty, they invariably viewed her as high risk.

However, in the 1980s and 1990s, women's lives were moving beyond these medical definitions. During the 1980s, when Dr. Kirz was first practicing obstetrics, the total number of births to American women over age thirty-five—the baby boomers—was increasing dramatically. Midlife pregnancy was becoming, at least from a social point of view, normal.

Dr. Kirz was both an obstetrician and a baby boomer, and the phenomenon of midlife pregnancy and age-related risks interested her. She decided to study midlife pregnancy and discover whether or not women over thirty-five years old were, in fact, at "higher risk" than women who were twenty to twenty-five years old. As she delved into the subject, Kirz found that medical researchers had previously defined risk imprecisely: Doctors in the eighteenth century defined it as risks to the mother, whereas doctors in the late twentieth century defined it as risks to the baby.

Kirz's three-year study, published May 1, 1985, in *The American Journal of Obstetrics and Gynecology,* found that older pregnant women were not at significantly higher risk than younger women were. Kirz concluded that:

"The obstetric literature is not only imprecise in its

definition [of risk], it is also somewhat pejorative in its attitude toward women bearing children in their 30s and 40s." She went on to point out the unflattering language used in earlier medical studies to describe women over thirty-five:

"The older pregnant woman has been variously referred to as post mature, obstetrically senescent, premenopausal, geriatric, gray, elderly, dangerous, and participating in childbearing in the twilight of the reproductive period."

Such pejorative terminology—and the attitude behind it—wrote Kirz, was "obsolete and, in fact, offensive." So she changed it: "A better choice of terms would be 'mature primigravida.' Mature is defined as 'having completed natural growth and development, having attained a final or desired state, condition of full development,'" wrote Kirz.

It has become increasingly common for women to get pregnant when they are "mature"—between the ages of thirty-five and fifty. Birth rates for women in their thirties have increased steadily since the mid- to late 1970s, according to the final national birth statistics for 1999 (these statistics were published in their final form in April of 2001). In the United States, between 1981 and 1999, the rate of births for women aged forty to forty-four increased by 95 percent. Record numbers of women aged forty-five through fifty-four were having babies. Because more women of the baby boomer generation were making babies in midlife, obstetricians were gaining more experience with women pregnant over age thirty-five.

As increasing numbers of these women had successful pregnancies and healthy babies, they provided their doctors with sufficient experience with "mature" pregnancy to erase some of the previous medical bias.

Medical studies supported the growing optimism about pregnancy and birth over age thirty-five. Older women had "good pregnancy outcomes" (which means healthy moms and healthy babies), although the studies showed that women over thirty-five had more complications of pregnancy and childbirth. A study by Dr. Gertrude Berkowitz et al. that was published in the March 8, 1990, issue of *The New England Journal of Medicine* compared birth outcomes in women over thirty-five years of age with those of women twenty to twenty-nine and thirty to thirty-four years of age and found that "advancing maternal age at first birth does not appreciably increase the risk of an adverse pregnancy outcome" (in women pregnant with only one baby) and that there were no significant problems for women aged thirty to thirty-four or thirty-five and over.

However, older mothers were more likely than the younger mothers to have more complications of pregnancy, more cesarean deliveries, and more babies admitted to the newborn intensive care nurseries.

Despite the possible complications, the message from the Berkowitz et al. article is an optimistic one: Even if you develop medical conditions such as pregnancy-induced diabetes and high blood pressure that you wouldn't have developed at age thirty, and even if you are two times more likely to have a cesarean section than a younger woman, you have excellent odds for a healthy pregnancy outcome.

The Berkowitz study sparked enthusiasm on the part of nationally known obstetricians such as Dr. Robert Resnick, who wrote in a 1990 letter to *The New England Journal of Medicine*:

The message is clear and highly optimistic. What should be emphasized is the fact that the few pregnancy-related problems in primiparous women who are 35 or older are readily manageable in 1990. Given sound genetic diagnosis, together with appropriate prenatal care and the judicious management of labor and delivery, the increasing number of women postponing first pregnancy can look forward to excellent outcomes. The

"Elderly Primigravida." The New England Journal of Medicine 1990; 322: 693–4.

Other studies supported the good news, although they also confirmed the increased rate of complications in older mothers. In 1991, a Washington State study by Gordon et al. compared pregnancy outcomes for women twenty to twenty-nine years of age with those thirty-five to fifty years of age and found an increased rate of diabetes and cesarean section in the older mothers. In 1996, a University of Utah study found "in women over 45 years old at delivery, maternal and fetal outcomes were generally good" but there was an increased incidence of chronic diabetes and hypertension as well as genetic abnormalities and GD.

On the whole, the news was good—late-in-life pregnancies were producing happy endings for women over age thirty-five and, much to the surprise of both doctors and women, to women over forty-five. "When it came to 'advanced maternal age,' doctors started seeing success. Now we have a body of experience," says Dr. Kirz.

While some physicians continue to see midlife pregnancy as high risk based on maternal age alone, others see risk not so much as a function of age but as a function of waning fertility. A high-risk pregnancy is often seen as a "high cost" pregnancy achieved at a high emotional, physical, and/or financial price. Such pregnancies are often called "premium" or "precious" pregnancies since they may represent a woman's last chance to have a baby. Although the precious pregnancy concept is grounded in good intentions, it is an attitude that can raise anxiety levels of both doctor and patient and subsequently lead to increased concern about fetal distress, to decreased patience with long labors, and to cesarean sections performed to alleviate anxiety.

Cesarean section rates are significantly higher in women over thirty-five than in women under thirty. In 1999, cesarean rates were 34.7 percent for women aged forty to fifty-four, 29.9 percent for women aged thirty-five to thirty-nine, and 21.8 percent for women aged twenty-five through twenty-nine. Although women over thirty-five tend to have more indications for cesarean birth, such as breech babies, diabetes, big babies, and other age-related problems (see Part 8), whether or not older women have a rate of birth complications high enough to justify their cesarean rate is the subject of medical debate. Some care providers believe that labors in older women tend to be dysfunctional and thus result in cesarean delivery of the baby. However, Dr. Kirz and other medical experts believe that the increased anxiety of both older patients and their doctors, as much as age-related complications of pregnancy and birth, lead to high cesarean section rates in women over thirty-five.

Kirz found that in her 1985 Long Beach study of over 1,000 pregnant women thirty-five or older, the rate of cesarean section was greater than the rate of indications for the surgery. Kirz suggested that the high rate was due to a "self-fulfilling prophecy" based on the physicians' attitude toward age:

The overwhelming majority of studies in the obstetric literature describe a significantly higher rate of cesarean births in older women. In this present study there was also an increased utilization of cesarean births for the older age group. It is unclear why this is so. No one specific indication for cesarean birth showed an increase in the pregnancies of women over 34 years. It may be that the increase in cesarean births for the older women is a self-fulfilling prophecy. Because the pregnancies have been considered to be at high-risk, the physicians may use a lower threshold for terminating pregnancy or the labor process [with a c-section].

According to Dr. Mark Sauer, for women who give birth over age fifty, cesarean rates are about 75 percent—more than three times the national average. Sauer also believes that physician/patient anxiety contributes to these high cesarean rates. "Many doctors are nervous and will section them [older women] at the drop of a hat. The diagnosis of dysfunctional labor may not be real," says Sauer. However, the true causes of high cesarean-section rates in older women are difficult to determine, Sauer explains. It is hard to estimate how many older women need cesarean sections due to increased birth complications, and how many women have cesareans due to anxiety about "premium pregnancies."

Possible Complications of Midlife Pregnancy

The term "high risk" can mean several different kinds of risk. It can mean genetic risks to the *baby,* such as the risk for Down's syndrome, which are among the first risks that many women over thirty-five consider when deciding whether or not to have a baby.

High risk can also mean *maternal risks* created by health problems that a woman develops as she gets older or health problems that are created by pregnancy itself. National health statistics show that forty- to forty-nine-year old women are twice as likely to have preexisting heart disease and four times more likely to have diabetes than twenty- to twenty-four-year-olds.

If you have diabetes or high blood pressure before you get pregnant, these preexisting conditions require that you and your baby be more carefully monitored for potential problems than if you did not have these conditions. Even if you are in excellent health before pregnancy, the state of pregnancy may create temporary health problems such as *gestational diabetes* (pregnancy-induced diabetes), preeclampsia (pregnancy-induced high blood pressure), back problems, or, in rare cases, eclampsia (a serious form of preeclampsia).

Under some circumstances, the mother's health problem may create problems for the baby as well. Maternal diabetes may result in *fetal macrosomia* (a very big baby), miscarriage, or other problems (see "Diabetes Mellitus Types I and II," this chapter), and maternal hypertension may result in small babies, preterm delivery, or placental abruption (see "Placental Abruption," this chapter). In the case of both diabetes and high blood pressure, delivery of the baby is often a "cure" for both mother and baby.

Fortunately, most of these potential complications of pregnancy can be safely managed with medications, diet, and/or rest, and most women who develop these conditions will go on to have healthy babies.

However, if you do have heart, kidney, or lung problems; cancer; an autoimmune disease; epilepsy; or any other serious or chronic medical condition, it is important to discuss your individual risks with your doctor before you get pregnant.

Genetic Risks

Around age fifty, the chances are one in ten of aneuploidy or Down's. Another way to look at it is: you have a 90 percent chance of having a normal baby.
—Dr. Murph Goodwin, perinatologist and Professor of Obstetrics at the University of Southern California

• • •

If you are over thirty-five, you can't help thinking about genetic risks since you will face having to make decisions about whether or not to get tests for genetic disorders during your pregnancy. The odds for genetic disorders increase dramatically between age thirty and age forty; consequently many women and their partners find themselves confronted with confusing lists of numbers that represent, in an impersonal and often frightening way, the odds of their baby being genetically damaged.

You may hear that at twenty-five your risks are "low," and at thirty-five they are "higher" or "high." But what do "low risk," "high risk," and "higher risk" mean in terms of your real-life situation? For some people, any risk for an abnormal baby is frightening and unacceptable; for them, only *no risk* is "low risk."

How you perceive risk also depends on how you read the odds and interpret the numbers. If you are thirty-five, for instance, your odds for having a Down's baby are less than 1 percent, which is higher than they were when you were thirty. In fact, the odds are very good that your baby will not have Down's—despite popular misconceptions that at midlife you run a high risk of Down's and related genetic problems. More specifically, your odds of having a child with Down's syndrome are 1 in 365 at age thirty-five; 1 in 32 at age forty-five; and 1 in 10 at age fifty. To hear that your risk increases exponentially or that you have a 1 in 10 chance of having a Down's baby may be distressing. But these numbers mean that even at age fifty, you have a 90 percent chance of having a non-Down's baby—the odds are 90 percent in your favor!

According to genetic counselor Michelle Trant, Down's is only one of several possible chromosomal problems that become more common with advancing maternal age. At age thirty-five, you have a 1 in 134 risk of having a baby with one of these chromosomal problems—but that is less than a 1 percent risk. "Your chances of having a healthy, normal baby are 99 percent," says Trant, a counselor with Perinatal Alliance Medical Group in Los Angeles. At age forty, your risks more than triple, leaving you with a 1 in 39 risk of a genetically unhealthy baby. However, there is still a 97 percent chance that your baby will not have a chromosomal abnormality. Although your risks of chromosome problems are considerably "higher" when you are forty than when you are thirty-five, they are not necessarily "high" from an absolute point of view.

Gestational Diabetes (GD)

Women get gestational diabetes. It's detectable and treatable and not an out-of-this-world problem.
—Dr. Donna Kirz

* * *

The incidence of gestational diabetes goes up considerably with age. At thirty-five, you might be at higher risk. But gestational diabetes can often be managed by diet alone.
—Dr. Allen Killam

* * *

Doctors estimate that 2 to 3 percent of pregnancies are complicated by diabetes mellitus; 90 percent of these cases represent women with GD. GD, otherwise known as pregnancy-induced diabetes, is not the same disease as chronic diabetes. Most physicians agree that GD is a *condition*—not an actual disease—that is generated by the metabolic changes of pregnancy and usually disappears after the baby is born.

GD is relatively common in pregnant women during the last trimester of pregnancy. Because GD is usually a condition of late pregnancy, the babies of women with GD are not exposed to extreme fluctuations of blood sugar or other chronic, diabetes-related problems during early pregnancy—

that vulnerable period when the baby's organs are forming. Consequently, the babies of mothers with GD are not at high risk for congenital abnormalities.

Unlike insulin-dependent diabetes, GD is not caused by an abnormally low production of insulin. Instead, GD is caused by changes in your metabolism of glucose (sugar) that normally occur during pregnancy and that promote the growth of your baby. If you develop GD, you still produce insulin, but the action of that insulin is suppressed by a pregnancy hormone, human placental lactogen (HPL), in order to free up sugar to feed your growing baby. In some pregnant women, the HPL suppresses insulin to a point where blood sugar remains abnormally high, and the woman is found to have "glucose intolerance"—in other words, GD. The elevated amounts of sugar in the blood of a pregnant woman with GD can "overfeed" her baby and produce a large baby that may (or may not) have trouble slipping through the birth canal. This large baby syndrome, known as fetal macrosomia, can cause problems for both a woman and her baby. Consequently, some doctors fear that leaving GD untreated could result in large babies, difficult births, and subsequent birth injuries to the baby.

What is reassuring is that many doctors say that even severe GD may be effectively managed. Careful monitoring of you and the baby and timely delivery of the baby minimize potential risks of macrosomia.

Also reassuring—at least in terms of women with pregnancy-induced diabetes—is that some studies indicate that the size of the baby is more closely linked to its mother's weight than to whether or not she has GD. Studies have shown that women who are obese or who have a combination of risk factors such as obesity and advanced maternal age are more likely to have a big baby, resulting in possible shoulder dystocia (which makes the baby's descent through the birth canal difficult or impossible), birth injury for the baby, or cesarean section for the mother.

Other factors such as age, race, and the number of babies you have had in the past may be more important factors than GD in determining your baby's weight. Thus, attaining a reasonable weight before you become pregnant and not gaining excessive weight during pregnancy may be important factors in preventing fetal macrosomia and the associated birth risks.

Developing GD does not pose any immediate risks to you, since the condition is usually temporary and thus does not result in the circulatory or kidney problems found in women who have chronic diabetes. However, some medical studies indicate that women who develop GD may have an increased risk of developing diabetes later in life. According to the American Diabetes Association, women with GD have an increased risk of developing Type II diabetes later in life, but women can reduce their risk of developing this disease by maintaining a healthy body weight and getting regular exercise.

Managing GD

Everything changed when I got GD—or when my midwife and doctor got concerned about GD. That resulted in a big change in my diet. I met with a nutritionist. I had some misconceptions about what kinds of foods I could eat. I thought things like fresh fruits and vegetables were fine: but things like carrots have sugars in them. I had to think about every morsel of food that went into my mouth. Is this a protein? Is this a high-sugar carbohydrate? This happened in the last part of my pregnancy. I thought, "If this is going to make some difference to my health or my child's health, I can tolerate this diet for a month and a half."
—Amanda, age thirty-six, gave birth to a healthy baby boy via a normal vaginal delivery.

* * *

"Oh, no—not chocolate!" was Anna's first response to her diabetic diet. She also had to dramatically change other parts of her daily food intake, which meant changing her lifestyle. "I knew I was really going to have to make a radical change in my eating habits, and in Los Angeles eating is a big thing." Anna remained disciplined about her new diet. While on vacation with her husband in Maui, Anna drank seltzer as Michael sipped a festive piña colada. Fortunately, Anna had to change her food routine for only two months, and her payoff for the change was worth it when she gave birth to a seven pound, four ounce baby girl.

For some women, the dietary treatment for GD puts them under additional stress. Anna, already on edge because she was considered high risk at age thirty-nine, felt even more at risk. The word "diabetes" made her feel frightened and potentially ill, since she feared developing true diabetes. "I was really devastated when I found out I had gestational diabetes. I was scared. My father had adult onset diabetes. What would happen to me? Would I remain diabetic?" Anna felt angry at her body for sabotaging her with GD, but she felt much better about her condition after seeing a nutritionist. "I was able to make things change by finding a nutritionist, changing my diet, and having it lower my blood sugar. I'm very thankful for that intervention. I think it changed my pregnancy. It was very helpful. I changed my diet and eating habits completely. I learned what I could do to help the situation." Anna's blood sugar levels returned to normal after the birth of her daughter.

Unfortunately, many women panic after being diagnosed with GD because they think they have a "bad disease" that will endanger their baby. This panic can interfere with their enjoyment of pregnancy and the happy anticipation of their baby's birth.

If you are diagnosed with GD, don't panic. Your body is

simply reacting to pregnancy. The good news is that your condition usually can be managed effectively with diet, both the diet and the diabetes are temporary, and serious problems for you and your baby are rare. The bad news is that temporarily you may have to give up pineapple, chocolate, and an array of other high-sugar foods.

The GD diet often consists of six small meals daily or three meals and two or three snacks designed to give you a good balance of proteins and carbohydrates. Check with your caregiver and nutritionist regarding the amount of food that is best for you, and the amounts of protein and carbohydrates you need. The diet will vary, depending on the severity of your GD and the number of babies you are carrying. For instance, you need more protein and calcium if you are carrying twins or triplets than if you are carrying one baby.

The timing and content of the six small meals is designed to keep your blood sugar relatively even throughout the day. The meals usually consist of protein, fiber, and complex carbohydrates—whole grains, rice, beans, potatoes, and fresh vegetables. The virtue of complex carbohydrates is that they are broken down slowly by your body and can thus provide you with energy that lasts for hours.

Although fresh fruit and fruit juices are good for you nutritionally, you may need to limit fruit in your diet since it contains fructose—a form of sugar. Fruit juice contains more concentrated sugar than a piece of fruit, so you may be allotted a whole piece of fruit but only half a glass of juice.

Although the diet is relatively rigid, there is room for imagination. Whole grain breads need not be boring since you can find a wide variety at your local bakery or health food store. Just make sure the bread is low in sugar. Similarly, lentils and peas can be flavored with spices and sauces. If spices don't work for you due to pregnancy-related indigestion, try flavoring dishes with low-sugar vegetables, fish, meat, hard cheese, a few drops of lemon or lime juice, or herbs like rosemary, thyme, or basil.

Oriental foods may serve as a useful model, since the Chinese, Korean, and Japanese diets feature rice (a complex carbohydrate) with stir-fried or boiled vegetables, fish, or meat. If you prefer pasta to rice, select whole grain pastas or rice noodles when you can, and check with your nutritionist or physician to see how much pasta (a carbohydrate) is acceptable for you. Avoid processed foods since they tend to be higher in simple carbohydrates and sugar. Read food labels carefully to see if the food contains added sugar.

The goals of a diabetic diet are to eat a source of protein (fish, chicken, turkey, eggs, beef, tofu, beans, peas, milk, yogurt, cheese, cottage cheese) and a source of complex carbohydrates (vegetables, whole grains, rice, rice cakes, whole wheat crackers, shredded wheat, bran flakes), and to drink adequate fluid (seltzer, herbal teas, water). If you find yourself craving sweets, humor yourself with one or two pieces of fruit a day (consult your nutritionist or doctor first) and wait until after the birth to indulge your sweet tooth. Amanda waited until after the birth of her son and then asked for "the sweetest drink in the whole hospital." The nurses brought her a large 7-Up.

Check with your care provider and nutritionist before undertaking any diet, since you need to base your diet on your specific health needs and food preferences.

Questions about Screening and Treatment

Since the mid-1980s, glucose tolerance blood tests have been used to routinely screen pregnant women for GD. Many American care providers recommend routine GD screening between the twenty-fourth and twenty-eighth weeks of pregnancy. The first screening test includes drinking a fifty-gram glucose drink—or eating a special carbohydrate meal—and then having your blood tested for "glucose tolerance or intolerance." If your blood results show 140mg/dl or above, you are considered at possible risk for GD and are given another, more sensitive, test to confirm diagnosis—a one hundred–gram glucose tolerance test—because the first blood test frequently results in false positives: Only about 20 percent of the women who test positive really have diabetes.

Some doctors recommend screening only for women who are at risk for GD due to weight, age, or diabetic symptoms and risk factors.

Those women who test positive are medically managed in ways appropriate to the degree of glucose intolerance. For mild GD, many doctors prescribe a diabetic diet. For more severe GD, some doctors use diet and/or insulin.

Some doctors treat pregnant women with GD for the same reason they treat pregnant women with chronic diabetes: in the hopes of reducing the rate of macrosomic babies, birth injury, and cesarean section. These doctors favor screening all pregnant women for GD, arguing that in women with diabetes severe enough to require insulin, the insulin has been found to decrease the rate of big babies from 20 percent down to the normal rate of 10 percent.

On the other hand, Dr. Murray Enkin and his coauthors of *A Guide to Effective Care in Pregnancy and Childbirth* (third edition) argue that although the use of insulin decreases the rate of fetal macrosomia (big babies), it does not significantly reduce other possible consequences of GD, such as "the use of cesarean section, the incidence of shoulder dystocia, or perinatal mortality." Dr. Enkin, as well as some of his Canadian and Dutch obstetricians, do not treat mild GD as aggressively as American obstetricians treat it. If you have GD that is not controlled by diet alone, discuss your treatment options with your physician.

Fortunately, both GD and diabetes mellitus can often be well managed during pregnancy.

Diabetes Mellitus Types I and II

Diabetes is one of the modern-day wonder stories of obstetrics.
—Dr. Donna Kirz

* * *

Preexisting diabetes makes the pregnancy higher risk, but lots of the complications can be prevented. If the diabetes is under control with diet or insulin, the woman's risk is the same as everyone else's.
—Dr. Donna Kirz

* * *

Both pre-existing diabetes and gestational diabetes (pregnancy-induced diabetes) become more common with increasing maternal age, but they are very different forms of diabetes. Preexisting diabetes (diabetes mellitus types I and II) is a chronic, systemic disease that can involve your circulatory system and kidneys, whereas GD is usually temporary and does not involve your kidneys or circulation.

Chronic diabetes once presented serious health problems in pregnancy for both women and their babies, but medical advances in diet and medication have made diabetic pregnancy relatively safe—as long as the disease is well controlled and your blood sugar does not become too high or too low.

Chronic diabetes (Type I or Type II) is now a treatable, although not yet curable, disease, and it is usually manageable during pregnancy through diet or insulin injections. If you have diabetes, consult with your doctor before getting pregnant to assess the severity of your diabetes and to arrive at a treatment plan: You may need to change your medications or your diet before pregnancy in order to keep your sugar levels steady and under control during pregnancy. Dr. Murray Enkin, a Canadian physician and pregnancy expert, advises women with diabetes to seek specialized care from "both obstetricians and physicians with special interest in this field" and to consult with a dietician.

Treatment of chronic diabetes both before and during pregnancy is very important, says Enkin, since severe or long-standing diabetes can create further health problems. In addition, untreated maternal diabetes can create problems for your baby by increasing its risks for congenital abnormalities, fetal macrosomia, and unexplained death. "The risks to the fetus are significant," writes Enkin in *A Guide to Effective Care in Pregnancy and Childbirth* (second edition), since "diabetes is associated with an increased incidence of congenital abnormalities up to three times as great as for the infants of non-diabetic mothers." However, he says that tight control of the diabetes before conception can significantly reduce this risk.

If your diabetes is particularly severe and involves significant vascular disease (problems with your blood vessels and circulatory system), talk to your doctor about pregnancy risks. Your doctor may or may not recommend that you avoid pregnancy, depending on your unique circumstances.

The mode of treating and controlling your diabetes may depend on whether you have Type I or Type II diabetes. Type I diabetes is caused by an insulin deficiency in which your pancreas doesn't produce enough insulin to adequately utilize the glucose (sugar) that you eat in the form of fruit, sugar, and carbohydrates. This insulin deficiency results in abnormally high amounts of sugar in your blood and urine and can create various systemic problems, depending on the kind of diabetes you have and the length of time you have had the illness. For instance, a forty-year-old woman who has had diabetes since childhood may have circulatory problems, kidney problems, and vision problems as well as elevated blood sugar. Any of these problems can worsen during pregnancy if the diabetes is not well controlled. Since Type I diabetes can cause extremes of both high and low blood sugar, and since these extremes can cause abnormalities in your developing baby, it is important that you get your disease under control before pregnancy and maintain control of your blood sugar during pregnancy.

Type II diabetes tends to develop after you've reached maturity. Although your pancreas still produces insulin, your body suppresses the effect of this insulin. Consequently, the insulin cannot break down the glucose in your blood, and your blood sugar becomes high. Type II diabetes also can affect your circulatory system and kidneys, although not as severely as Type I. Often this form of diabetes can be treated with diet, although sometimes it requires insulin as well.

With either Type I or II, the key to a safe pregnancy is management, which means taking the time to plan appropriate meals, blood tests, ultrasound scans, and frequent visits to your care provider. Consequently, pregnant women with diabetes should be cared for by an obstetrician or perinatologist experienced in the care of diabetic pregnancy.

Nowadays, women with diabetes can—and do—have safe pregnancies and healthy babies.

High Blood Pressure

If you're forty-five and hypertensive, your heart is under stress from both the pregnancy and the hypertension. Renal disease can be aggravated; you can be more prone to placental abruption. You also have a higher chance of a small baby or preeclampsia.
—Dr. Donna Kirz

* * *

We see obstetrical complications in 50 percent of women over forty-five. Twenty to 30 percent of older women develop high blood pressure. But the likelihood of an untoward event is only 1 percent.
—Dr. Mark Sauer

* * *

Blood pressure that is 140/90 or higher for two recordings taken at least six hours apart is considered high. If the systolic pressure (the top number) is elevated thirty or more points from your normal baseline pressure, this, too, may be considered high for you. The condition may be managed with rest or blood pressure medications (check your medications with your doctor and pharmacist since some hypertension medications are toxic to developing babies).

Hypertension can take several forms: *pregnancy-induced high blood pressure; preeclampsia* or the *toxemia of pregnancy;* chronic, preexisting high blood pressure; *superimposed preeclampsia* (a combination of preexisting hypertension and preeclampsia); or *eclampsia,* an advanced and dangerous stage of preeclampsia.

If you have high blood pressure before or during your pregnancy, you will need to be closely monitored since you are at higher risk for developing preeclampsia or other hypertension-related conditions.

Pregnancy-Induced Hypertension

Pregnancy-induced hypertension is high blood pressure that appears during the course of pregnancy and disappears after the baby is born. This type of hypertension does not include edema and protein in the urine, which develop with preeclampsia (see below). However, if you develop this kind of high blood pressure during pregnancy, you will need to be monitored, since you are at risk for developing preeclampsia.

Preeclampsia

Preeclampsia is more common with first babies—or in a first baby with a new partner, your risk is as if you are having a first baby.
—Dr. Murray Enkin, Professor Emeritus of Obstetrics and Gynecology at McMaster University in Ontario, Canada

●　●　●

Medical studies indicate that pregnancy-induced high blood pressure affects between 3 and 10 percent of all pregnant women. Your risk of developing high blood pressure increases as you get older. Your risk also increases if you are a first-time mother, are pregnant with multiples, or have a history of prepregnancy hypertension. Fortunately, this rise in blood pressure is temporary and can usually be well managed with proper prenatal care, diet, and rest.

Women over age thirty-five have an increased risk of developing a more specific and serious form of pregnancy-induced hypertension called preeclampsia. Preeclampsia is a disease of pregnancy that is often accompanied by *proteinuria* (protein in the urine) and can have far-reaching effects that involve your kidneys and liver. High blood pressure may or may not be an early warning sign of a developing preeclampsia, but high blood pressure in combination with edema and protein in your urine is a sign that you already have preeclampsia and that your caregiver needs to carefully monitor you during your pregnancy. The advanced form of this disease—eclampsia—can cause seizures, coma, or death, and it is important to catch preeclampsia early in order to prevent it from developing into eclampsia. Call your care provider immediately if you develop any of the following symptoms of preeclampsia:

- Swelling of your hands or face
- Sudden weight gain
- Increased fluid retention
- Dizziness
- Headaches
- Unusual drowsiness
- Mental confusion
- Blurred vision or other vision problems
- Stomach upset or pain
- Nausea or vomiting
- Rapid heart rate
- Difficulty breathing
- Fever
- Decrease in urination
- Protein in your urine (which can be detected in a urine dipstick test)

These may be relatively advanced signs, but they may be the first things you notice. Many women with early preeclampsia *have no symptoms,* which is why some doctors suggest frequent obstetric visits for women late in their pregnancy.

Fortunately, in most cases, preeclampsia can be effectively managed. When preeclampsia occurs before your baby is mature enough to be born, a common treatment is rest—sometimes strict bed rest at home or in the hospital and sometimes limited activity. Although bed rest is not a proven cure for this condition, some caregivers believe that it helps manage some of the symptoms and helps prevent the condition from worsening. Because strict bed rest may carry a risk of circulatory problems, do not prescribe it for yourself. Consult with your doctor about the pros and cons of bed rest versus limited activity.

The best treatment of all for preeclampsia is delivery of the baby; delivery relieves your symptoms and is healthier for the baby, since it removes the baby from the hypertensive environment of your womb in which she may be receiving less oxygen and nourishment due to decreased blood flow to the placenta. If your preeclampsia is severe and your baby is old enough to be delivered, your caregiver may either induce labor or, in some cases, deliver your baby by cesarean section.

The cause of preeclampsia is not well understood. There is, as yet, no cure—except delivery of the baby: "There is no pill, no shot, and blood pressure meds don't help it. Bed rest may ameliorate it," says Dr. Kirz. Resting in bed, preferably on your left side, may increase blood flow to your uterus and placenta and thus, to your baby. Lying flat on your back, however, may actually limit blood flow since some major blood vessels are compressed by this posture.

Sometimes doctors argue that preeclampsia may be treated with blood pressure medications or medications given to prevent blood clotting. The more advanced form of the condition, eclampsia, is treated with drugs used to treat convulsions. Discuss possible treatments with your care provider, since treatments tend to change as new studies are published, as current treatments are reevaluated, and as new drugs come into the market.

Preeclampsia may occasionally cause placental abruption— a *rare condition* in which the baby's placenta may separate from your uterine wall. A major symptom is bleeding, which may or may not be painful. Sometimes this separation of the placenta is severe enough to necessitate emergency delivery of the baby. Like preeclampsia, placental abruption can be "sneaky and unpredictable," says Dr. Allen Killam. Fortunately, the risk of abruption is small—even if you are over forty. According to Dr. Killam, "These are serious medical problems that occur in younger people less than 1 percent of the time. They can be doubled in older people, especially with high blood pressure or previous surgery of the uterus. But it is still a small number; you are doubling a number that's smaller than 1 percent."

Chronic Hypertension with Preeclampsia

Preeclampsia may be as much as 20 percent more common in women who have high blood pressure before they become pregnant. If you are already hypertensive, you may develop superimposed preeclampsia, which may involve your liver and kidneys. Both preeclampsia and hypertension involve your circulatory system, which can affect other organ systems sensitive to blood flow (such as the kidney) and can interfere with blood flow to the baby's placenta.

Eclampsia

Eclampsia—we don't see it often now. I suppose we pick it up earlier.
—Dr. Murray Enkin

∗ ∗ ∗

Although there is an age-related increase in the incidence of high blood pressure, the most serious form—eclampsia—is a rare condition that is found more frequently in very young mothers.

Eclampsia is a *rare,* dangerous, and usually preventable condition that causes convulsions. The convulsions can lead to coma and, very rarely, death. Surprisingly, the rate of this potentially life-threatening complication of pregnancy is highest in women under age sixteen, occurring in 0.53 percent of these youthful pregnancies. However, among American women between age thirty and age thirty-four, the risk of developing preeclampsia is only 0.28 percent, and for women forty to forty-nine it is 0.44 percent, according to 1998 *National Vital Statistics Reports* listing pregnancy complications in women who had given birth. (These figures refer to women who had live babies; since high blood pressure may sometimes lead to miscarriage or other problems, the numbers for all pregnant women, regardless of their pregnancy outcome, would be higher.)

If you should develop eclampsia, you will need experienced medical care from a seasoned obstetrician or a perinatologist who is familiar with the current therapies for this condition. Although eclampsia has been treated with medications such as magnesium sulfate or anticonvulsant drugs, drug therapies may change as new information or medications become available.

DES Daughters

If your mother took the synthetic hormone DES (diethylstilbestrol) while pregnant with you, you are considered a DES daughter. DES was a widely prescribed "anti-miscarriage" drug in the United States and Europe from the 1940s to the early 1970s, and if your mother took this drug during her first trimester of pregnancy, you may face some increased risks during your pregnancy. You may also have some difficulty getting pregnant.

DES daughters are at an increased risk for miscarriage and premature delivery due to uterine and cervical abnormalities caused by their prenatal exposure to DES, especially if they were exposed to the drug when they were four- to ten-week-old fetuses (a critical period for the formation of the reproductive system). If you have a T-shaped uterus or a shortened or weakened cervix as a result of your drug exposure, you may be at increased risk for miscarriage or premature labor. See a doctor who has experience with DES daughters and their potential pregnancy risks; often this will be a high-risk pregnancy specialist or a seasoned obstetrician.

Since DES daughters are also at higher risk for vaginal cancer, breast cancer, and other physical problems, make sure you get a thorough physical exam when you start to consider pregnancy. If you have encountered fertility problems, seek out a fertility specialist familiar with DES-related hormonal imbalances (see Part 3).

High Fever and High Body Temperature

A high maternal fever or body temperature may create problems for your baby, especially if your temperature is high for a long period of time.

If you have a high temperature, drink plenty of fluids but hold off on the Tylenol or other medications until you have consulted with your care provider. Remember that high body temperature can easily be created by long exposure to hot tubs, saunas, steam baths, or even very hot baths. Avoid exposing a developing baby to such extremes of temperature.

IVF Pregnancies

Women with IVF pregnancies often are referred by their fertility doctor to a high-risk pregnancy specialist, since these doctors may regard such long-awaited, expensive pregnancies as particularly "precious."

Whether or not IVF mothers face more risks in pregnancy has not been determined. There is some speculation that IVF pregnancies have higher rates of placenta previa—a placenta lying close to, or on top of the birth canal, making a vaginal delivery either difficult, dangerous, or impossible. If you have an IVF pregnancy, discuss your birth philosophy and your individual health considerations with your infertility specialist in order to get a referral to the most appropriate care provider for you. Some women with IVF pregnancies go to nurse-midwives or general obstetricians while others would feel comfortable only with a perinatologist.

Placenta Previa

Placenta previa increases tenfold in older women. But ten times

a rare thing is still a rare thing.
—Dr. Watson Bowes Jr.

❖ ❖ ❖

Placenta previa is a relatively rare condition that occurs in only 1 out of every 200 pregnancies—about 0.5 percent. In this condition, your placenta is implanted over or near the cervix and lies between your baby and the birth canal. It is more common in multiple pregnancies because there are more placentas present.

Although the condition may be detected by ultrasound, sometimes the only warning of placenta previa is painless vaginal bleeding. Usually this bleeding occurs in the last trimester of pregnancy. The bleeding may be intermittent or steady; in either case, report vaginal bleeding immediately to your health care provider.

Do not drive to work or hop on a plane thinking that painless bleeding can be dismissed. Your care provider may need to promptly examine you and use an ultrasound to determine if you have placenta previa or other problems. If you do, you need to rest, and you and your baby should be carefully monitored for the rest of your pregnancy. Placenta previa often requires a cesarean birth since the placenta may create an obstacle between your baby and your birth canal. Consequently, if you are diagnosed with this condition, you may find it helpful to join a childbirth class or a support group that offers preparation for cesarean birth. Planning for the possibility of a cesarean can reduce stress should you require one.

Placental Abruption

There is a one out of one hundred risk of abruption in the general population.
—Dr. Katherine Shaw

Placental abruption, the complete or partial separation of the placenta from the uterus before your baby's birth, is another relatively rare condition occurring in approximately 1 out of 100 to 200 births—which means you have approximately a 0.5 percent chance of having this happen to you. Women who have chronic high blood pressure, preeclampsia, or the circulatory and blood pressure problems that can result from long-standing diabetes are at greater risk for abruptions. Women who drink alcohol, smoke, or take drugs like cocaine are also at increased risk of placental abruption. Women who have had several children are also at risk for abruption.

Abruption may occur spontaneously and unpredictably at any stage of pregnancy. Symptoms include vaginal bleeding, a hard or tender abdomen, abdominal distension, and severe abdominal or back pain. Call your caregiver immediately. Placental abruption is an emergency that can result in maternal hemorrhage and fetal oxygen deprivation; it requires immediate treatment and sometimes immediate delivery of the baby.

If the separation of the placenta from the uterus is small, bleeding may be minimal or even not apparent, but it is still potentially dangerous since the separation could increase in size. In this case, your caregiver may need to watch you carefully, put you on bed rest or limited activity, allow you to continue in labor if you are already in labor, or perform a cesarean section.

Treatment for abruption depends on the degree of placental separation from the uterine wall. If your bleeding is profuse and the abruption or separation is severe, you may need an immediate cesarean section. If your caregiver is not available, call an ambulance. Go to an emergency room if you are close to a hospital. If the abruption is moderate, your physician may hospitalize you and prescribe limited activity or strict bed rest at home or in the hospital. In the case of a mild placental abruption, your symptoms may eventually resolve, although your doctor may want you to rest.

Ectopic Pregnancy

At 12:30 I left work and was heading to my truck—and all of a sudden I was crippled with pain. That's when my tube burst (but I didn't know it).
—Rhonda was able to conceive again three months after emergency surgery to remove her affected tube.

❋ ❋ ❋

In an ectopic pregnancy, the fertilized egg (embryo) implants itself within the fallopian tube before it reaches the uterus. (Sometimes the embryo will be unable to pass through the fallopian tube because the tube is obstructed by structural abnormalities, scarring, or endometriosis.) The most common signs and symptoms of an ectopic pregnancy are a missed menstrual period, vaginal bleeding, sharp abdominal pain, low blood pressure, or an hCG level that is high enough to test positive on a pregnancy test but not high enough to correlate appropriately with your week of pregnancy.

Signs and symptoms of an ectopic pregnancy may appear early on in pregnancy—in fact, they may appear before you realize that you are pregnant. When detected early, some ectopic pregnancies can be treated with medications. However, surgery to remove the part of the tube affected, and sometimes the entire tube, is sometimes the only solution.

Do not ignore the warning symptoms of a possible ectopic pregnancy since it can eventually rupture your fallopian tube and become a life-threatening emergency. Ectopic pregnancy is responsible for 10 percent of maternal mortality.

Rhonda tried to ignore her symptoms and drive home

(instead of stopping at the hospital) because she didn't want to be tagged "a whiner" by the hospital staff:

"The pain was so bad I thought I was going to pass out. I pulled the car over to the median. I got out of the car and was on my hands and knees in pain. I couldn't hold out my hand to wave someone down. Two cars pulled over. I asked, 'could someone give me a ride home? I just want to lie down on my couch.' I was worried about getting charged if they called an ambulance. I had no idea what was going on with me. I already had my miscarriage. [She had miscarried a few weeks earlier, but she hadn't realized that she was pregnant with twins. One of the twins had implanted in her fallopian tube.] Ectopic never entered my mind. Finally the paramedics came and had me try to sit up. 'I'm taking you to the hospital right now—no ifs, ands, or buts,' the man said. Twenty-four hours after surgery I still had grass in my hair from the median strip."

After the paramedics brought Rhonda to the hospital, she was rushed to surgery where doctors removed her tubal pregnancy and fallopian tube. Rhonda was determined to have a baby. Months later, Rhonda became pregnant again—even though she had only one fallopian tube. She had a normal pregnancy.

If you experience severe abdominal pain during your pregnancy, do not attempt to drive yourself to the hospital. Call 911, and call your doctor.

Treating Ectopic Pregnancy

Some ectopic pregnancies may be treated as an outpatient, but only after a thorough evaluation with an ultrasound and only under strict medical supervision as some ectopic pregnancies can be fatal [if surgery is not available to remove the ectopic and control bleeding].
—Dr. Allen Killam

Fortunately, it is now possible to diagnose and treat an ectopic pregnancy before it becomes an emergency by performing a series of blood tests or by using a transvaginal ultrasound to visualize your fallopian tubes. Ectopic pregnancies may be successfully treated surgically or medically. Some of the surgical options consist of salpingectomy (removal of all or part of the affected tube) by laparotomy, an operation that involves an abdominal incision and anesthesia, or a salpingectomy by laparoscopy, an operation that involves a tiny incision and less anesthesia, pain, and recovery time than a laparotomy. Not all surgeons are trained in laparoscopy, so the treatment you receive may be determined by either the training of your surgeon or your individual circumstances regarding bleeding, low blood pressure, and the stage of your ectopic pregnancy. Ask your doctors about the options most suitable for you

Medical treatment means avoiding surgery but taking a powerful drug called methotrexate that stops the ectopic pregnancy from growing. The drug allows you to avoid the risks of surgery and anesthesia. If you have an ectopic pregnancy, your physician may wish to hospitalize you for observation if you have persistent pain or other symptoms.

What Kind of Doctor Do You Need?

If you develop a condition such as preeclampsia, placental abruption, or severe GD that makes your pregnancy "high risk," you may need to see a perinatologist or internist during the course of your pregnancy. In some cases, you may need to see this specialist only once or twice—for a second opinion—and then return to your regular physician. In some cases, such as uncontrolled diabetes, you may need to be seen by both your specialist and an obstetrician for the duration of your pregnancy.

Chapter 12

Genetic Testing, Genetic Counseling, and Other Forms of Prenatal Diagnosis

If you are a woman over thirty-five, you may worry about your genetic risks as well as the risks of tests—amniocentesis and chorionic villa sampling (CVS)—that are used to diagnose genetic problems. This chapter introduces you to the various tests and the risks and benefits involved in each. It also addresses the emotions you may have when deciding whether to have a test and when you are waiting for the test results.

Because not everyone sees these risks in the same way, I present several perspectives best summed up by Dr. Allen Killam and Dr. Katherine Shaw, both high-risk pregnancy specialists who have counseled midlife mothers on genetic risks. Dr. Killam urges women to get pregnant by age forty, since their risks increase dramatically after that age. "Before forty, incidence of Down's is 1 in 1,000; after forty it is 1 in 100. By age forty-six, it is 1 in 17. . . . We're building an argument about getting pregnant before forty." However, Dr. Shaw believes that the risks can be seen from a more reassuring, though still realistic, perspective: "Most older women have these horrible thoughts about their risk of birth defects. At age forty, the Down's risk is 1 in 100. The risk at age forty-nine is 1 out of 12." That means you have a 90 percent chance of having a baby that does not have Down's syndrome.

Genetic Counseling: Understanding the Risks

There are people who are forty-one and as physically healthy as most thirty-five-year-olds. The thing a person can't get around by keeping healthy is genetic risk.
—Dr. Allen Killam

      ❋ ❋ ❋

The "magic" about age thirty-five is that the risk of a chromosome problem becomes equal to the risk of amniocentesis. They are both small risks.
—DeeDee Lafayette, genetic counselor and labor assistant

      ❋ ❋ ❋

You can obtain information about your baby's genetic health by selecting some form of prenatal diagnosis—amniocentesis, CVS, triple-screen blood tests, ultrasounds—to learn, within widely varying degrees of certainty, whether or not your baby is genetically normal. You can use this knowledge to prepare yourself emotionally or financially for the birth of an abnormal child, or you can use the information to terminate the pregnancy.

The uncomfortable question facing expectant mothers and their partners these days as they choose whether or not to pursue prenatal diagnosis is: What will we do with the information once we have it? It is in helping expectant parents answer this question that genetic counseling is useful, says Dr. Allen Killam. "The skill in genetic counseling is in helping the woman decide for herself what is best for her. A woman with IVF and a lot of expense to get pregnant may have only noninvasive tests such as ultrasound and blood [AFP triple screen] tests."

Counseling can help you evaluate your risks and your options, and identify the issues and emotions involved in aborting a long-awaited baby or raising a Down's baby or a baby with other birth defects.

Many expectant parents are overwhelmed by the implications and possible risks of genetic testing and the uncertainty involved in making such momentous choices. They find the process of sifting through all the information and making informed, rational choices too complex and anxiety provoking to do on their own. It is in situations such as these that genetic counselors can help parents sift through all the technical jargon about Down's rates and the comparative risks of amniocentesis and CVS in order to make difficult decisions.

Perspectives on Risk

When you compare your risks of having a genetically abnormal baby with the risks of women younger than you, the striking differences in the numbers may be misleading. It is more accurate—and far more reassuring—to look beyond these relative or comparative risks to see more clearly what your "real" or absolute risks are of having a normal or an abnormal baby.

For instance, being at "higher risk" (compared to a twenty-five-year-old) does not mean you are at "high" risk. Your risk of having a baby with any of several chromosomal abnormalities may increase from 1 percent to 3 percent between the ages of thirty-five and forty, which means that, although your risk may triple, it still is not high.

Age-Related Genetic Risks of Midlife Pregnancy

Age Thirty-five:
1 in 134 risk = a less than 1 percent risk of chromosomal abnormality.

This also means that your baby has a 99 percent chance of *not* having a chromosomal abnormality.

Age Forty:
1 in 39 risk = a less than 3 percent chance of chromosomal abnormality.

This also means that your baby has a greater than 97 percent chance of *not* having a chromosomal abnormality.

Age Forty-five:
1 in 11 risk = about a 10 percent chance of chromosomal abnormality.

This also means that your baby has about a 90 percent chance of not having a chromosomal abnormality despite the fact that you are reproductively—and genetically—"mature."

If you are forty, your absolute, or "real," risk of having a baby with chromosomal problems may be 3 percent—compared to a thirty-five-year-old's 1 percent. By age forty-five, your risks have tripled compared to those at age thirty-five, but the odds of having a genetically normal baby are still 90 percent in your favor. Although your genetic risks have increased dramatically, they may be less than what you had previously believed.

Whether a risk is too high or not, however, is never merely a matter of numbers. What is important is what risks are tolerable to you as an individual. Perhaps a 1 percent risk is intolerable to you—and not a "low" risk at all. On the other hand, perhaps a 10 percent risk is perfectly acceptable.

Part of your response to the numbers that define your odds will be based upon your personal perception, although your perception may be influenced by your care provider's or genetic counselor's interpretation of risk. Their perception of risk may, in turn, be based upon what their peers in the medical community think about risk—and such perceptions are subject to change.

Tests to Screen for Fetal Abnormalities

If you decide to have your baby tested for fetal abnormalities, you have an array of choices available to you at different stages of your pregnancy:

- Triple screen
- Ultrasound
- Amniocentesis
- Early amniocentesis
- CVS
- Percutaneous umbilical cord sampling

Triple Screen Blood Test

The triple screen is a blood test that involves an analysis of your blood done at fifteen to twenty weeks of pregnancy to test your levels of alpha-fetoprotein (AFP), hCG, and estriol. High maternal blood levels of AFP may indicate neural tube defects such as spina bifida or anencephaly. Neural tube defects are not an age-related phenomenon, since 0.1 percent (1 in 1,000) of all babies will have a neural tube defect (40 percent of these defects will be anencephaly and 60 percent will be spina bifida). However, the risk of neural tube defects for babies of women who already have had a child with a neural tube defect is 3 to 5 percent (30–50 in 1,000 babies).

Luckily, many neural tube defects can be prevented if you take folic acid both before and during pregnancy. Studies show that 0.4 mg of folic acid per day for three to six months taken before you conceive and continued through three months of pregnancy may reduce the occurrence of neural tube defects by 60 percent. The baby's neural tube—what later becomes its spinal cord—is formed very early in pregnancy. Consequently, you need to have folic acid from food or vitamin sources in your body before you know you are pregnant.

Spina bifida sometimes can be seen on an ultrasound, but the triple screen blood test can screen for the disorder more reliably than ultrasound. However, an amniocentesis is the most reliable way to diagnose neural tube defects, since it is accurate about 98 to 99 percent of the time.

The triple screen is the only preliminary, noninvasive test that can sometimes indicate the existence of Down's syndrome. By identifying the pattern of two hormones—hCG and estriol—in your blood, a triple screen test can sometimes detect a pattern typical of Down's syndrome. Although the triple screen test cannot test definitively for Down's syndrome (since it is only 60 percent sensitive), it can be used as a preliminary test for Down's.

The triple screen also tests for the chromosomal disorder trisomy 18, a disorder that is less common than Down's but often more severe. However, because it is a screening test, not a diagnostic test, results are not concrete and are subject to some false positives and false negatives. "Of all the babies with Down's, 60 percent are caught by the triple screen and 40 percent are missed," says Melissa Trant, a genetic counselor with a Los Angeles perinatal center.

Diagnostic tests like amniocentesis and CVS offer more concrete results for chromosomal abnormalities such as Down's syndrome. However, of these two diagnostic tests only amniocentesis detects AFP.

Ultrasound

In the ultrasound he was like a blinking light on a Christmas tree—a little light in a sea of black.
—Holly's description of the first time she saw her son, Soren

* * *

Ultrasound can give you an early picture of your baby. You can see its heart beating, and sometimes you can see the baby sucking its thumb. The ultrasound can help your care provider see structural abnormalities of the baby's heart, spinal cord, head, intestinal tract, or bones and pick up fetal abnormalities that are typical of Down's syndrome, spina bifida, and several rare disorders. In addition, some pregnancy experts believe that early ultrasound exams may reduce the rate of inductions for apparent postterm labor, since the ultrasound may help establish the baby's gestational age.

Ultrasound is a noninvasive procedure that generates heat and sound—the effects of which appear to be safe for you and your baby. However, some health experts think ultrasound screening should not be routine but rather used as needed, since any medical procedure could have potential side effects. Consequently, some experts recommend that ultrasounds be done for diagnostic purposes only and not to help a woman bond with her baby or to give parents a first picture of their unborn child. If you are concerned about ultrasound, some care providers suggest that you ask your doctor to limit the time of exposure by freezing an image on the screen while you are discussing your baby instead of keeping the machine running.

Amniocentesis

Of the available diagnostic tests, amniocentesis provides the broadest spectrum of information with the most accuracy. It can detect neural tube defects with an accuracy of about 98 to 99 percent and chromosomal disorders with an accuracy of about 99 percent. The test indicates the amount of AFP found in the amniotic fluid (rather than in your bloodstream), which may indicate neural tube defects. It also can pick up chromosomal disorders including trisomy 21 (Down's syndrome), trisomy 18, and trisomy 13.

In cases of familial genetic diseases or diseases related to your ethnicity, such as cystic fibrosis or sickle-cell anemia, special tests of your amniotic fluid can be used to diagnose these diseases. Additional examinations of the fluid can be done, if necessary, to detect some fetal infections such as herpes, rubella, or toxoplasmosis.

One of the prevailing myths about amniocentesis is that a needle is passed through your belly button. This is not true.

A fine, thin needle is carefully guided through your abdominal wall and then through your uterine wall until it reaches the sac of amniotic fluid that covers your baby. The doctor uses an ultrasound image of your baby and its placenta and sac to guide the needle toward the sac and away from the baby and the placenta. When the fluid sac is penetrated, the doctor withdraws a small amount of amniotic fluid, withdraws the needle, and the procedure is over. The test itself usually takes about thirty seconds, although you may be in the examining room for twenty to thirty minutes during which time an ultrasound test will be performed to locate the position of your baby.

Many women consider the test uncomfortable but not painful. When the needle first pierces your skin, you may feel a small pinch, as you would in a blood test. Your doctor may numb the skin on one side of your belly with some anesthetic first, so you won't feel the amniocentesis needle. However, sometimes anesthetic is not used since the numbing process may be as painful as the amniocentesis.

When the needle enters the uterine muscle, some women experience some cramping. Few women experience severe pain. If you know any calming visualization or meditation techniques, it is useful to practice them before and during the procedure to minimize your discomfort and your anxiety.

The primary downside to amniocentesis is that it is an invasive procedure, and all the invasive prenatal diagnostic procedures (such as CVS and early amniocentesis) carry with them a potential risk of miscarriage.

The procedural-associated risk in the case of standard amniocentesis (carried out after the fourteenth to sixteenth week of pregnancy) is small when the test is done by a skillful and experienced doctor. For a standard amniocentesis done by a skilled physician around the sixteenth week of pregnancy, the miscarriage rate is about 1 in 200, giving you an approximate 0.5 percent to 1 percent risk of miscarriage. However, such risk may not be small to you if you have had previous miscarriages, if you are older and pregnant with a long-awaited baby, or if you already are very bonded to your developing baby. At this point you need to carefully weigh the benefits of the procedure against its physical and emotional risks (see "Making a Decision about Amniocentesis").

After the test, you should not experience any discomfort. If you experience bleeding, pain, severe cramping, fever, or leakage of amniotic fluid after the amniocentesis, call your doctor immediately. Such symptoms do not necessarily indicate miscarriage, but it is always safer to consult your doctor. Your doctor may recommend that you rest or come in to the hospital for an ultrasound or, in the case of infection, for medication.

Your test results will be ready between seven days and two

weeks after the procedure. Many women experience this waiting period as excruciating, although some manage to handle it with relative calm. Another downside to amniocentesis (as with other prenatal diagnostic procedures) is the anxiety associated with waiting for test results.

Use whatever strategies you have found effective in past stressful situations to help minimize your anxiety—listening to music, focusing on work, surrounding yourself with good friends, taking walks.

Another way to both minimize your anxiety level and your risk is to find a skilled physician to do your amniocentesis. You decrease your risk of problems by finding a doctor who does the procedure frequently, who is either an obstetrician or a perinatologist or a specialist in amniocentesis, and who is not an obstetrics resident or fellow who is just learning to do the procedure. Ask your care provider whom he or she recommends; in some cases, the person who does your amnio will be your care provider. Other sources for recommendations for doctors experienced in amniocentesis are nurses at well-respected hospitals and nearby university obstetrics departments or departments of maternal-fetal medicine.

However, some level of anxiety is unavoidable, given the questions you will ponder as you wait for results.

Early Amniocentesis

Early amniocentesis, carried out around ten to twelve weeks, gives you the advantage of knowing earlier, rather than later, if your baby has a chromosomal defect or serious abnormality. You can terminate the pregnancy, if you choose to, at a point when the abortion procedure is physically easier on you. However, the miscarriage rate for early amniocentesis is greater than at sixteen weeks, and sometimes your baby does not have sufficient amniotic fluid for a successful test. Consequently, some doctors are uncomfortable with early amniocentesis. "Early amniocentesis [at twelve weeks of gestation] may be associated with more miscarriages than if it is done after fourteen weeks' gestation," cautions Dr. Allen Killam. Amniocentesis before twelve weeks is discouraged by many care providers unless the benefits clearly outweigh the risks (if, for example, a baby has a one in four chance of having a serious genetic disease). Recent studies reviewed by Enkin et al. in *A Guide to Effective Care in Pregnancy and Childbirth* (third edition) indicate that early amniocentesis at ten to twelve weeks has a higher miscarriage rate than either CVS or midtrimester amniocentesis. Consequently, many doctors strongly discourage early amniocentesis and favor CVS if early diagnosis is needed.

Making a Decision about Amniocentesis

When you are deciding whether or not to have an amniocentesis, you may face a complex, challenging decision—depending on your past experience and on how you view the test and the pregnancy. As in all medical decisions, you need to balance the benefits and risks of having the procedure with those of not having it.

With amniocentesis, you have the benefit of knowing, in advance, whether or not your baby has certain medical problems. This may give you the relief of knowing that your baby does not have one of the more common chromosomal or neural tube defects (which is the most likely result—even if you are over forty). It may also give you the opportunity to plan and take some forms of action if your baby is abnormal. For instance, if your baby has Down's or spina bifida, knowing in advance can help you (1) plan for the birth and ongoing care of a child with Down's or spina bifida, (2) terminate the pregnancy before the cutoff point for legal abortions, or (3) plan for continuing the pregnancy and then placing the child in the care of a halfway house or care facility for children with disabilities.

Your risks include the possible, though relatively slight, rate of miscarriage due to the procedure. Miscarriage risks for women during midtrimester (after week 16) amniocentesis are 0.5 percent, if done by an experienced medical practitioner. You will have to decide if that is a tolerable risk and worth the benefits of knowing more about your baby's health.

If you feel overwhelmed by the choice or by the consequences of a choice you have already made, discussing your thoughts and feelings with a genetic counselor may provide you with valuable information and support. Many counselors are trained to be nondirective and to support any choice you have made. The process and the consequence of deciding whether or not to have an amniocentesis may call up for you profound emotional, social, and even spiritual associations. It is a decision that may have a significant impact on you, your children, and your partner and may cause considerable anxiety.

The decision to have an amniocentesis may also affect the way you experience motherhood until the amnio results are in. Many women feel detached from their baby and from their pregnancy until the pregnancy is pronounced healthy by amnio results. For Joanne, it wasn't until after her results came back normal that she felt like she was "really pregnant." She describes the experience:

"Waiting for results seemed to be forever. Dr. Dwight called me at 4:00 in the afternoon before a three-day holiday weekend to tell me that the test was OK. That's a moment in time that was amazing. I took him and Dr. Bates flowers. Then I felt, 'OK. Now I'm pregnant.' I told my family and colleagues at work."

Although many doctors recommend amniocentesis for women over thirty-five, the procedure is not mandatory. Women are free to choose it or not. "One of the biggest misconceptions is that a woman has to have amniocentesis," explains Melissa

Trant, a genetic counselor. Rhonda, after going through a traumatic miscarriage, refused amniocentesis because of the miscarriage risks. She also came to terms with the possible consequences of giving birth to an abnormal baby and came to this conclusion: "I thought there was no way I was going to terminate this baby—no matter what was wrong with it."

CVS

The risk depends to a fair degree on the skill and experience of the person doing it. It is 1 percent more risky for pregnancy loss than amniocentesis and there is some fear of limb reduction.
—Dr. Allen Killam

• • •

The main advantage of CVS is that you need not wait for sixteen weeks to find out if your baby is abnormal. CVS can be done between ten and twelve weeks of pregnancy, which gives you the benefit of terminating the pregnancy relatively early on when termination may not be as physically or emotionally difficult. However, CVS does not test for AFP, although it does diagnose chromosomal abnormalities like Down's syndrome and trisomy 18.

To perform a CVS, the doctor uses a thin needle or catheter to take a tiny tissue sample from the chorionic villi—little projections of tissue that eventually will become the baby's placenta. Since this tissue develops from the fertilized egg, it shares the baby's genetic makeup.

The procedure can be done one of two different ways: by a transabdominal method or a transcervical method. The transabdominal method involves the doctor's guiding a fine needle through your abdominal wall. The placement of the needle is directed by an ultrasound that determines the exact location of the placenta. The transcervical method is done with a thin catheter that is inserted through the cervix to obtain a sample of the chorionic villi.

Currently, the major disadvantages of CVS are that it gives you less information at more risk when compared to amniocentesis. CVS involves a miscarriage rate of 1 to 2 percent (1 or 2 in 100) compared with the 0.5 percent risk of amniocentesis, although some of the increased risk of CVS depends on "who's doing it and how aggressive they are," says Dr. Killam.

Another disadvantage of CVS is that the procedure has been associated with certain fetal birth defects such as fetal limb reduction, leading some doctors and genetic counselors to perceive the risks of CVS as outweighing the benefits (except under some special circumstances). The procedure is also associated with more bleeding, more false positives, and more pregnancy loss than second-trimester amniocentesis, according to the review of medical studies by Dr. Murray Enkin and his coauthors in *A Guide to Effective Care in Pregnancy and Childbirth* (third edition). Because of the increased risks associated with CVS, some university obstetrics departments have stopped it altogether.

Preimplantation Diagnosis

If you are having a baby via IVF—whether it is ZIFT, GIFT, ICSI, or egg donation—you potentially have another option in terms of prenatal testing: preimplantation testing. In this case, the embryos formed from your IVF procedure can be tested for genetic abnormalities before they are implanted in your uterus. Thus, your doctor can select only the healthy embryos for implantation. Currently, this is an expensive procedure, and it is offered in only a handful of medical centers. But it is the wave of the future. Scientists speculate that the human embryo someday may be treated for illnesses and cured while still in a petri dish.

Other Tests

Doctors no longer use percutaneous umbilical cord sampling (PUBS) for diagnosing certain genetic problems as frequently as they once did. Genetic amniocentesis and CVS are often used instead.

Age-Related Chromosomal Problems

Normally, you have forty-six chromosomes in every cell—except in egg or sperm cells. Your eggs have only twenty-three chromosomes, since these will match up with the chromosomes in a sperm cell after fertilization occurs. As a result of fertilization, the twenty-three chromosomes from the sperm and the twenty-three chromosomes from the egg pair up to form a forty-six-chromosome zygote.

Chromosomes ordinarily come in pairs, but in the case of Down's and other age-related chromosome disorders, certain chromosomes form groups of three. This kind of "genetic mistake" is more likely to happen if the egg comes from a woman over thirty-five years of age. Women are born with a lifetime supply of eggs, and as these eggs get older they are likely to "make mistakes" during the pairing up of chromosomes that occurs after fertilization. Age-related chromosomal abnormalities like Down's and trisomy 18 and 13 are such "mistakes."

Trisomy 18 and 13

Down's syndrome makes up about 50 percent of the age-related chromosomal disorders, and trisomy 18 and 13—both more severe than Down's—together make up the majority of the remaining 50 percent. Trisomy 18, which occurs in 1 in 6,000 births, often involves severe heart and kidney defects and brain malformations so severe that the baby dies within the first year of life. Trisomy 13 also is rare, occurring in 1 in 5,000 births. These babies have severe disabilities including retardation, cleft palate, and heart problems, and may live about three years.

Down's Syndrome
There is no particular age at which the risk [of Down's] jumps dramatically, but rather a steady increase. For a woman at age 30, the chances are roughly 1 in 1,000, at age 35, 1 in 350, and at age 40, 1 in 100.
—Barbara Katz Rothman, *The Tentative Pregnancy: How Amniocentesis Changes the Experience of Motherhood*

* * *

Down's syndrome is caused by an "extra" chromosome in chromosome pair #21, a genetic mistake that creates cells with forty-seven instead of forty-six chromosomes. Although all babies with Down's have the same chromosome pairing problem, they do not all have the same level of retardation or physical disability.

People with Down's may be moderately retarded or severely retarded. Some graduate from high school, and some are employable as adults. Others are dependent on their families for their entire lives. People with Down's may have minor physical problems, or they may have serious heart disease. Some people with Down's syndrome have obvious physical abnormalities such as a flat nose, sloping forehead, and small stature. Some do not. Some people with Down's live relatively long lives; some die young. It is hard to predict. Even more difficult to predict is the effect of a Down's child on your life and your family's life. Some parents see their sweet-natured Down's child as a cheerful blessing; other parents may not feel so blessed as they are burdened by the costs in time, emotion, and money that can go into the care of a severely ill and retarded Down's child.

The diagnosis of Down's results in complex feelings and choices. If your baby tests positive for Down's after a diagnostic test or on a screening test, you may find it helpful to discuss your reactions and your choices with a genetic counselor who has helped other parents in similar situations.

Dr. Susan Porto counsels her patients by telling them, "There is a very wide spectrum of Down's children. Some are minimally retarded and highly educable and may lead normal lives. Others are severely retarded and need lifelong assistance. Some have major medical problems that shorten their life span." Porto explains that the degree of anatomical abnormality in a Down's baby does not determine the degree of retardation—so there is no way to predict where a Down's fetus will fall in the spectrum of retardation. Such uncertainty, of course, makes the decision all the more difficult. "As parents, you have to decide what you are able to cope with," advises Porto.

Correctable Birth Defects

Some heart, kidney, and gastrointestinal abnormalities— even severe ones—are surgically correctable after birth. The future holds possibilities such as diagnosing and curing fetuses in the womb of genetic diseases like Tay-Sach's, sickle-cell anemia, and cystic fibrosis.

Chapter 13
Coping with Pregnancy Loss

After age thirty-five, the spontaneous miscarriage rate is between 35 percent and 50 percent. Since women over thirty-five are more likely to miscarry or to lose a baby to complications than younger women, a book on late-in-life pregnancy would be incomplete without a section on pregnancy loss and how to cope with such a loss.

Statistics indicate that up to 20 percent of all pregnant women lose a pregnancy, especially an early pregnancy, through miscarriage. According to a standard textbook, Gabbe's *Obstetrics: Normal and Problem Pregnancies:* "Of clinically recognized pregnancies, 10 to 15 percent are lost. Of married women in the United States, 4 percent have experienced two fetal losses and 3 percent have experienced three or more." The numbers are even higher if you look at the rate of "subclinical pregnancies"—pregnancies that begin just after ovulation but that end within ten to fourteen days. In the case of a subclinical pregnancy, the woman might not even know that she is pregnant since the only symptoms may be a late or heavy period. Sometimes there are no symptoms at all.

Fortunately, for pregnancies that get past the first trimester, loss rates are only 1 percent in women who are confirmed by ultrasound to have a viable pregnancy at sixteen weeks.

Mourning a Pregnancy Loss

If you have lost a baby, you are not alone. Unfortunately, many women may feel alone because those close to them—husbands, partners, friends, family—may not understand the nature of their loss or know what to say to comfort them. After Rhonda miscarried at age thirty-seven, she felt that her miscarriage was a taboo subject that nobody wanted to talk about. Leda, a DES daughter, had five miscarriages due to DES-related abnormalities of her cervix and uterus. She felt that people tend to minimize miscarriage because they fail to understand the impact it may have. "People think miscarriage is like a bad flu. It's not."

When Anna miscarried at age forty-two, she told herself that the pregnancy was not meant to be. Her doctor told her, "Sometimes your body has a way of dealing with what's best for it." However, not all women find such reassuring words comforting.

Many women experience miscarriage, even if it is a very early one, as a death, and well-intended words of comfort may do little good if they fail to acknowledge the depth of a woman's grief. Unfortunately, our culture does not automatically provide women with either an acknowledgment of their grief or a formalized way for them to express it. We have few funerals or wakes for miscarried babies. For some women, the absence of ritual is appropriate, since they find it maudlin or embarrassing to commemorate their grief over a child that was never a "real" person. Other women, like Holly, feel that the absence of support and ceremony creates a void that makes the loss more difficult to bear.

Holly miscarried when she was pregnant with her second

baby. She told only her closest friends that she had miscarried. To her other friends, she simply said she was "going through a hard time," and she'd tell them about it later. It was two years later that she finally elaborated. The loss had hit Holly hard, even though she had a healthy son, a good marriage, a challenging job, and a "can do" approach to life. She also had an understanding husband and compassionate doctors who supported her throughout the miscarriage. "The two doctors were very sensitive. They said they could give me a sedative, but that I should feel my feelings. They explained what was going to happen. One of the doctors held my hand. My husband held the other hand."

But during the weeks and months following her miscarriage, Holly grieved her loss without the support of her community or the comfort of a ritual to give the death meaning. "My biggest regret is that we didn't commemorate that loss in some meaningful way," says Holly. "There is no way to mourn that loss—to plant a tree or formally acknowledge the loss. You have nothing left. Most women don't even tell people that they're pregnant."

Fortunately, Holly was able to find comfort and acknowledgment years later in a special Quaker meeting for women who had suffered losses. Many of these women, it turned out, had lost a child.

Susan gave birth to one baby but lost two. When she got pregnant the first time, she was thirty-five. She worked full-time and proceeded with life as usual. When she started feeling fatigued at work, she kept going. She knew of no other way, since she saw the pregnant women around her working through their pregnancies. In her eleventh week she began to bleed and eventually lost her baby to a placental abruption.

For Susan, the profound sadness following her miscarriage late in pregnancy had a positive side: She realized how much she wanted a child and how important it was to make the needs of her developing baby her first priority. Susan got pregnant again when she was forty and gave birth to a baby boy.

At age forty-four, Susan was pregnant again. This time, she lost her baby at nine weeks. She mourned her loss with her husband and close friends. Since Susan was a practicing Buddhist, the baby was given a Buddhist funeral. She found solace in giving the baby a ceremony to honor it. She felt that having a memorial helped her say good-by.

Susan encourages other women to allow themselves to mourn and to commemorate the loss:

"The best thing you can do is to let yourself mourn it. It helped me a lot to have a memorial, to give the baby a name, to give it a place, and to give it a figure and a stone and a place to be remembered and a ceremony. The ceremony was a real closure. It wasn't an end but a way to do honor. I guess that is what memorials are—a way of saying good-by."

To help women say good-by to miscarried or stillborn babies, many caregivers encourage their patients to hold a funeral. In the case of a stillborn baby or a baby that is unlikely to survive, caregivers often suggest that parents hold and touch the baby. Both the physical contact and the ceremony provide more closure for grieving parents and help them cope with the loss.

Experts say that women who lose a pregnancy go through the same emotional process as anyone experiencing a death—denial, anger, guilt, grief, bargaining, and acceptance—because the emotional investment in pregnancy, even in its early stages, is great. Consequently, caregivers often encourage grieving parents to join bereavement groups to help them cope with their feelings. (See appendix for support groups.)

Your Next Pregnancy

Experts say it is important for women to deal with the feelings elicited by miscarriage before they get pregnant again, so that they don't end up frozen in fear during a subsequent pregnancy or haunted by unresolved anger or guilt.

Preventing Miscarriage

"I learned that if I wanted to have a child, I had to devote myself to that child—even in utero," says Susan, who focused on nourishing her developing baby by eating well, drinking enough water, getting plenty of rest, and avoiding stress.

In addition to these basics, you can help protect your pregnancy by:

- Getting good and appropriate prenatal care (e.g., seeing a high-risk pregnancy specialist if you are high risk)
- Calling your doctor immediately in the event of vaginal bleeding, abdominal pain, or any other unusual symptoms
- Controlling your diabetes or high blood pressure
- Avoiding environmental and occupational toxins known to cause miscarriage
- Avoiding extremes of temperature and altitude
- Exercising moderately but not excessively
- Modifying your work routine to accommodate your pregnancy needs
- Avoiding smoking

When you are pregnant, you need more rest than usual, because growing a baby is hard physiological work. To give yourself the best chance for maintaining a healthy pregnancy, avoid long shifts in stressful environments, hard physical labor, or long hours on your feet. If you feel fatigued, take time to rest—even if you are in the middle of a workday.

Unfortunately, some miscarriages are not preventable because they are due to chromosomal abnormalities, and no amount of nourishment or rest can change a chromosomal problem.

Bed Rest

Susan's doctor put her on bed rest when she developed a placental abruption during her pregnancy. Since she had miscarried a previous baby, and she was willing to do anything to save her pregnancy. "I spent seven months on bed rest. We did everything—everything—to let this child be born. And he was. I remember that time as being a very quiet, meditative, preparatory time. It took me two or three months to get to the point where I really accepted it. I realized that if I wanted a child, I had to put aside everything else," remembers Susan.

"For the first two or three months my biggest difficulty was wrestling with guilt. I thought, 'Thousands of women have babies, but who's lying in bed all day?' However, I knew that if I wanted a baby, I had to be totally responsible. I was reading a lot, and I was devoting myself to prepare for this child. Life took on a different rhythm and a different pace." Susan gave birth to her son when he was thirty-six weeks gestational age.

Bed rest was once the standard "treatment" for a pregnancy in danger of miscarriage, but nowadays doctors do not recommend it as frequently. However, your care provider may recommend strict bed rest or "minimal activity" if you are at risk of miscarrying due to bleeding, placental problems, degenerating fibroid tumors, incompetent cervix, pregnancy with multiples, high blood pressure, and some other problems.

If you are resting in bed, do not lie on your back for long

periods of time, since in many cases this can decrease blood flow to your baby. Lie on your side, and change positions from time to time. (For more detailed information on bed rest, see Part 6.)

Causes of Miscarriage

Chromosomal Abnormalities

"Most miscarriages are due to a faulty egg where the chromosomes are wrong. Nothing is going to change that," says Dr. Allen Killam. Fifty percent of all miscarriages are due to chromosomal abnormalities, especially if the miscarriage occurs within the first trimester. Sometimes the egg simply doesn't fertilize properly, a condition known as a blighted embryo. These are the kinds of pregnancies that some caregivers describe as "nature's way" of taking away babies that aren't meant to be. Of course, even though a genetic reason for miscarriage may explain why your pregnancy didn't take—and may represent a fluke of nature that may not happen again—it doesn't take away your sadness.

LPD

In summary, LPD [luteal phase defect] probably exists, but it is far less common than once believed. . . . Treatment should be initiated only if the diagnosis is firmly established, and only if couples are apprised of the unfounded claims of progesterone teratogenicity. Patients should probably be informed that therapeutic efficacy is unproved.
—Dr. Joe Leigh Simpson in Gabbe, *Obstetrics: Normal and Problem Pregnancies*

❋ ❋ ❋

Once LPD was well accepted as a cause for miscarriage, but this is no longer the case. "LPD seems to be considered an uncommon cause [of early miscarriage]," writes Dr. Joe Leigh Simpson in his chapter of the medical textbook *Obstetrics: Normal and Problem Pregnancies.* Furthermore, says Simpson, there are no randomized studies verifying the efficacy of treatment for LPD with the hormone progesterone.

However, many obstetricians believe that an inadequate luteal phase may be responsible for miscarriage in some women, especially in women over thirty-five who have decreasing progesterone levels. A luteal phase defect may also be caused by decreasing levels of progesterone in the corpus luteum—the ovarian follicle from which the egg emerges. The corpus luteum remains on the ovary and secretes progesterone until the implanted embryo can produce enough progesterone to maintain the pregnancy—around five weeks after conception. However, the amount of progesterone it produces varies. In a woman with luteal phase defect, some theorize, the lining of her uterus (the endometrium) may not be prepared sufficiently for the implantation of an embryo due to this progesterone deficiency. Consequently, the treatment for LPD has been the hormone progesterone taken in vaginal gel or suppositories.

Those who do not support the common existence of LPD point to the fact that some women who have lower-than-normal progesterone levels get pregnant and successfully maintain their pregnancies without needing progesterone treatment.

If you are diagnosed with luteal phase defect, you face a difficult decision—whether or not to take progesterone therapy. Although progesterone is a naturally occurring hormone, some researchers believe that it may pose some risks to the baby (see Chapter 7). Some researchers believe the drug is safe, that it treats a true luteal phase defect, but that it does not work effectively to prevent miscarriage. Discuss your individual medical circumstances with your caregivers to help you arrive at a decision.

Diabetes Mellitus

Women with poorly controlled diabetes are at an increased risk of miscarriage, particularly of early pregnancy loss. If you have diabetes, get your condition under control before becoming pregnant and carefully stick to your treatment plan once you are pregnant. If you have GD, you are not at increased risk of early pregnancy loss.

Thyroid Disease

Thyroid disease—either hyperthyroidism or hypothyroidism—has been associated with decreased conception rates and increased miscarriage rates. Some doctors run thyroid blood tests as part of a medical workup in women over thirty-five who wish to become pregnant, in order to screen for and treat this disorder.

Maternal Infection

Some infections may cause miscarriage. Chlamydia trachomatis, ureaplasma urealyticum, typhoid, toxoplasmosis, and malaria have been known to cause miscarriages, although chlamydia and ureaplasma are the most common causes.

Incompetent Cervix

If you have a weakened or shortened cervix or have had prior cervical surgery, you may have what is called an incompetent cervix—one that can't remain closed for the duration of pregnancy. Your cervix may be weakened from previous abortions, from birth injury, from prenatal exposure to DES, or if you have had a cone (a slice of cervical tissue) removed due to cervical cancer—circumstances more common in women over thirty-five than in younger women. Consequently, your cervix may start to dilate during your second or third trimester and your water may break prematurely, placing you at risk for miscarriage or delivering early.

To prevent your cervix from dilating, your doctor can put in a *cerclage*. A cerclage is a purse-string type suture placed in the cervix in order to prevent further dilation. Some doctors recommend strict bed rest to prevent miscarriage in women with an incompetent cervix in order to prevent gravity from pressing the baby against an already weakened cervix.

Placental Insufficiency

High blood pressure, smoking, cocaine use, heart disease, asthma, chronic lung disease, and severe diabetes that involves the circulatory system can increase your risk of placental insufficiency—a condition in which the baby's placenta doesn't provide it with adequate oxygen and nourishment due to limited blood flow. If the blood flow to the baby is not restored, the baby may not grow or you may miscarry.

You can improve placental efficiency by taking care of the hypertension or diabetes and/or by bed rest. Bed rest, under these circumstances, may involve lying on your left side—an optimal position for placental-fetal blood flow. (See the section on bed rest in Part 6.)

Smoking

If you smoke during pregnancy, you face increased risks of miscarriage.

Environmental Chemicals

Chemicals associated with miscarriage are anesthetic gases, arsenic, aniline dyes, solvents, benzene, ethylene oxide, formaldehyde, some pesticides, lead, mercury, and cadmium. If you have come into contact with any of these chemicals or suspect that you have, talk to your caregiver. If you encounter these chemicals at work, discuss with your employer the importance of limiting your contact during pregnancy.

Exposure to high-dose radiation and chemotherapy may also cause miscarriage.

Maternal Illness

If you have a life-threatening disease, your miscarriage risk may be increased by the presence of your illness. Discuss your individual circumstances and options with your caregivers.

Uterine Fibroids

Fibroid tumors rarely cause miscarriage. If fibroids do cause miscarriage, it is due to their location—not necessarily their size. Submucosal fibroids, the kind of fibroid most likely to cause miscarriage, are tumors that lie just beneath the endometrium, or lining of the uterus. These tumors may cause a thinning of the endometrium, which prevents secure implantation of the embryo. Miscarriage may result.

If your fibroids grow during pregnancy (and not all of them do) and if they lie close to your uterine cavity or protrude into the cavity, the fibroid(s) can impinge upon the cavity of your uterus and reduce the space required by your developing baby. This can result in late pregnancy loss or early delivery of the baby. A fibroid can also grow so rapidly that it competes with the baby for its blood supply, which may also result in miscarriage.

Many physicians recommend that your fibroids be removed only if they cause repeated miscarriage or chronic bleeding and anemia, since women can have successful pregnancies despite the presence of numerous or large fibroids.

Immune System Problems

Various immune and autoimmune conditions may interfere with pregnancy and cause miscarriage, although these conditions are complicated and many of them are not well understood. If you are Rh-negative or have lupus erythematosus or any other rheumatoid or connective tissue disease, consult your doctor about possible effects on the baby. Other immune system problems may contribute to miscarriage, although the "immune therapies" are still controversial.

Part Six

Pregnancy with Twins, Triplets, and More

Chapter 14
The Ups and Downs of Pregnancy, Birth, and Parenthood with Multiples

Twins and triplets have been the subject of fascination since ancient times, and multiple births have often been viewed as special, magical—even divine.

Although we no longer think of twins as divine, we still view pregnancy with twins or triplets as special, though it has become increasingly common over the last decade. With the increased use of ovulation-induction drugs and assisted reproduction, pregnancy with twins, triplets, and high-order multiples (now called triplet/+) has increased exponentially—especially in women over thirty.

Such abundance may be exciting at first, although giving birth to four or more babies may be risky for mothers and babies and may bring medical, financial, and emotional burdens.

This chapter addresses the ups and downs of pregnancy, birth, and motherhood with multiples—especially twins. It draws from the experience of parents and physicians in order to help you choose an appropriate care provider, make informed choices regarding your medical and childbirth options, learn strategies for nursing and bonding with your babies whether they are premature or full term, and meet the challenges of a very special kind of motherhood.

Who Has Twins and High-Order Multiples?

Women over thirty-five having a pregnancy using the assisted reproductive technologies ought to prepare themselves for pregnancy with multiples.
—Dr. Louis Keith, Professor of Obstetrics at Northwestern University and expert in pregnancy with twins

❋ ❋ ❋

Currently, women in their thirties, forties, and fifties have the highest multiple birth rates in the United States. According to the *National Vital Statistics Reports'* final birth statistics for 1998, "multiple birth rates rise with increasing maternal age until age group 35–39 years, dip slightly for women aged 40–44 years, and then peak sharply for women aged 45–54 years. This is a change from earlier years when rates were highest among women aged 35–39 years."

Even before fertility treatments such as ovulation induction, IVF, and egg donation became popular, women in their late thirties conceived twins more frequently than younger women due to midlife hormonal changes that cause the release of two eggs, instead of one, during a menstrual cycle. But twins were still not the norm for women aged thirty-five and over, and triplets and quadruplets were rare. All that has changed dramatically since the early 1980s as treatments for infertility have become increasingly popular. In the last two decades, the rates of multiple births have skyrocketed: The twin birth rate has risen 49 percent and the triplet and triplet/+ birth rate has risen 423 percent. Most surprising has been the increase in multiple births to women over forty-five. By 1998, one in every six babies born to women forty-five to fifty-nine years of age, and one in every three babies born to women fifty to fifty-four years of age, was born in a multiple delivery, according to national health statistics reports. In 1999, twin births continued to rise, although the triplet/+ births declined.

Most doctors are uncomfortable with the increased rate of multiples, especially triplets, quadruplets, or more, since such pregnancies pose risks to both mother and babies. To prevent pregnancies with triplets or more, many infertility specialists now transfer fewer embryos during IVF and egg donation procedures, and they closely monitor and control ovulation induction therapy. This more conservative approach to assisted reproduction contributed to decreases in the rate of triplet/+ births in 1999.

Figure 14-1. Numbers of twin, triplet, quadruplet, and quintuplet and other higher-order multiple births: United States, 1989–1999

Year	Twins	Triplets	Quadruplets	Quintuplets & other higher order multiples[1]
1999	114,307	6,742	512	67
1998	110,670	6,919	627	79
1997	104,137	6,148	510	79
1996	100,750	5,298	560	81
1995	96,736	4,551	365	57
1994	97,064	4,233	315	46
1993	96,445	3,834	277	57
1992	95,372	3,547	310	26
1991	94,779	3,121	203	22
1990	93,865	2,830	185	13
1989	90,118	2,529	229	40

[1]Quintuplets, sextuplets, and higher-order multiple births are not differentiated in the national data set.

The number of multiple births has been escalating rapidly since 1989. However, there was an overall decline in triplet/+ births in 1999.

From: Births: Final Data for 1999, *National Vital Statistics Reports*, Volume 49, Number 1, April 17, 2001 (from the Centers for Disease Control and Prevention, National Center for Health Statistics, National Vital Statistics System).

Types of Twins

There are two kinds of twins, identical and fraternal. Identical twins are *monozygotic* since they result from the fertilization of one egg by one sperm. The resulting zygote (fertilized egg), by some quirk in the fertilization process, divides into two genetically identical parts and then splits in half. The two halves subsequently become genetically identical babies.

Fraternal twins are *dizygotic* since they come from two genetically different zygotes that develop from two eggs and two sperm. Dizygotic twins are associated with ovulation-induction drugs, race, and age. Most of the twins conceived as a result of ovulation-induction drugs (which push the ovaries to produce many eggs instead of just one per menstrual cycle) are fraternal twins. Black women have twins more often than white women, and a Nigerian group called the Yorubas have a frequency of 45 twins per 1,000 births; most of these are fraternal twins. Maternal age also influences a woman's odds for conceiving fraternal twins; women aged thirty-five to forty have a much higher rate of fraternal twins than women under age twenty.

Expecting Multiples

My doctor said that I should transfer three fertilized eggs [in an IVF procedure] and that there was a 10 percent chance of all three fertilizing and a 30 percent chance of two fertilizing. At

first, all three fertilized. After that, having twins didn't freak us out so much.
—Sharon's third embryo never developed, leaving her with twins.

* * *

I was absolutely thrilled when we had the ultrasound. It was one baby—yeah! Two babies—yeah! We were glad it wasn't three. I was excited to have two: two for the price of one.
—Stacy, at twenty-eight, conceived twins after an IVF procedure.

* * *

Although some women share Stacy's glee with a twin pregnancy, many women and their partners are unnerved and overwhelmed by the news that they are expecting two or more babies since few parents plan to become pregnant with multiples. There is even a name for this state of surprise—twinshock.

For women expecting triplets or more, the news may be even more overwhelming.

If you are pregnant with twins, triplets, or higher-order multiples, you may feel overcome by fearful visions of the near and distant future, asking yourself: "How can I cope with the effort of carrying and birthing two babies? How can I return to work with two infants at home? How can I afford not to work, since the financial responsibilities will be great? Will this pregnancy be risky for the babies and me? Will I need a cesarean section? Will my babies spend weeks in a preemie nursery? Will I be able to breastfeed? How will I care for my other children?" These are common fears that haunt women pregnant with multiples.

On the bright side, pregnancy with twins is a fascinating experience. You may feel fertile and full of life. You will have the excitement of two babies who interact with one another as they move within your womb. Your pregnancy will "show" sooner, and people will respond to you as a pregnant woman early on. There is something special and compelling about a woman pregnant with twins, and people you barely know may become interested in your pregnancy and may offer to help. After the babies are born, you will have two or more babies—an entire family—from only one pregnancy.

Other benefits to having twins or triplets are that your children will always have playmates their own age. After the babies are born you will have the unique experience of watching twins bond with one another. "They're individuals who are born with a really special relationship to each other. It seems like they communicate really well—they look at each other and crack up. They amuse each other when they're playing," says Sharon, who has watched with fascination as her girls developed their relationship as babies and now as toddlers.

Although getting pregnant with more than one baby may seem like a time-efficient way of having your whole family all at once, more is not necessarily better. Pregnancy with multiples carries with it inherent risks for mother and babies. Mothers of multiples—even young mothers—are more likely to miscarry and are more susceptible to high blood pressure, gestational diabetes, and other pregnancy-related medical problems; more likely to end up in bed during their last weeks of pregnancy; and more apt to undergo cesarean section due to breech or transverse presentation of one of the babies.

The babies, especially in the case of triplet/+, face higher risks of low birth weight, prematurity, and death. Some of these babies spend their first weeks or months in intensive care nurseries relying on respirators until their lungs are sufficiently developed to function on their own.

Special Preparations

Women pregnant with twins or multiple babies need special preparation for pregnancy, birth, breastfeeding, and early motherhood. Since your babies may be premature, it is best to start preparing earlier than you would with a single baby. Find a childbirth preparation class that caters to mothers expecting multiples or that includes preparation for cesarean section. Although you may not require a cesarean, your odds for having a cesarean section are increased if you are pregnant with multiples. Some doctors will deliver twins vaginally (if the first baby is in the vertex or head-down position); others will not. Most doctors will opt for cesarean section in the case of triplets or more. Consequently, your needs as a woman pregnant with multiples will be best served by a class that prepares you for cesarean surgery and for the recovery period that follows.

Join a mothers of twins club and go to meetings *before* you give birth. Hearing the stories—and the coping strategies—of women who gave birth to multiples may help you formulate plans for child care, returning to work, remaining at home, and so forth. Such groups may provide you with lasting friendships and a support system that offers everything from advice to used baby clothes. If you intend to breastfeed your babies, attend a La Leche League meeting before you give birth to get contacts to call during your first weeks (or months) of breastfeeding. La Leche League is a group that teaches women breastfeeding techniques and offers a twenty-four-hour help line to women to guide them through whatever problems they might encounter. Breastfeeding twins and multiples is a challenge that may require some coaching from a La Leche League member or a lactation consultant (see Chapter 21).

Preparing for two or more babies also means eating for two or more. Consequently, you need to eat well and get enough proteins, carbohydrates, calcium, and iron for growing healthy babies. Some experts recommend a daily intake of 4,000 calories and 140 to 150 grams of protein for a twin pregnancy. Although opinion on the ideal pregnancy diet differs greatly, many experts agree that a mother of twins should gain from forty to fifty pounds, mothers of triplets fifty to sixty pounds, and mothers of quads sixty-five to eighty pounds. In *When You're Expecting Twins, Triplets, or Quads,* Dr. Barbara Luke, registered dietician and Professor of Obstetrics at the University of Michigan, recommends that mothers of multiples eat three meals a day plus four substantial snacks. For Dr. Luke, a snack is a mini-meal such as cereal with milk and bananas, a sandwich, macaroni and cheese, or peanut butter on whole grain bread or crackers.

Get a variety of nutrients that includes the basics:

1. *Carbohydrates*: fresh fruit and vegetables, whole grains
2. *Protein*: fish, fowl, milk, meat, eggs, soybeans, lentils, split peas, black-eyed peas, seeds/nuts, tofu
3. *Fats and oils*: especially soy, olive, and other vegetable oils
4. *Fluids*: water (eight large glasses or more) plus other beverages
5. *Minerals:* calcium and iron

Since twins and multiples put a greater strain on your legs, feet, back, and abdominal muscles than a single baby, you need to maintain or increase your muscle tone and to enhance your circulation with mild exercise (see Chapter 9).

Choosing a Doctor

The most important step you can take to minimize risk is to select a doctor experienced enough to anticipate these potential

problems [of multiple pregnancy], detect them early, and treat them in the best way possible.
—Dr. Barbara Luke and Tamara Eberlein, *When You're Expecting Twins, Triplets, or Quads*

❖ ❖ ❖

If a woman is having multiples, she should look for a higher standard of prenatal care from a doctor who understands multiple pregnancy.
—Dr. Louis Keith

❖ ❖ ❖

Women pregnant with multiples should take special care in choosing a doctor who has enough experience with multiple pregnancies to detect and treat potential problems. You need a doctor who is willing to monitor you closely for problems that may arise (preeclampsia, gestational diabetes, premature labor, breech presentation, growth discordance, and the rare but serious twin to twin transfusion syndrome (TTTS), who has seen many women through pregnancy and birth with multiples, and who is sufficiently comfortable with multiple births to reassure you.

Most (but not all) doctors will perform cesarean sections for triplet deliveries, and some prefer to deliver twins by cesarean section. If you are pregnant with multiples and interested in a vaginal birth, shop for a doctor who is skilled in delivering multiples and in performing breech delivery and external or internal cephalic version—a procedure in which the doctor turns a *breech* (bottom-first) baby to a *vertex* (headfirst) position (see Chapter 29).

Some doctors will deliver vaginally a second breech twin, but many doctors will perform a cesarean section if the first twin is breech or *transverse* (lying on its side). You may not easily find a doctor who is willing to do a vaginal breech delivery, since many doctors have been trained to do cesarean, not vaginal, delivery of breech babies (see Chapter 29). The mode of delivery of breech twins is controversial, and there is not one "right way" of delivering twins. Medical texts suggest either vaginal or cesarean delivery of second breech twins, depending on your particular situation and the skills and training of your particular physician.

Do not press a doctor to perform a kind of delivery that she or he is not comfortable doing. If you want to find a doctor willing and able to deliver vaginally, call a nearby medical school for a referral or call some of the doctors in your area who trained as obstetricians in the 1960s or 1970s, and discuss with them their approach to multiple births. It is possible that most of the doctors you contact deliver multiples by cesarean, and you may require a cesarean birth anyway—especially if the first baby is breech or in another awkward position.

When you choose a doctor, it is important to consider the hospital with which your doctor is associated. If you are expecting multiples, choose a doctor who can admit patients to a hospital with a neonatal intensive care nursery (sometimes referred to as an NICU). NICUs are categorized as Level I, Level II, or Level III according to their ability to deal with the special needs of very premature babies. A Level III nursery (often associated with a university medical center) is equipped to care for the smallest preemies, who may need considerable support for breathing and feeding. A Level II nursery can accommodate some of the feeding and breathing needs of a preemie but does not have the sophisticated equipment of a Level III hospital. Level I nurseries, offered by most small, community hospitals, are designed to manage uncomplicated births. If your town has a community hospital but not an NICU, the hospital may take premature babies to a nearby NICU by ambulance or helicopter.

If you are pregnant with triplets or triplet/+, it is to your advantage to choose a hospital with a Level III nursery, since high-order multiples frequently are premature. Otherwise, if your preemies need special care, they may be transferred to a Level III hospital after birth, potentially placing you and your babies in different hospitals. You can always request to be transferred with your babies should the need arise, but the transfer will depend upon whether there is an available bed for you.

If you live in a small town with a community hospital, your baby should be taken to a NICU in a nearby town if the baby requires special care.

At Work and Pregnant with Multiples

I was huge. I would be sitting in meetings at work, and I would watch some men just staring at my belly. I was working twelve-hour days. In the beginning, I would wear very professional clothes. Later, I was wearing stretch pants and Birkenstocks. The bad thing about carrying twins, you end up having swollen feet.
—Stacy

* * *

Carrying multiple babies does not necessarily mean that you need to stop working, but it does mean that you need to use good judgment about how much energy you expend at work and how much stress and strain you are exposed to. Remember that working stressful twelve-hour days when you are pregnant with multiples has different consequences than working twelve-hour days when you are not pregnant or are pregnant with only one baby. Try to construct a pregnancy/work strategy that allows you to do your job without jeopardizing the growth and health of your babies. If you are tired, set aside time for rest breaks each day and take them no matter what: lie down on the office floor, relax in your chair with your feet up, stretch out on a couch in the break room, or bring a fold-up cot to the rest room. You may wish to job share or to take an early pregnancy leave if your job is extremely physically demanding. If your job requires lifting or long hours on your feet, ask your doctor about how to best fit your work to your pregnancy.

Women who work at stressful jobs when they are pregnant with multiples increase their risk of premature delivery, says Dr. Barbara Luke, an expert on multiple pregnancy. In their book, *When You're Expecting Twins, Triplets, or Quads*, Dr. Barbara Luke and Tamara Eberlein write:

Those [women] who work in physically and/or emotionally stressful jobs, studies show, are two to three times as likely to deliver prematurely. Most at risk are nurses, doctors, saleswomen, cleaning staff, assembly line workers, and military personnel; people who work with chemicals, vibrating machines, or in a cold, noisy or wet environment; anyone who works a rotating shift; and any woman who puts in more than 45 hours per week.

Consequently, it is important to limit unnecessary sources of fatigue and stress when you are pregnant with multiples and at higher risk for premature labor. Limit your time standing at work to no more than one or two hours at a time, depending on your stage of pregnancy and your health. Discuss a reasonable work plan with your care provider, since you may need to modify your work activity even more if you are at high risk for premature labor or high blood pressure. Avoid physical exertion that brings on uterine contractions. If you experience uterine contractions or a backache at work, lie down on your side immediately and call your care provider: You may be having preterm labor.

Some care providers suggest that women pregnant with multiples cut back on work hours and take a leave from work between the twenty-fourth and twenty-eighth week of pregnancy if at all possible.

If you cannot take a leave, either cut back on your hours or take rest breaks during the day.

Preventing and Managing Preterm Labor

I caution women who are pregnant with twins that they are at more risk of preterm labor—and they have to be more conscious when deciding what is a contraction and what is not.
—Dr. Susan Porto

◦ ◦ ◦

The girls were born premature. They were born at three pounds each. My water broke eight weeks before my due date. I was in bed in the hospital and stayed still for five days. Then I went into labor.
—Sharon

◦ ◦ ◦

Many women pregnant with twins and triplets have healthy, full-term pregnancies. For instance, Dion, at age forty-five, delivered two robust—and full-term—boys. However, her doctors monitored her closely for preterm labor, just to be on the safe side: They wanted to detect any potential problem early enough to manage it. Dion also learned the subtle warning signs and symptoms of premature labor so that she could seek medical assistance if necessary.

Although you cannot always prevent premature labor or delivery, some experts believe that you may decrease your babies' risks of prematurity by drinking enough fluids, eating well, avoiding excessive stress, and getting enough rest. To decrease your risk of premature labor, incorporate the following into your daily schedule:

1. Drink fluids and stay hydrated.
2. Eat nutritious meals.
3. Engage in at least one relaxing activity per day (swimming, reading, meditation, listening to music).
4. Get enough rest.
5. Avoid excess physical and emotional stress.
6. Keep diabetes or high blood pressure under control.
7. Avoid physical strain.
8. Monitor your baby with a home monitor (if appropriate during your pregnancy) and maintain sufficient contact with your care provider.
9. Learn the signs of premature labor and promptly call your doctor if they occur.

Some experts on multiple birth say that good nutrition, adequate rest, and adequate fluid intake are essential in preventing preterm or low birth weight babies.

Recognizing Symptoms and Seeking Treatment

Unfortunately, many mothers of twins and almost all mothers of supertwins cannot detect contractions at all. . . . It is better to check with your doctor when in doubt (and don't be put off with "You're just carrying twins—of course it's a bit uncomfortable") rather than waiting until it is too late and labor is established.
—Elizabeth Noble, *Having Twins*

The symptoms of preterm labor in a pregnancy with multiples may be so subtle that you do not recognize them. Your uterus may be so stretched that the contractions do not feel the way they might have felt with a previous singleton pregnancy.

The Subtle Signs of Preterm Labor

1. Menstrual-like cramps that are constant or rhythmic
2. Rhythmic or constant pressure that may extend to your thighs
3. Regular contractions (painless or painful) occurring every fifteen minutes or fewer that make the uterus tighten, harden, and become globular in shape
4. Gas pains, diarrhea
5. Vaginal discharge of mucous, blood, or waterlike fluid
6. Low backache—continuous or coming and going—that may extend to your sides or front
7. A feeling that something is "different" or not quite right

If you have any of the symptoms of premature labor, call your doctor. If you do not reach your doctor, call his or her partner or go to an emergency room. Plan a just-in-case premature labor scenario with your doctor and decide upon the appropriate hospital for you.

If your premature labor is diagnosed early enough, it sometimes can be stopped in order to give your babies more time to develop in your womb. Possible treatments for preterm labor include drugs that relax the uterine muscle and stop contractions (these are most effective if administered before labor is well established), rest, and increased fluid intake.

Home Monitoring

Sometimes your doctor will give you a home monitor in order to keep track of your contractions and your babies' well-being. You will strap on the monitor for a given period of time and then transmit the information by phone to the doctor. Home monitoring may help you know when it is time to go to the hospital—and whether or not you should have your babies at a hospital with a NICU.

Bed Rest

If you develop complications of pregnancy that could jeopardize your health or your babies' health, your doctor may recommend *strict bed rest* either at home or in the hospital. Although bed rest was once widely recommended to prevent miscarriage and preterm labor in women pregnant with multiples, nowadays doctors do not recommend it as frequently. For some pregnancy complications that are not severe, your doctor may recommend "limited activity" at home rather than strict bed rest. Bed rest is not a cure-all, and it is not without risks. A woman on strict bed rest has an increased risk of developing *deep vein thrombosis* in her legs—a condition that may lead to serious blood clots. For a pregnancy with multiples, many doctors believe the safest approach is to increase your periods of rest and to resort to strict bed rest only if your care provider recommends it. Talk to your care provider about the best ways to prevent preterm labor given your individual circumstances.

If you are put on bed rest, it is important to know that staying in bed all day may create stress or depression. To keep your spirits up, bring all the things you need to entertain yourself or relax within easy reach of your bed. Create as positive and aesthetically pleasing an environment as possible. Bring in supplies such as:

- Favorite photos or pictures
- Stacks of engrossing books and magazines
- Television (sign up for interesting cable channels)
- A telephone—and a list of phone numbers of bed-rest support groups you can call if you get too restless (see appendix)
- Your favorite music on CD, tape, or radio
- Relaxation tapes
- A laptop for work, school, or surfing the Net
- Cards and letter-writing materials
- Crayons, coloring books, pastels
- Knitting
- Crossword puzzles
- Games
- Favorite fragrances or massage oils
- Comfortable lounging clothes that are not pajamas
- Healthy snacks, drinks, water

Invite your friends over to visit you to avoid isolation and the doldrums that come with being cut off from friends, coworkers, and family. If you have children, bring some of your children's toys into your room in order to create a family environment—or set up shop in the living room or den where you can rest but still feel a part of your household. To stay productive, bring a laptop computer to bed: catch up on work, write that master's thesis, join a chat group, or shop online.

When you are in bed, you need to keep your limbs moving—and your feet circling—in order to maintain good blood circulation and muscle tone. It may be helpful to meet with a physical therapist who specializes in pregnancy-related issues and is familiar with bed rest and safe bed exercise. An occasional massage from your partner or a professional may help relieve stiff muscles and promote circulation and tone.

If you are single, bed rest may force you to call on all your resources—friends, family, acquaintances, church groups, or members of La Leche League or Mothers of Twins. You will need to invite—or hire—someone to stay with you or go to stay with friends or family. Strict bed rest is extremely difficult if you are alone. With a flexible bed-rest routine, you may be able to get by on your own, but talk to your care provider before you embark on solo bed rest.

Doctors sometimes recommend partial bed rest or limited activity. If your doctor makes such a recommendation, you may find yourself wanting to negotiate for more time being upright. Stick to your doctor's prescription, even if it causes you temporary frustration and loss of time at work. This is your only time to grow your babies, and you can return to work after the babies are born.

Risks for Mothers

Every multiple pregnancy is a high-risk pregnancy.
—Dr. Louis Keith

* * *

This is a high-risk situation no matter what. But we had a woman who, at age fifty-one, delivered triplets. She did well.
—Dr. Mark Sauer

* * *

Pregnancy with multiples may be considered higher risk than pregnancy with singletons, but you can still have a healthy pregnancy—even if you are well into midlife. However, when you are pregnant with two or more babies, your risks of the complications of pregnancy go up. You are at higher risk for anemia, pregnancy-induced hypertension, preeclampsia, gestational diabetes, placental problems, and pregnancy loss. Fortunately, many of these problems can be treated or at least managed. Anemia, a lack of iron in your blood, can be treated with iron tablets or by eating iron-rich foods. Gestational diabetes can be controlled with diet or insulin or both, and it usually disappears after the babies are born.

Preeclampsia, a syndrome that involves high blood pressure accompanied with protein in the urine and swelling of the hands and feet, develops more frequently in women pregnant with multiples than in women pregnant with one baby. "There is a 40 percent risk of preeclampsia in first-time mothers. With each additional fetus that risk expands," explains Dr. Allen Killam. Preeclampsia usually can be managed with rest or, if necessary, with the delivery of the baby. If preeclampsia turns into eclampsia, the resulting problems may be treated with medications, although the only real cure is delivery of the baby. Eclampsia is a very rare but dangerous condition (see "Possible Complications of Midlife Pregnancy" in Chapter 11).

A pregnancy with multiples is three times more likely than a pregnancy with a singleton to result in placental abruption— a situation in which the placenta separates from the uterine wall and causes bleeding; this bleeding may endanger both the mother and the baby if the baby isn't delivered immediately (usually by cesarean section). However, if the abruption is small, the bleeding may stop, and an immediate cesarean may not be necessary.

Call your doctor immediately if you start bleeding during pregnancy. If you start bleeding after office hours, call your doctor, the obstetrician covering for your doctor, or the hospital emergency department.

Women pregnant with two or more babies also are more prone to get some of the minor, yet annoying, problems: varicose veins, hemorrhoids, heartburn, mild shortness of breath, swollen feet and legs. For varicose veins and swelling, the usual remedies apply: wear support hose, don't spend long hours on your feet, elevate your legs when possible, and do ankle circles to increase circulation. Heartburn may be eased by mild foods and crackers. Mild shortness of breath will go away after the baby is born. However, for sudden or troublesome shortness of breath, call your doctor immediately, call 911, or go to the nearest emergency room.

Risks for Babies

With twins there is five times the perinatal mortality rate as singletons; the rate is 1 percent in singletons and 5 percent in twins.
—Dr. Katherine Shaw

* * *

Prematurity is the greatest risk for twins, triplets, and higher-order multiples. Fifty percent of twins are born preterm.
—Dr. Louis Keith

* * *

The older preemies, born at thirty-six weeks or even at thirty-three or thirty-four weeks, often do well. In fact, thirty-six weeks gestational age is often considered "normal" for twins, and many of these babies do very well. Discuss your babies' gestational age and well-being with an obstetrician who has extensive experience with multiple gestations.

The younger the baby, however, the greater its risk of various handicaps such as cerebral palsy, blindness, deafness, and developmental disabilities. Nowadays, babies may survive at twenty-five or twenty-six weeks old, but they are at risk for handicaps and developmental problems. Due to stunning advances in neonatal medicine, some very premature babies may survive and flourish, although there is often a price to pay in daily anxiety as the baby (and thus the parent) faces various crises due to respiratory distress or other problems. Very premature babies may have underdeveloped lungs or gastrointestinal tracts and are at risk for numerous medical problems until their bodies develop with time—and a lot of support from medical technology.

Because current neonatal medicine can do extraordinary things to simulate the nurturing environment of the womb, many very premature babies who would not have survived ten years ago can now grow up to be healthy "veterans" of NICUs. Some do not survive, especially if they are extremely premature.

Even if they are only slightly premature, multiples tend to have lower birth weights than singleton babies. To some extent, it is "normal" for multiples to be low birth weight, although the lower the weight, the greater the potential risks for the baby.

Other possible complications for multiples develop when one baby grows larger than the other. This condition is called growth discordance, and it complicates 15 to 30 percent of twin pregnancies. TTTS (Twin-Twin Transfusion Syndrome), a serious complication, occurs in about 5 to 10 percent of twin pregnancies when the placenta is shared by identical twins. In this syndrome, the twins share their circulation through blood vessels in the placenta, and one baby develops at the expense of the other. Fortunately, the transfusion syndrome does not occur frequently, says Dr. Susan Porto. "In ten years of practice, I've seen four cases of bona fide twin-twin transfusion syndrome, and I've taken care of a lot of twins."

High-Order Multiples: A Lifeboat Scenario

It's totally unrealistic to think you'll end up with seven live babies. . . . Statistics favor selective reduction at four or more

[quadruplets or more]. You don't reduce triplets, because there is a 12 percent risk of losing the other babies.
—Dr. Allen Killam

* * *

Although premature twins and triplets stand a good chance of surviving and growing into healthy children, quadruplets and quintuplets may endanger one another, resulting in what embryologist Stan Beyler calls a "lifeboat scenario." Mothers and fathers of high-order multiples may face a heart-wrenching dilemma: whether to continue the pregnancy and risk the lives of some or all of the babies or "reduce down to twins" early on by aborting one or more of the fetuses. This scenario has prompted many infertility specialists to transfer fewer embryos from the "test tube" to the womb—three instead of four or five—in order to avoid the disquieting and controversial possibility of "reducing down."

Birthing Multiples

I gave birth to both twins vaginally. The babies were both head-first. The labor wasn't bad at all. I had been having contractions for a while, but I didn't realize they were contractions. I went into the hospital when the contractions were six minutes apart. I had a ten-hour labor . . . Elizabeth was the first one born. They were both healthy. Thirty-six weeks is generally considered full term for twins. They went to the regular nursery. I held the babies for a little bit, and then they took them right away. Jeff was with them.
—Stacy had an epidural, went to sleep, and woke up when her cervix had dilated to seven centimeters. She turned on her side and dilated to ten centimeters. Two days after the twins were born, Stacy and her husband took them home.

If you are having twins, prepare for a normal vaginal birth, since a vaginal birth is possible if you and your babies are healthy, your babies are in a good position, and your care provider is comfortable with the vaginal delivery of twins. Also prepare for a cesarean birth, since twins are frequently delivered by cesarean section.

With twins, your birth options tend to be more varied than they are with triplets or high-order multiples. With twin deliveries, doctors may offer you the option of vaginal or cesarean delivery, depending on the position of the baby and the doctor's philosophy regarding delivering multiples. However, most doctors deliver three or more babies by cesarean section.

Whereas the birth of twins may be more complicated than the birth of a singleton baby, labor with twins may be much the same (see Part 7). The only notable difference with a multiple birth is that labor may come on more subtly, making it easy for you to mistakenly think you have just a backache or cramps.

Twins: Headfirst or Bottom First?

Multiple gestations have more risk for abnormal position; earlier they are more likely to be breech. As long as the first one is head down, it's OK to do a vaginal delivery. If not, you go to a c-section.
—Dr. Katherine Shaw

* * *

In 35% to 40% of twin gestations presenting in labor, the first twin will be in vertex presentation and the second twin will be in breech presentation or transverse lie.
—Lynn L. Simpson and Mary E. D'Alton, "Multiple Pregnancy." *Management of Labor and Delivery*

Twins assume certain positions to accommodate one another within your uterus, and some of these positions allow for an easier vaginal birth than others. The easiest position for a vaginal birth, at least from the point of view of many doctors, is the *vertex/vertex* position. In this case, each twin is in the headfirst (vertex) position and may be well positioned for a vaginal delivery. If the babies are in the *vertex/breech* position—with the first twin headfirst and the second twin bottom first or *breech*— it may also be possible for you to have a vaginal delivery, especially if the second baby (the breech baby) is the same size or smaller than the first baby. However, if the first baby is breech, or if one or both babies is *transverse* (lying sideways in your uterus), many doctors will advise a cesarean section (see Chapter 29).

How to deliver twins when the second twin is breech or transverse is the subject of considerable controversy, according to Lynn L. Simpson and Mary E. D'Alton in their chapter on multiple pregnancy in the obstetrics textbook *Management of Labor and Delivery.*

Doctors disagree as to the best mode of delivery—cesarean or vaginal—depending on the babies' positions, the doctor's experience, the size of your pelvis, the size and condition of your babies, and your doctor's birth philosophy. Some doctors deliver all twins and triplets by cesarean section. Some doctors will deliver twins vaginally, but only if the babies are in the vertex/vertex position. Other doctors, who are skilled at breech birth deliveries, will deliver twins vaginally if the babies are in the vertex/breech position and the second baby is the one that is breech.

Even if your babies are in a breech or transverse position as your due date approaches, they may move before or during labor to a more advantageous position for birth. The position of the second twin may change in up to 20 percent of women after delivery of the first twin.

Triplets

Triplets: If you get over two, the overwhelming majority deliver by cesarean section. The risk of having a complicated labor is much greater.
—Dr. Watson Bowes Jr.

• • •

If you are having three or more babies, you most likely will have a cesarean section. Prepare for your cesarean section by attending a childbirth class that addresses cesarean section, offers support from other women who are birthing babies by cesarean section, and provides you with positive ways to view birth by cesarean section. You will also need to plan for your recovery (see "Surgery and Recovery: What to Expect" in Chapter 28), since you will be healing from surgery while adjusting to mothering twins or triplets. Even the most energetic and self-sufficient woman will need help under these circumstances. Plan on getting help for at least two weeks (preferably more) from friends, family, or neighbors, or hire someone to cook, clean, shop, and care for your other children. Consider hiring a postpartum doula who can help you develop strategies for caring for three babies (see appendix).

Bonding and Breastfeeding

I nursed them together. I needed help when they started getting heavier. I could lay them down in a "football hold" at first. After the first few months, I needed help.
—Sharon

• • •

I had to leave the babies in the hospital for six weeks and bring them pumped breastmilk. They were too small to breastfeed. . . .

In the beginning they were being fed through a tube in their mouths. . . . I would pump every two or three hours during the day and during the middle of the night, but nothing is as efficient as a baby sucking.

My primary relationship with breastfeeding was with my pump [when the twins were still in neonatal intensive care]. I was pumping at home around every three hours. I physically couldn't spend twenty-four hours a day in the hospital, though my bonding was intense for a couple of hours every morning and evening. I had a little section in the nursery refrigerator and freezer that was mine. The nurses never had to give the babies formula.

—Sharon's HMO hospital encouraged breastfeeding and gave nursing mothers the option of refrigerating and freezing their pumped milk, so the babies could be nourished on their mother's breastmilk even while in the NICU.

* * *

When your babies are ready to be held, you can bond with them in the age-old way by holding them skin-to-skin and by gently touching them and talking to them. They already know your voice—they've been hearing it for months from inside your womb—and they know your smell. If the babies are in the NICU, ask the nurses about bonding with the babies or feeding them in a way that is safe for them. You may wonder if you can breastfeed multiples. Many women successfully breastfeed their twins. Even if your babies are premature, it is possible for you to feed them breastmilk: The nurses may initially feed your preemies your breastmilk through a tiny tube in their mouths, but the babies can shift to your breast as they learn how to suck. As they develop, their ability to suckle will develop. Spend time with each baby—holding it, nursing it, and getting acquainted with it as an individual.

When twins are mature enough to nurse, it is possible, and sometimes advantageous, to nurse them both at once. Many mothers try to feed their twins simultaneously and keep the babies on the same schedule, so they are ready for feeding—and for sleeping—at the same time. You may need some help situating the babies at the breast, especially when they grow older and heavier.

If you find the nursing process awkward or you are worried that you won't have enough milk, call La Leche League or a lactation consultant. Most women can nurse their infants with the help of some good coaching and a lot of patience. Remember that the more you nurse, the more milk you will produce. Most important for your babies' nourishment and your comfort, learn how to help your baby latch on appropriately.

You may worry that breastfeeding is impossible if your babies are very premature, but you can "teach" preemies to breastfeed and prepare them for it, even if they are unable to suck efficiently at first. "You go through the motions," says Sharon, whose babies were three pounds each when they were born at thirty-two weeks. "You put them on a breast, and they try to suck. We had to teach them to nurse. They were fed breastmilk through a gavage tube in their throat. They'd nurse before and after, so they'd associate feeding with the nursing."

The NICU

There were a lot of days when there were mini-crises. The nurses would be poking the babies for one thing or another. Every day you're freaked out about how the test will come out. Monitors are constantly going off. It's a constant din. You're always looking at the monitor to see if it's your baby. . . . But nothing bad happened. The girls are really healthy. . . . We had a really

good experience with the nurses. We learned a lot. They taught us how to do things so we felt pretty experienced by the time the girls came home.
—Sharon's twin girls, Rachel and Maia, were relatively healthy even though they were small. The twin girls are now healthy two-year-olds.

※ ※ ※

Only some hospitals have NICUs. The NICUs with the most sophisticated respiratory support and state-of-the-art equipment are Level IIIs. Level II units have less high-tech kinds of respiratory support.

The NICU can be both a blessing and an emotional roller coaster for anxious parents of newborns. NICUs utilize advanced medical technology to provide for the needs of premature infants. For very premature babies, the Level III nurseries provide respirators to help the babies breathe until they are able to breathe on their own. To keep the babies warm, the NICU provides heated beds or incubators. For a baby whose sucking response has not yet developed, the NICU provides a tiny feeding tube that is used to guide expressed breastmilk or formula toward the baby's throat until she is able to suckle and feed.

Many NICUs work wonders in helping babies develop and survive, even if the babies are very premature. However, until your babies have grown strong and become official NICU "graduates," you may spend nerve-wracking days or weeks hovering over infants.

Bonding with preemies may seem difficult at first, since they seem so fragile as they lie curled up in plastic isolettes or sprawled out on warming beds surrounded by high-tech equipment. However, even though preemies may have some special needs for assistance in breathing or feeding, they share common needs with all infants: They need to hear your voice, feel your touch, and smell the unmistakable scent of their mother. The staff can teach you how to bathe, hold, and comfort your premature infants so by the time you leave the hospital you will be relatively experienced in caring for them—and confident that you can continue to nurture them at home.

NICUs can become a home away from home as you sit long hours with your babies and develop relationships with the nurses and doctors. Most units have twenty-four-hour visiting, and they provide rocking chairs so parents may rock their babies at any time of the day or night. Some units encourage ongoing ties between parents and staff by holding yearly reunions for the "graduates" as they grow up.

Since premature babies in an NICU may need many high-tech interventions—at least in their first few days or weeks—make sure the staff clearly explains the reason for the procedures and the benefits and risks involved. You need to be given the opportunity to make informed decisions in the best interest of your babies. Sometimes sustaining a baby's life can extend its suffering, and determining the best interests of the baby may be a complex and emotional process.

Some NICUs offer support groups for parents or follow-ups for the babies with specialists in child development. Make use of such services when you can, since sharing experiences and coping strategies often can provide much-needed comfort and advice.

Coming Home

They were five pounds when we left the hospital; it was very scary. But we had a lot of practice over the six weeks with great nurses.
—Sharon

• • •

I went home on Christmas, and the nurses brought the twins to me in little stockings. It was a weird feeling, coming home with two babies.
—Stacy brought her healthy baby girls, Elizabeth and Katherine, home only two days after their birth.

* * *

Going home with twins or more is both exciting and scary. You can make the experience more manageable by adjusting your expectations to fit your new situation. Aspire to contained chaos instead of a tidy house. For instance, large, attractive baskets can pleasantly hide mounting piles of bedding and clothes. Stock up on fruit, cheese, frozen food, and menus from restaurants that deliver: Do not plan on doing much cooking. If friends offer to help, you may want to suggest they bring food or that they watch the babies while you take a bath. You will probably need to get some help taking care of your multiples, at least for the first few months. "Enlist as much help as you can. Get as much family help as you can. Be ready for life to be a blur. Be ready to be going, going, going and not to have time for yourself," advises Stacy.

Count on fatigue, especially for the first several months, unless your babies adopt a simultaneous feeding and playing schedule. Encourage them to adopt similar schedules, although this may be difficult with triplets or more since it may be impossible to feed all the babies at once (unless of course you get outside help). When nursing two babies, you may need help placing the babies at the breast, especially after they start to gain weight. Feeding the babies often requires the involvement of your partner if you hope to get enough sleep at night. Even with a good feeding schedule, Stacy and her husband felt sleep deprived: "We tried to keep them on the same schedule. We'd each take one and give them a bottle. We were both incredibly exhausted. It would have really been difficult had I not had a supportive husband. My husband got up at night and fed the babies for two weeks. Then one night he broke down at two A.M. and said, 'I can't do this any more.' I said, 'That's OK. Thanks for helping the way you have.'"

Many parents say that raising twins is a job almost impossible to plan for and that they do best when they "go with the flow" of their new life. For instance, Sharon never expected that going to the grocery store would be difficult with twins. But shopping with the girls before they started walking turned out to be a two-person job that required some lifestyle changes for both Sharon and her husband. "It was almost impossible for me to go out with them alone. When I got groceries, we needed to have two carts with me pushing two babies," says Sharon. "My husband and I did all the shopping together. It was physically impossible to do all the things you can do with one child. I couldn't carry these girls at the same time up the stairs, and I couldn't physically get them out of the house at the same time. I couldn't bathe them at the same time alone."

Mothers of twin infants may benefit from the moral support and collective wisdom of other women who are learning to care for twins. Many parents of twins feel anxious about taking care of their tiny and seemingly fragile babies. You may find yourself fretting about all the things that could go wrong—from nursing problems to fevers to worst-case scenarios like SIDS. To allay your anxieties and get additional support, try to find a pediatrician with a home health nurse who will come to your home if problems should arise.

If you are worried about SIDS, ask your pediatrician about prevention techniques. Some experts believe that babies who are exposed to other people's breathing throughout the night are less likely to develop SIDS, since others' regular breathing stimulates their own. Consequently, these experts recommend that babies sleep in or near their parents' bed at night so they can respond to the rhythmic breath sounds and chest movements of the parents until they are no longer at risk for SIDS. However, most proponents of "cosleeping" or "family bed" arrangements recommend that the bed be a large one and that the babies not be placed on or next to pillows (to prevent possible suffocation). Parents who are restless sleepers may want to avoid cosleeping and seek other SIDS monitoring or prevention techniques.

The combination of postpartum blues, sleep deprivation, isolation at home, and/or returning to work can take its toll on a mother of twins or triplets. However, a mothers-of-twins support group can also offer coping strategies to get through the first few months of parenthood.

Raising Twins

You can pick up only one at a time, and that's really difficult if both are crying. You can't always be there the way you are for a single child. They're going to learn a lot about sharing and waiting.
—Sharon

* * *

It got easier [taking care of twins]—when I went back to work and had a nanny. By eighteen months or two years they [the babies] were comforting each other. . . . They learn from each other: that's neat to watch. It's really neat watching two different personalities develop at the same time. They're very concerned about each other. Elizabeth was sick. I think she had a high fever. Katherine started crying. I asked her why. She said she was worried about Elizabeth.
—Stacy

"Raising twins is very special and unique and wonderful. It's also very hard," says Sharon.

Dividing attention between two children is one of the many challenges facing parents of twins, especially when the twins are infants. A baby's cry is a piercing thing designed to get parents' attention. Most mothers are attuned to their baby's cry to the point that it will wake them out of a sound sleep. With twins or more, those cries may be multiplied by a factor of two. This is where a twins and/or multiples support group can be extremely helpful, since you can learn from others' experiences in coping with the needs of two or more babies—and you do not need to reinvent the wheel.

The good news is that many parents of twins say life with twins gets easier as they mature. "It gets better and better," says Sharon of her two-year-old girls. "Their play is very interactive, and they get along very well all the time. It makes it easier for us to go out and do things, and it makes it easier for me at home."

Part Seven

Giving Birth

I tell women that their bodies know what to do and that labor is hard, it's time limited, and the rewards are great.
—Pam Spry, CNM, Ph.D., Assistant Professor of Nursing at the University of Colorado

※ ※ ◆

"My body knows how to do this. Women have been birthing babies for thousands of years," is a useful affirmation to repeat to yourself before and during childbirth. Prepare for a normal birth, learn about all your birth options, have faith in the birth process, and do not give up on your ability to have a normal birth—no matter what age you are. Your preparation and attitude are important factors in determining your experience of childbirth and influencing how well you cope with contractions.

Even if your labor is long, it can still be a normal labor that responds to simple methods of moving labor along such as walking, using birthing positions that work with gravity, and relying on supportive and encouraging companionship throughout labor and birth.

Fortunately, as a woman over thirty having a baby in the twenty-first century, you have access to a variety of approaches to help you birth your baby.

In Part 7, I focus on the process of normal childbirth and the many ways in which you can facilitate that process and prepare for the birth of your baby. I discuss a spectrum of preparation approaches that includes childbirth classes; birthing positions; hypnosis; continuous emotional support during labor by birth partners, doulas, or midwives; and strategies to cope with the various stages of childbirth. I also explain various pain management techniques, including epidural anesthesia and pain medications as well as natural methods such as showers and Jacuzzis.

Chapter 15
Preparing for Childbirth

*The older woman is up against a challenge—the medical estab-
lishment sees it as a risk. She needs more than anyone a course
to increase her self-confidence in her body and her birth process.*
—Michelle Brill, MPH, Doula and Childbirth Educator,
Birthworks

* * *

As your due date nears, joyful anticipation of the baby's
arrival mounts as you choose a crib, hang colorful mobiles, and
accumulate stuffed animals and tiny clothes. Anticipation of the
birth itself, however, may bring with it a spectrum of emotions:
excitement, awe, anxiety, and fear. "Yes, birth is a miracle," you
may say to yourself, "but how will I manage the potential uncertainties—and pain—of labor and delivery?"

As a mature woman with considerable life experience, you
may be accustomed to having some control over your life. But
how can you control your baby's unique reaction to labor, and
your body's reaction to labor?

When it comes to having the kind of birth you want, "there
is a lot you can do to tip the scales in your favor," says Kathleen
Gray Farthing, a childbirth educator, doula, and mother of

three. You cannot control all the potential unknowns of your birth experience, but you can give yourself more options, and thus more control, if you plan for some possible birth scenarios.

"The choices you make and the things you do will greatly affect your birth experience," says Farthing. Your choice of health care provider, hospital, childbirth class, birth plan, and childbirth support person can greatly enhance your odds for having the kind of birth you want. It is important to be realistically prepared for labor and delivery, to know what you want, and to make sure that your beliefs and your caregivers' beliefs are in sync regarding labor and birth.

To tip the scales in your favor for a normal labor and birth, prepare yourself for childbirth by learning about pregnancy, nutrition, breastfeeding, birthing positions, relaxation techniques, medications used to induce or enhance labor, anesthesia options, and surgical interventions such as episiotomy, forceps delivery, and cesarean section.

Avoid categorizing yourself according to your age—and keep the faith in your body's ability to give birth. Do not assume that because you are over thirty-five you will have a difficult labor or need a cesarean section. Such assumptions may become a self-fulfilling prophecy, creating unnecessary fear and anxiety.

Whether your labor is long or short, uncomplicated or complicated, your attitude can make a critical difference in the kind of birth experience you will have. Enlist a supportive partner or friend to encourage you and help you maintain a positive attitude, and consider hiring a doula to support you through labor and birth.

Choosing Childbirth Preparation Classes

Our childbirth teacher explained a lot of options and told us, "Pick one that works for you." The breathing techniques work.

If you're thinking about breathing, you're not tensing up.
—Sharlene gave birth when she was forty-eight and fifty-two

* * *

Women who are well informed about the birth process before labor begins and who have good relationships with their doctors or midwives tend to feel less anxiety, less muscular tension, and, consequently, less pain.

Since anxiety releases stress hormones called catecholamines that may increase pain and slow labor, anything that reduces your anxiety—whether it is a supportive partner, good childbirth preparation, or a positive attitude—may enhance your childbirth experience.

Dr. Allen Killam, an obstetrician for many years at Duke University Hospital, found that his patients who had childbirth preparation and a supportive birth partner experienced decreased pain and anxiety: "If a woman has a supportive partner who has gone to childbirth classes with her, and the woman and her partner are trained to listen to each other, that is very, very valuable. If there is an involved partner in the birth process, preferably a close person such as a marriage partner or significant other, that support helps her. The childbirth training raises her pain threshold, it lowers her anxiety, and I'm convinced that labor goes much better with a woman who is not pouring out epinephrine and catecholamines that inhibit labor."

Numerous studies confirm that childbirth preparation classes have positive effects on a woman's birth experience and that women who take preparation classes have reduced pain, reduced use of pain medications, and fewer "instrumental deliveries" by forceps or vacuum extraction.

Childbirth classes will provide you with general information about pregnancy, labor, and birth, and they will teach you breathing and relaxation techniques that can minimize labor

pain. Most classes familiarize you with medication and anesthesia options for pain relief. In addition, birthing classes offer
you the support and experience of other women. Friendships
formed in these classes often serve as lasting resources for play
groups or breastfeeding support long after you give birth. Such
contacts with other mothers and babies may be particularly
helpful if most of your friends have grown children and are no
longer in the child-rearing mode.

If you are over thirty-five, choose a birth class that teaches
you techniques to make labor easier but also prepares you for
the possibility of cesarean section, since a woman in your age
group is twice as likely to have a cesarean as a woman in her
twenties. Although some health care experts argue that the
cesarean rate in the United States is unnecessarily high, cesarean
section is a reality that must be considered by all pregnant
women and especially those pregnant in midlife.

Choose a class that matches your birth philosophy, your
personality, and your circumstances. For instance, some classes
may address the needs of older mothers, single mothers, or
mothers pregnant with multiples.

How do you find the right childbirth class for you? Ask
other women and your care provider for references. Call local
midwives, birthing centers, or women's centers. Interview the
instructors by phone. Of the childbirth classes, Lamaze, Bradley,
and Birthworks are the best known, although you will probably
find a variety of independent and hospital-run classes that offer
a smorgasbord of techniques. Courses that offer a variety of
techniques or "bag of tricks" for childbirth may increase your
odds of finding a technique that works for you.

Midwives often suggest that women take independent
rather than hospital-run courses, since the independent courses
are apt to focus on the unique needs of each woman.
Independent classes tend to be consumer oriented and are more

apt to teach you to be your own advocate, to articulate your needs, and to negotiate with your doctor and hospital in order to have the kind of birth you want. The instructor of a class that is not sponsored by a hospital may be more apt to point out what hospital policies you may wish to question. For example, some hospitals separate mother and baby after birth by taking the baby to the nursery for a bath, eye drops, and exam. If you do not want your baby taken from you during the first hour or two after birth—or at all—you must be prepared to negotiate in advance with your doctor and hospital.

Although hospital-run courses may offer excellent education and preparation for the birth process, some of these courses may emphasize hospital rules and protocol and teach women and their partners how to comply. "Don't do it [childbirth classes] through your hospital," advises Ceal Bacom, a nurse-midwife at Chicago's Alivio Clinic. "They'll just tell you what the rules are."

However, there are times when your best strategy may be to take the hospital course. If your care provider prefers the hospital class and you see eye to eye with her or him on childbirth philosophy, take the hospital course.

Start the class at least two months before your due date.

Lamaze and Psychoprophylaxis

I never lie about labor. I say, "There's pain. Let's do something about it." You never lose by learning how.
—Elizabeth Bing, a physical therapist who brought the Lamaze technique to America from Europe, is Emeritus Director of Lamaze International

∘ ∘ ∘

By psychologically and physiologically preparing a woman for birth, the Lamaze method seeks to reduce the "unnecessary pain" caused by fear and tension. Practitioners call this approach psychoprophylaxis, since it enlists both a woman's psyche and her body in the reduction of pain. Central to the Lamaze technique is a kind of *reconditioning* in which women learn to change their perception of and response to pain.

In her book, *Six Practical Lessons for an Easier Childbirth*, Elizabeth Bing writes of the Lamaze goal "to recondition ourselves and to create a new center of concentration, thereby causing the awareness of pain to become peripheral." To recondition yourself, you must concentrate on your own breathing and change your breathing as the process of labor moves from one stage to another. Bing likens this to shifting gears on a car.

Lamaze has changed with the times and now offers a smorgasbord of techniques to help women prepare for labor with as little anxiety and discomfort as possible. The organization also embraces the role of midwives and doulas in the birth process.

The Lamaze method offers you breathing, visualization, and massage techniques that distract you from labor pain. You learn how to focus on an external object (anything from a candlestick to a doorknob), to change your breathing to accommodate each stage of labor, and to use gentle massage for relaxation and distraction. The techniques can induce a kind of trance that helps you remove yourself from the pain and "allow your labor to do its work."

Contrary to popular myth, Lamaze is a technique in "prepared childbirth" rather than "natural childbirth." Although the Lamaze Method had once been associated with a doctrinaire advocacy of medication-free "natural childbirth," the contemporary Lamaze philosophy accepts pain medication as a valid individual choice and considers medication-assisted births as "successful" as those without medication.

Lamaze teachers are trained in the basic Lamaze philosophy, but the flavor and flexibility of the classes differ from instructor to instructor. Shop around and sample a few classes to find one that suits you.

The Bradley Method

The Bradley Method teaches slow, relaxed, deep breathing intended to help a laboring woman relax and work with her contractions.

The Bradley Method focuses the laboring woman and her partner on the experience of giving birth and on positive feelings of love and accomplishment. According to the Bradley philosophy, a woman's emotional, physical, and mental relaxation are key to reducing and managing pain. Bradley teachers encourage women to believe in the capacity of their own bodies to give birth, to design their own birth plan, to find relaxing positions during the early stages of labor, to breastfeed their babies immediately after delivery, and to bond with their babies without any interference for two hours after birth.

Dr. Robert Bradley, the Denver obstetrician who developed this technique of natural childbirth in 1947, thought that medications, including epidurals and spinals, were harmful to both mother and child. He believed that women, with their mates as "coaches," could successfully deliver babies about 94 percent of the time without medical intervention

Bradley moved fathers from the waiting room and bar into the delivery room. He encouraged husbands to coach their wives, and he taught couples to rely on the love bond between them to enhance the birth experience. Making fathers participants in the birth process, once a radical aspect of the Bradley philosophy, is now part of standard obstetrical practice. But nowadays, the "coach" is not necessarily a husband or a man.

With the emphasis on the team of the woman and her coach, the doctor takes a back seat. Dr. Bradley envisioned himself merely "as a lifeguard at a pool" and referred to delivering babies as "catching babies." He argued that anyone can "catch a baby properly pitched." Many conventional obstetricians were displeased with Bradley's attitudes. Some doctors still consider the Bradley approach "antidoctor" and see Bradley instructors as too militant and too willing to defy hospital policies. However, other doctors prefer the Bradley approach, because it often produces confident, well-educated patients.

Although the Bradley Method does encourage you to assert your preferences in a birth plan, it also promotes positive, diplomatic communication with care providers. The *Bradley Method Student Workbook* advises you and your coach to:

- Tell the doctor or midwife how special they are as a source of support
- State preferences that apply to a normal, uncomplicated labor and birth in "a positive and polite way rather than making it just a list of demands"
- Give your care providers a chance to state their responses to these preferences

Whether or not the Bradley Method takes an adversarial or advocacy stance often is determined by the style of the particular instructor. Look for a class and an instructor that suit your personality.

Dr. Grantly Dick-Read—"Natural Childbirth"

Both the Lamaze and Bradley techniques found their early inspiration in Dr. Grantly Dick-Read, who believed, rather idealistically, that the pain of childbirth could be reduced or totally eliminated by educating women about birth and helping them to see it as a normal process.

Dr. Grantly Dick-Read invented the term "natural child-birth." He thought childbirth was a normal, natural, physiological process, and in his book *Childbirth Without Fear,* he argued that the pain of birth was due to social conditioning, ignorance, tension, and fear. Dick-Read believed labor pain could be reduced—even eliminated—if women understood the birth process and relaxed.

Although Dick-Read's philosophy has been greatly modified in most childbirth preparation classes, his ideas on education and relaxation have had a strong influence on contemporary approaches to childbirth preparation.

Birthworks

Birthworks uses physical and psychological approaches to reduce a woman's anxiety and fear, to give her confidence in her ability to bear a child, and to offer her techniques to use during labor that will reduce pain and stress. Techniques include slow, relaxed abdominal breathing; positional changes to facilitate labor; visualization; massage; baths and showers; and positive ways of perceiving the birth experience.

In addition to labor techniques, Birthworks encourages women to access their inner knowledge about birth. "Within every woman is the knowledge of how to give birth," explains childbirth educator Kathleen Gray Farthing.

Birthworks classes teach women to identify fears about childbirth that may interfere with the birth process, and then replace the fears with beliefs that can give confidence in birth.

As for women over thirty-five, Birthworks teaches that women should not be considered high risk because of age alone.

Other Alternatives

Active Birth

Janet Balaskas, in her book *Active Birth: The New Approach to Giving Birth,* offers an active method of childbirth preparation in which women can move around, change positions, and give birth however they wish. Part of Balaskas's preparation routine involves yoga and stretching to get women in shape for labor and birth.

Balaskas argues that an active birth is safer than a passive birth, basing her argument for upright posture on studies showing that walking increases the strength of uterine contractions, increases cervical dilation, and contributes to shorter labor, less pain, greater comfort, and increased psychological benefits to the woman (who feels that she has contributed to her own labor). She also believes that an upright maternal posture is better for the baby.

Balaskas thinks that stretching for pregnancy helps prevent backache, improve circulation, prevent varicose veins, and increase energy levels. She also thinks that stretching helps you stay in touch with your body's spontaneous response to birth and to "surrender to the powerful forces within your body during labor," to get in touch with your body, and to feel comfortable with how your muscles work with gravity during childbirth.

In an active birth, you will walk, kneel, squat, sit—in short, assume any position that you find comfortable during the first and second stage of labor. The yoga facilitates comfortably assuming these positions.

Combined Approaches

Health educators, including doulas and midwives, may offer childbirth classes that combine aspects of Bradley and Lamaze with other less structured approaches to relaxation and birth. Some courses add techniques of alternative medicine and midwifery—massage, aromatherapy, visualization, and birthing balls—to create a woman-centered approach to birthing.

If you are interested in alternative approaches to birth or approaches that complement Western medicine, call your local midwives, doulas, birthing centers, or women's centers.

Hypnosis

A hypnotically prepared patient can expect to use considerably less medication, reducing the depressive effects of narcotics on the baby.
—Dr. Larry Goldman, "The Use of Hypnosis in Obstetrics," *Psychiatric Medicine*, Vol. 10, No. 4, 1992

◆ ◆ ◆

Hypnosis is used in two ways to control pain perception in childbirth: self-hypnosis and post-hypnotic suggestion. Most hypnotherapists teach self-hypnosis, so that women may enter a trance during labour and reduce awareness of painful sensations. Other techniques used are relaxation, visualization (helping the woman imagine a pleasant safe scene and placing herself there, symbolizing her pain as an object that can be discarded, or picturing herself as in control or free of pain), distraction (focusing on something other than the pain), and glove anaesthesia (creating a feeling of numbness in one of her hands through suggestion and then spreading that numbness wherever she wishes by placing her numb hand on the desired places of her body). The woman is taught to induce these techniques herself; only rarely do hypnotherapists accompany their clients in labour. Other therapists rely almost entirely on post-hypnotic suggestion.
—Dr. Murray Enkin et al., "Control of Pain in Labour," *A Guide to Effective Care in Pregnancy and Childbirth* (second edition)

◆ ◆ ◆

Some women have found hypnosis useful in lessening the fear and pain of childbirth. The most effective kind of hypnosis for childbirth involves the pregnant woman's learning hypnotic techniques from an experienced practitioner (a hypnotherapist or doctor who is trained in hypnosis) and then practicing the techniques for several months before her baby's birth.

The hypnosis used in labor is primarily a method of relaxing and distancing from pain; sometimes the self-hypnosis is facilitated by a doctor or birth partner, and sometimes it is guided by the woman herself. Frequently, the hypnosis used for labor closely resembles techniques taught in childbirth classes or in biofeedback, especially techniques that involve deep relaxation, visualization, and repeated suggestions given in a soothing tone by a partner or birth attendant. Suggestions such as "let go," visualizations such as "envision a circle widening," and deep relaxation of various muscle groups are techniques that may be utilized by doulas, midwives, and childbirth educators as well as by hypnotherapists.

"The lines between good coaching and good training and hypnosis merge," explains Dr. Allen Killam. "People may be using the principles of hypnosis and working with them and not calling them hypnosis. In childbirth classes, the training that people do—'breathe in and out,' 'relax,'—sounds similar to what you hear if you listen to someone being hypnotized."

Some women report that hypnosis dramatically reduces their pain and increases their sense of self-control. Of course, hypnosis is neither effective nor appropriate for everyone. Some women do not find it useful for controlling pain. Other women, especially women with a history of severe trauma such as rape or abuse, may find themselves confronting traumatic memories and should undergo hypnosis only with an experienced psychotherapist.

Hypnosis is not widely used in labor, and its pain-reducing effects in labor have not been thoroughly researched. Perhaps the many misconceptions about hypnosis prevent pregnant women and their doctors from taking it seriously as an effective method of pain control. For instance, hypnosis has long been viewed as a magic trick performed on stage in front of large audiences or as an intrusive method by which psychiatrists probe the depths of their patients' psyches. However, hypnosis is neither magical nor intrusive if practiced by a responsible professional. It is merely a state of deep relaxation that many people can attain with practice, rather like meditation. In fact, many of us briefly enter mild trancelike states when watching television, running, or swimming laps.

Hypnosis and biofeedback have been successfully used as pain control techniques in medical settings. However, because hypnosis in childbirth has not been extensively studied, you may wish to include it among your pain management strategies—but not make it your only strategy.

Preparation for Breastfeeding

I had failed breastfeeding with my first child. When I decided to breastfeed my second baby, my friends told me about La Leche League. Preparing for breastfeeding by going to La Leche meetings gives you good role models and good information about what you're going to encounter—-and you're going to encounter something. Sometimes women give up if they encounter problems—even simple problems. One of the common myths in the United States is that some women can't breastfeed, but it would be a rare woman who can't. However, it helps to get off to a good start. I found La Leche people to be compassionate and not the least fanatical. I took the classes before I gave birth. Then I

had a network, since La Leche has a twenty-four-hour call line that you can call if you have a problem.
—Linda-Carol

* * *

The first few days after your baby's birth may be overwhelming, especially if you are changing diapers, bathing a newborn, and nursing—all for the first time. As a new mother, you may find yourself additionally stressed if you baby doesn't "latch on" well or nurse effectively.

Fortunately, there is much you can learn by taking a breast-feeding preparation class or by attending a breastfeeding support group before the birth to help you and your new baby adjust to one another, to prepare you for nursing, and to reduce any anxiety you might have.

Studies have shown that women who are prepared for breastfeeding experience more success and avoid many potential problems when breastfeeding their babies.

Breastfeeding preparation may be offered as part of a childbirth education class, as a separate class, or as part of an ongoing support group such as La Leche League. La Leche League is a national organization that offers support groups for women who intend to breastfeed or who are already breastfeeding their babies. La Leche instructors are experienced, well-trained women who will sometimes act as doulas for the women in their group.

If you are interested in learning more about breastfeeding, shop for a La Leche group just as you would shop for a childbirth class, since group leaders differ in their level of enthusiasm and flexibility. Although some La Leche groups have the reputation of being over-zealous, others offer a relaxed approach—it all depends on the personality of the leader and the group.

Such resources are useful for both first-time mothers and

for mothers who have had previous children but have not been successful at breastfeeding. Your hospital may provide a lactation consultant to talk with you after the birth of your baby and to help you get started with breastfeeding. You may benefit from her advice, although it is always a good idea to get a head start and to learn about breastfeeding before the birth of your baby. Other organizations also offer breastfeeding classes and support groups. Check your local hospitals, birth centers, and women's centers. (For more resources, see the appendix.)

If you are approaching menopause, consult your doctor to discuss proper nutrition and calcium intake. Sharlene became pregnant with a donor egg when she was fifty-two—and menopausal. She decided that fifty-two wasn't too old for breastfeeding, and she successfully breastfed her baby.

However, the effects of breastfeeding on premenopausal or menopausal mothers are not well understood, since these women are more vulnerable to calcium loss and bone density problems than are younger women. If you are in or approaching menopause and planning to breastfeed your baby, consult with your care provider about your calcium requirements. Discuss with your doctor your family history of osteoporosis, and ask your doctor whether you should have a bone density test.

The Doula: Ongoing Education and Support

Doula is a Greek word referring to an experienced woman who helps other women. The word has now come to mean a woman experienced in childbirth who provides continuous physical, emotional, and informational support to the mother before, during, and just after childbirth.
—Marshall H. Klaus, M.D.; John H. Kennell, M.D.; and Phyllis H. Klaus, M.Ed., C.S.W., *Mothering the Mother*

A revival of a centuries-old tradition, the use of an experienced, supportive female birth companion, or doula, has become increasingly popular as a way to complement the birth partner and the childbirth educator. A doula becomes part of the birth team, and she supports both you and your birth partner.

A doula "mothers the mother" in a nondomineering way that allows the laboring mother to be active and in charge. The doula's role is to support the mother and her partner in whatever birth plan they have chosen—and to respect their birth plan whether or not it includes pain medication or medical interventions. The doula is not a coach; instead, she takes her cues from the mother (rather than requiring the laboring woman to do specific breathing patterns or follow specific regimens). "The labor doula does not tell the mother what to do but follows the individual mother's pace," writes Marshall and Phyllis Klaus and John Kennell in their book *Mothering the Mother*.

Recent medical studies show that doulas benefit women in childbirth. Women who have doulas by their side during childbirth have shorter labors, fewer medical interventions (such as forceps or cesarean deliveries), less pain, and healthier babies. According to Dr. Marshall Klaus and his coauthors, "the presence of a doula reduces the overall cesarean rate by 50 percent, length of labor by 25 percent, oxytocin use by 40 percent, pain medication use by 30 percent, the need for forceps by 40 percent, and the requests for epidurals by 60 percent." Women who have doula support are also more successful at breastfeeding than women who do not have doulas.

Some doulas offer you support before you give birth, visiting you at home several times before the baby's due date and then again when labor begins. Your doula may stay in contact with you by phone during early labor, meet you at the hospital when labor intensifies, and stay at your side until you give birth.

During the childbirth, the doula encourages you during

contractions, shows you birthing positions that facilitate birth and reduce pain, anticipates your needs, reassures you, and thus takes some of the pressure off your birth partner, who no longer needs to be "coach," masseuse, hand-holder, and emotional support person all at once. Many birth partners are themselves inexperienced and in need of support during labor and birth; consequently some laboring women feel compelled to take care of their family members or partners as well as deal with their own needs during labor. A doula frees you to focus on your own needs and conserve your energy for the birth process (see "Labor Support" in Chapter 17).

Postpartum doulas may help you care for your baby in the week or two following birth (see appendix for "postpartum" doulas).

If you decide to have a doula present during your labor, ask your childbirth educator, midwife, or local birthing center for references. Some women ask their childbirth educator to be their doula, some ask their mothers or friends who have experienced pregnancy. You should start shopping for a doula several months before your due date in order to find a good match for your personality and your birth plan. Whomever you decide upon, make sure that you feel comfortable with her and with her ability to communicate tactfully with your partner and with the hospital staff. Since her purpose is to stay with you throughout your labor and birth, it also is important that she be available to you and not committed to several other women with similar due dates. For more information, contact Doulas of North America (see appendix).

Finding a Pediatrician

Late pregnancy is a good time to start shopping for a pediatrician. If you are anticipating a cesarean section, and you will not have family or friends to help you take care of yourself and the baby for your first two weeks out of the hospital, try to find a doctor with a pediatric nurse who makes house calls. Having a nurse come to your home will save you the strain of driving to a doctor's office with a healing cesarean incision.

Childcare

If your community childcare centers have long waiting lists, it is wise to enroll your child in a childcare center before you give birth—sometimes up to three months before you give birth. Although enrolling your unborn child may seem bizarre, it may be the only way to get childcare if you plan to return to work within three months. Call your local childcare centers to get specific information on the waiting period.

Your last several months of pregnancy are also a good time to find names of women who do childcare in their homes or in yours. If you are going back to work in two or three months, you may want to have your childcare prearranged. If you are pregnant with multiples, you may want to find someone who can come into your home and help with the babies, since there are times you may need help feeding them or grocery shopping (see Part 6 and Chapter 32).

Chapter 16

Creating a Birth Plan

During your prenatal visits, take the time to talk to your care provider about your preferences for the kind of birth you want as well as your anxieties about pregnancy and birth. Write a birth plan and share it with your care provider as a way to clarify your preferences. Use your birth plan as a starting point; expect the plan to evolve to fit the changing circumstances of your pregnancy and birth and the judgment calls of your care provider.

Writing Your Birth Plan

A birth plan is a point of dialogue. I don't think patients ought to present it as nonnegotiable and binding as a contract. But it is a real good place for a woman to think things through and write down her preferences and to talk with her doctor about what the doctor's views are on important topics and see if there's a problem or mismatch. It's a good communication tool.
—Dr. Donna Kirz

• • •

Your birth plan is a list of your preferences for your labor, your baby's birth, and the time you spend with your baby after it is born. The birth plan often becomes a work-in-progress that develops during the course of your pregnancy as your conversations with your caregivers, your understanding of birth, your feelings, and your medical circumstances evolve. Your birth plan is an easy, direct way of communicating your wishes to your care providers after you've already had some preliminary discussions with them about pregnancy and childbirth

Give one copy of your birth plan to your care provider, one to the hospital, and one to the labor and delivery nurse (because it may be hours before your doctor arrives at the hospital). Keep one copy for yourself.

Creating Your Birth Plan

When writing your birth plan, state your preferences and wishes in a polite and positive way; avoid becoming defensive or adversarial. Your birth plan can set the tone for your birth experience.

Include the following items in your birth plan:

1. *The place.* What kind of room would you like? A private room for labor and delivery and for postdelivery? A birthing suite? A shower? A fold-out bed for your partner, doula, or family member?
2. *The people.* Who would you like to have access to your room? Do you want to limit this number to "known" caregivers (unless an emergency arises) and birth companions? Do you wish to be informed of and introduced to any unfamiliar people such as neonatal nurses and doctors who might need to come in to examine your baby? Do you want your partner or doula to have access to you at all times, even in the event of surgical interventions? If you go to surgery for a cesarean, whom do you

want with you—your partner, family member, doula?

3. *Environment and mood.* What kind of environment do you want to create to support you in labor? Music? Candles? Soft lighting? Aromatherapy essences? Massage oils? Do you want a birthing ball? Birthing stool? Birth pool or Jacuzzi?

4. *Prepping procedures.* How do you feel about enemas, shaving, IVs, hospital gowns?

5. *Food and fluid intake.* Is it important for you to eat and drink during your labor? Is it safe, given your preexisting medical conditions or the condition of your baby? How do you feel about getting your fluids and nourishment intravenously?

6. *Pain medication.* How do you feel about pain medications? Under what circumstances might you accept medication (in the case of back labor? breech? prolonged labor?)? If you require a cesarean section, what kind of pain medications would you prefer during and after your surgery?

7. *Monitoring.* How do you feel about being physically restricted during labor by a fetal monitor? Do you wish to move around freely during labor and assume whatever positions are comfortable to you? Do you wish to avoid continuous fetal monitoring? Would you prefer intermittent monitoring that allows you to get up and move around from time to time? There are times when continuous fetal monitoring may be the safest thing for your baby. Discuss with your caregiver under what circumstances he or she recommends continuous fetal monitoring.

8. *Fetal scalp sampling or scalp stimulation.* If your baby shows signs of distress during intermittent or continuous monitoring, do you wish for a confirmation of the diagnosis of distress by fetal blood scalp sampling or tests of

the baby's responsiveness to stimulation?

9. *Interventions to enhance the progress of labor.* You may be offered drugs, like Pitocin, to help strengthen your contractions in cases of prolonged labor. How do you feel about the induction or augmentation of your labor with Pitocin (oxytocin)?

10. *Alternative methods for support in labor.* What alternative techniques do you wish to support you in labor? Massage? Acupuncture? Hypnosis? Support from doula or labor coach?

11. *Positions.* Is it important for you to move around as you wish, and to find positions that are comfortable to you during labor and birth?

12. *Age bias.* If you are over thirty-five, do you wish to be treated the same as a woman under thirty-five and not be categorized as high risk due to your age alone? Do you want to ask your caregiver not to lean toward a cesarean section just because you are forty, forty-five, or fifty?

13. *Episiotomy.* Would you prefer to avoid episiotomy? Under what conditions would you accept an episiotomy (e.g., would you accept one in the case of fetal distress or to avoid a vaginal tear)? Sometimes an episiotomy is the best thing for your baby if the baby needs to be delivered quickly. Discuss with your caregiver under what circumstances an episiotomy may be in the best interests of you or your baby.

14. *Forceps or vacuum extraction.* Would you prefer that your care provider explain possible medical interventions such as forceps and vacuum extractions during an office visit— and weeks before you go into labor? Do you wish to know under what circumstances your care provider would recommend such interventions? Would such interventions be acceptable to you in the case of an emergency or to

minimize risks for your baby? (See Part 8.)

15. *Cesarean section.* Would you prefer to avoid cesarean section unless absolutely necessary? If you have a cesarean, do you wish to remain awake and not grow sleepy from pain medications? Do you want music during the surgery? Videotaping? Whom do you wish to include or exclude—family members, medical students, partners? Do you want your caregiver or partner to bring you the baby after delivery, and do you want private time with your baby? Do you want to nurse your baby as soon as possible after your cesarean?

16. *VBAC.* If you have had a previous baby by cesarean section, do you want to attempt to deliver your baby vaginally? Do you meet the criteria for VBAC? Under what circumstances would you consent to a repeat cesarean section? Discuss your questions with your care provider as you write your plan.

17. *Decision-making/informed consent.* Do you wish to be consulted about your caregivers' decisions to perform a cesarean or to induce labor, to have procedures explained to you before they are performed, and to have an opportunity to discuss such procedures with your caregiver and/or partner? Do you want to be informed in advance of any medical procedures involving your baby?

18. *Special needs or precautions.* Do you have any medical problems or drug sensitivities that your caregivers need to be aware of? For instance, are you hyperglycemic, easily exhausted, sensitive to pain medications? Do you have psychological predispositions that your caregiver needs to be aware of, such as previous pregnancy loss, claustrophobia, fear of hospitals or of anesthesia? If you have fears based on negative past experiences such as a traumatic illness or sexual abuse, tell your caregiver. (In

such cases you may benefit from the continuous supportive presence of a doula.)

19. *Blood transfusions.* How do you feel about blood transfusions? Under what circumstances would you accept
one? Ask if you can donate your own blood in advance if
you are uneasy about blood bank supplies.

20. *Bonding time with your newborn.*

   a. What are your preferences about bonding with your
   baby in the first two to twenty-four hours after birth? Do
   you want uninterrupted skin-to-skin contact with your
   baby in the first one to two hours after birth? Would you
   prefer that you and your partner be left alone with your
   baby before caregivers give your baby eye drops or a
   bath? Would you prefer that caregivers perform any necessary medical tasks in your presence and that you not be
   separated from your baby? Would you accept periods of
   separation during which the baby would be taken to the
   nursery for eye drops and a physical exam?

   b. If you have a cesarean section, do you prefer that your
   baby be left with you and your support person or with
   your partner or doula and not be taken away to the
   nursery after its birth? If so, ask your caregiver how—or
   if—this may be arranged.

   c. How much time do you wish to spend with your baby in
   the hospital? Do you want your baby with you at all
   times, or would you prefer that your baby spend some
   time in the nursery? Do you want your baby in the
   nursery at night?

   d. If your baby requires some time in the NICU, how would
   you like to enhance bonding with your baby? Discuss
   with your caregivers a visitation schedule that best meets
   your needs and the developmental needs of your baby.

21. *Breastfeeding*. Do you want to breastfeed your baby? If so, do you prefer trying to nurse your baby in the first hours after birth? May the hospital staff supplement your breastmilk with sugar water or formula during the baby's hospital stay, or would you prefer that your baby be given your breastmilk? (There may be some circumstances under which your baby may need supplementation to maintain its health. Discuss such circumstances with your caregiver.) Do you wish to speak with a lactation consultant during your hospital stay?

22. *Circumcision*. How do you feel about circumcision? If you have a boy, do you want him circumcised? If so, do you want him to have a local anesthetic? Would you prefer that the circumcision occur in the hospital or at home?

23. *Transfer*. If you need to be transferred from a birth center to a hospital in the event of a complication, what hospital do you wish to be taken to and who do you wish to accompany you? A hospital may have stricter limitations than the birth center on the number of people allowed at your birth, and you may want to choose in advance one or two people who you definitely wish to be with you at the hospital. If your baby needs to be transferred from a birth center or from a Level I hospital to a Level III hospital to receive special care, do you wish to be transferred with your baby if at all possible? If not, do you wish your partner or friend to accompany your baby to the hospital?

If you are having twins, triplets, or high-order multiples:

1. *Vaginal or cesarean birth*. Under what circumstances would you like to attempt to deliver twins vaginally or by cesarean section?

2. *Intensive care: Bonding and breastfeeding.*

a. If your babies must go to the NICU, would you like to

"bank" your breastmilk for your babies?

b. If your babies need to be transferred to another hospital, do you wish to accompany them if possible?

3. *Rooming in*. If your babies are in your room, what kind of support system do you need in place in order to care for them in the hospital setting? Would you prefer that your partner, family members, and/or doula assist you with infant care during your first twenty-four to forty-eight hours in the hospital?

Plan A

"Every woman should have a flexible birth plan," says Penny Simkin, childbirth educator, author, and doula. Consider your plan for a normal, uncomplicated birth as Plan A, since the odds for a normal birth are in your favor. But write a Plan B to allow for possible variations from your ideal. Plan A is your "best-of-all-possible-worlds" birth. It might include a peaceful walk on the beach or in the woods during early labor; a warm, relaxing bath (if your membranes have not ruptured); a birthing suite with soft lighting and your favorite music; and two blissful, uninterrupted hours of bonding with your baby. Your ideal birth may or may not include pain medication or breast-feeding, depending on your individual preferences.

If you and your doctor cannot reach an agreement about your birth plan, find another care provider whose views are closer to yours (although you may want to ask a friend to read your plan to make sure it is a reasonable one before you change care providers). Kathleen R. had disappointing discussions about her birth plan with her doctors. "They couldn't match me point by point," she said, so when she was thirty-four weeks pregnant, Kathleen switched to a midwife. The midwife and hospital honored her plan, except for a few unanticipated circumstances.

Kathleen's Plan A

Check in:

1. We prefer a labor and delivery room with a shower if available.
2. We prefer a private room postdelivery.

Labor:

1. Kathleen is very sensitive to narcotics/sedatives and cannot take codeine.
2. Kathleen has a high metabolism and runs out of energy quickly when "athletically active" unless she is taking in enough calories (she's "hit the wall" athletically).
3. We would like to be able to move about freely and eat and drink freely.
4. We would like intermittent fetal monitoring.
5. We don't want vacuum or forceps to extract the baby unless absolutely necessary.
6. We want to avoid all medications and epidurals but will do anything to avoid c-section.
7. Kathleen does not want a blood transfusion unless absolutely necessary for the continuance of life.
8. We would like to be informed in advance of all impending procedures for Kathleen and the baby and be given time to talk about them.
9. We think we want to see the placenta.

Postdelivery:

1. Please check the baby for Rh factor.
2. Immediately after the delivery, we want the baby skin-to-skin with Kathleen for at least one hour.
3. We do not want the baby to be bathed, just wiped off.

4. We want rooming in with the baby.
5. We do not want any bottle feeding/sugar water given to the baby.

Kathleen organized her birth plan according to stages in the birth process. She was clear about her preferences. She got most of what she wanted, and she was flexible enough to adapt when parts of her birth did not go according to her ideal plan.

Holly's Plan A

Holly, a lawyer, wrote a more detailed plan. Generally:

1. We prefer an atmosphere that is private, calm, and quiet, if possible, with the light and sound levels low. Minimal interruption, preceded by a knock.
2. While we prefer no medication and a spontaneous labor/delivery, we are willing to accept changes in our plan if medical problems arise. We trust that you [the doctors] will present our options clearly and assist us in selecting the least invasive/restrictive procedures.

Preferences for Labor:

1. Privacy: the freedom to create a comfortable environment and wear own clothing.
2. Mother's movements unrestrained by IV or fetal monitor; mother free to choose most comfortable positions and to move about.
3. No medication, except upon request or strong medical indication. If used, minimum dosages with effects on mother and baby made clear.
4. Drink fluids; eat as desires (instead of IV).
5. Fetal heartbeat monitored by stethoscope or Doppler

ultrasound.

6. No catheterization; as few vaginal exams as possible; enema only with mother's consent.
7. Spontaneous, all-natural labor. Prefer waters to break naturally.

Preferences for Birth:

1. Choice of position; freedom to move.
2. No catheterization and frequent voiding in first stage.
3. Allow for longer second stage and position variations to enhance progress.
4. Lower lights and quiet.
5. Mother follows urge to push; avoid prolonged breath holding and bearing down.
6. No episiotomy: compresses, slower delivery. If necessary, late episiotomy, preferably without medications that could affect baby.
7. Spontaneous delivery rather than forceps or vacuum extraction.
8. Father participates to maximum degree: helps catch baby, cuts cord, etc.

Preferences after Birth:

1. Lowered lights and quiet.
2. Gentle handling of baby with as much done by parents as possible.
3. Baby care done on mother's abdomen. Baby placed, skin-to-skin, on mother's abdomen after birth, with blanket over both.
4. Baby's cord cut, if possible, when pulsing slows.
5. Delay in nonessential routines. Wait at least two hours for eye drops, vitamin K shot, weighing, measuring. Prefer these occur in room, that baby and mother not

be separated during this time. Prefer no bath in first twelve to twenty-four hours.

6. Allow baby to nurse immediately. Avoid plain or sugar water; no formula.
7. Allow longer time for birth of placenta.
8. Ice on episiotomy, if performed, first eight to twelve hours.
9. Perform single PKU test no sooner that twenty-four hours after birth or at three-day check.
10. Total rooming in.
11. No circumcision!
12. Early discharge from hospital.

The Unexpected:

1. Cesarean only if emergency.
2. Allowed to go into labor before surgery begins.
3. Father present to support mother.
4. Epidural.
5. Screen lowered at time of birth; mother allowed to see baby immediately if baby is not in distress.
6. Father allowed to hold baby if baby is not in distress.
7. Mother allowed to breastfeed as soon as possible.
8. Infant in distress: parents maintain maximum contact.

Plan B: Your Backup Plan

Writing a backup birth plan is a way of thinking through your options in the event that some unexpected, but possible, scenarios arise. Think through your preferences should you need a cesarean delivery, pain medication, or epidural anesthesia. Learn about the pros and cons of these interventions weeks before you go into labor. If you understand your options in advance, then you need not grapple with risk/benefit questions when you're in active labor (a time when you are not able to sort through complex decisions), and you improve your chances of having the kind of birth experience you want.

Holly had an idealistic Plan A for the birth of her son: a serene, walk-in-the-woods kind of labor and a natural, drug-free birth. Instead, she attended a grueling executive meeting and then experienced prolonged labor and a forceps delivery. She could have taken Pitocin, a drug commonly used in cases of prolonged labor, to strengthen her contractions and move her labor along. Holly resisted Pitocin, however, because she didn't know much about it. "I wish I knew more about Pitocin," Holly says, realizing a more comprehensive Plan B might have included medical interventions to shorten labor and facilitate birth.

Holly put the "unexpected" in her birth plan only because her childbirth instructor told her to. In retrospect, Holly advises that women over thirty-five should spend more time learning about having a pregnancy where they might be faced with the unexpected. She hadn't listened when her doctors went over the benefits of medical interventions with her during office visits, because she felt such things would never apply to her: "I, who did not take an aspirin, was certainly not going to take Pitocin or anything else. I wasn't going to have Soren [her son] grogged out," Holly said.

When the birth didn't go as smoothly as planned, Holly panicked. When her doctor explained to her the necessity of a forceps delivery during the pushing stage of labor, an exhausted Holly no longer could think clearly. "I'm sure the doctor asked me if I was OK [with the procedures]. I'm sure I was incoherent. I was crying. I was very concerned." Worst of all, she felt like a failure.

Fortunately, the forceps delivery went smoothly. The baby popped out easily, and Holly needed no episiotomy. The story ended well: The baby was given to her, placed skin-to-skin on her belly, allowed to nurse, and slept in her bed or in a crib next to it. He received only breastmilk, and he was never separated from her.

Since you never know in advance exactly how your labor is going to proceed, a flexible birth plan can help you feel like you succeeded under a variety of circumstances. Even if you don't get your ideal birth, you will achieve a sense of control that comes with anticipating alternatives and planning for them.

To avoid disappointment, accept that some circumstances will be beyond your control (even if you do everything "right"), and focus on outcome: a healthy mother and child.

Sharlene's Plan B

When Sharlene was pregnant with her second baby, she wrote a new birth plan and went over it with her doctor, because she wanted to discuss what was satisfactory and unsatisfactory about her first birth experience. Sharlene wanted to feel less overwhelmed by hospital staff and protocol during her second birth. Consequently, her new birth plan stipulated that she did not give permission for "nonessential personnel" such as medical students to be in her room during labor and birth.

Even though Sharlene hoped for a natural, vaginal birth, her birth plan anticipated the possibility of cesarean section and laid out very specific preferences (since she realized after her first baby that a cesarean section was a real possibility). Consequently, Sharlene wrote the following Plan B:

1. Spinal or epidural anesthesia will be used if possible. There will be no preoperative medications.
2. The father will remain with the mother at all times regardless of the circumstances. Even if, and specifically

if, the mother should receive general anesthesia for the birth, the father will witness the birth.

3. The parents will love and nurture the baby while the incision is being closed.

4. The baby will not spend a mandatory period in the nursery. Rooming in will be immediate and continuous unless there is a genuine problem with the baby. Parents and baby will be in the recovery room after delivery.

5. There will be no supplemental feedings of the baby.

If you are having a cesarean birth, discuss with your caregivers your specific wishes regarding bonding time with your baby. Proponents of breastfeeding believe that immediate mother-child contact greatly improves the child's ability to breastfeed and enhances bonding.

To try to avoid separation from your infant after a cesarean section, thoroughly discuss a cesarean scenario with your doctor, and call the nursery to discuss hospital policy. Negotiate in advance, if possible, with recovery room staff and anesthesiology as to when and how you can spend some of your recovery time with your baby. Since you may be weak or groggy, you may wish to arrange for your birth partner or doula to hold and care for the baby—but at your bedside.

If you wish your partner or birth companion to stay at your side during a cesarean birth, discuss this possibility in advance in order to arrive at an acceptable solution. If your birth companion does not want to see the actual surgery, he or she can look at your face during the surgery and look at the baby after it emerges from your belly, thus avoiding seeing the actual surgery or incision.

However, even the most meticulous of plans will not ensure that you will get the birth you intended, since you cannot control nature, hospital policy, or which caregiver is on call or even an individual nurse's or doctor's reaction to your birth plan once you are in a hospital. Given such limitations, plan to be flexible.

Chapter 17

Exploring Your Options

"Women should communicate their anxieties to their doctor. They should go over the questions they have. It's really best for a woman to thrash out those important issues—doulas, medication, epidurals, monitoring—before she goes into delivery," advises Dr. Allen Killam. A significant part of your job as an informed, active participant in your baby's birth needs to be done long before you feel your first twinge of labor. Become sufficiently informed to ask your caregiver questions. If you are well informed about birth options, you will feel more able to participate in important decisions once you are in labor.

"If you don't know what your options are, you don't have any," says Diana Korte, author of *The VBAC Companion* and *A Good Birth, A Safe Birth*. Anticipating your childbirth options is a means for feeling more relaxed, confident, and in control during the birth and during the weeks preceding the big event. Educate yourself (through reading, classes, conversations with other women) about all your birth options and what you, your partner, and your caregiver can do to best meet your needs during labor and delivery.

To ensure that your caregivers understand your preferences and that you arrive at a mutually agreeable birth plan, make your wishes crystal clear and pay attention to how your care-givers respond to your requests. Try to reach agreements before labor begins, since it is difficult to learn your options for the first time and make complex decisions once you're in the middle of having contractions. Discuss with your caregivers the factors involved in making decisions about a cesarean section, forceps delivery, episiotomy, continuous fetal monitoring, and the use of medications for pain or for the enhancement of labor, before your last month of pregnancy. "It's not a decision made in the labor suite but a trust that's built up over several weeks of conversation," says Dr. Edward Quilligan, Director of the Center for Health Education at the University of California, Irvine, who advises that a pregnant woman develop a good, open relationship with her care provider before she goes into labor.

By the time you get into labor, you need to trust your care-giver and make sure your beliefs are in sync. It is important to know your caregiver's birth management philosophy before you find yourself in the seventh or eighth month of pregnancy. This is what the initial interview is for (see Part 2). There are times, however, when your initial interview with your doctor or midwife fails to screen out someone whose philosophies differ radically from yours. If irresolvable differences between you and your caregiver come to light once you are in the third trimester of pregnancy, you will find yourself faced with two less-than-ideal options: either stay with a health care provider who does not see eye to eye with you on important issues, or change to a new provider toward the end of your pregnancy. It may require some effort to find a new doctor in the weeks or months before you give birth.

However, it may be better for you to change caregivers—even though shopping for a new one may take time and research—than to remain with one you no longer trust.

"There's a lot of trust that needs to be built up over several months. If a woman can't feel that there's mutual trust and understanding about her goals and the goals of the physician, she's in the wrong relationship," advises Dr. Quilligan.

If you need to change care providers during the course of your pregnancy, act quickly and efficiently. To get references for doctors or midwives: ask nurses, other women, your primary care physician, the staff at a local birthing center, the labor and delivery nurses in the obstetrics ward of a good local hospital. Be a good consumer. Do your research. Do not panic. You are now better equipped to find an appropriate caregiver than you were early in your pregnancy.

If you cannot change care providers, bolster your support system during pregnancy and childbirth. Enlist your friends and family or a doula to be your advocates and cheering section.

Labor Support: Midwives and Doulas

Many women are not aware of an important childbirth option: the *continuous support* of a midwife or doula during the course of labor and birth. Even women who know about the existence of doulas and midwives do not know what medical studies have shown: that women supported by doulas and midwives have less pain and shorter labors than women who are not supported during childbirth.

If you have a normal pregnancy and are considered low risk for complications of pregnancy and birth, one of your options for medical care—and labor support—is a midwife. Midwives are trained to medically manage normal pregnancy and birth; if you develop complications that call for certain surgical or medical interventions, the midwife must turn your care over to her backup physician. However, some midwives will "labor-sit" and stay with you throughout labor and birth—even if you have been transferred to their backup physician.

The doula's only job is to offer you continuous support during childbirth whether you are low risk or high risk (that is, if your hospital or birth center allows a doula to be present). Doulas do not offer medical care, and they are not medical personnel. However, they may complement the medical care of physicians and midwives by offering you emotional and physical support before, during, and after childbirth.

Nurse-Midwives

What midwives are about are options and choices. We listen to women. What is it this woman wants in labor and birth? We facilitate it.
—Laraine Guyette, CNM, Assistant Professor of Nursing, University of Colorado

* * *

"Those women who want to be treated like pregnancy is normal choose midwives," says Pam Spry, nurse-midwife and Assistant Professor of Nursing at the University of Colorado. Nurse-midwives tend to view pregnancy and birth as normal conditions, not as illnesses.

Some midwives are trained as nurses and then take postgraduate midwifery courses and a national midwifery certification exam.

A nurse-midwife is trained to medically manage normal pregnancy and childbirth. By treating childbirth as a normal process, many nurse-midwives seek natural means such as positional changes, walking, relaxation exercises, and Jacuzzis to ease pain and promote progress during labor. Frequently, these simple techniques provide options that may help women avoid invasive procedures such as cesarean section, forceps or vacuum extraction, and episiotomy. In fact, medical studies show that nurse-midwives increase a woman's odds of a vaginal delivery if her labor is normal and her baby is not in distress.

Such seemingly homey midwife remedies as walking and taking Jacuzzis make good medical sense and are more sophisticated than you might think. For instance, walking promotes progress in labor by increasing the dilation of the birth canal and helping the baby assume an advantageous position for its descent. Warm showers are relaxing and ease pain by distracting the nervous system. According to the "gateway" theory of pain, the nervous system cannot transport two kinds of messages at the same time. Consequently, the sensation of the water from the shower beating on your abdomen and back helps block the message of pain from getting from your belly to your brain (at least not in its full intensity) and thus helps "close the gate," says Laraine Guyette.

Continuous encouragement during childbirth also contributes to a reduction in pain and anxiety, which can, in turn, decrease pain and enhance the process of labor.

If you are over thirty-five, your odds of having a cesarean, forceps, or vacuum delivery are greater than those of a younger woman. Although you are at an increased risk of conditions such as preeclampsia and prolonged labor, for which cesarean section may be the safest type of birth, you are also at increased risk for cesarean section due to "physician/patient anxiety" about a late-in-life "premium pregnancy." In the latter case, a relaxed, normalized view of pregnancy could mean the difference between a cesarean section and a vaginal birth.

If you are over thirty-five and are having a healthy pregnancy with no major complications, most midwives will boost your self-confidence about your ability to birth a baby—even if your labor may take a little longer than a thirty-year-old's. "Women need to believe in themselves and their ability to birth their child. If they believe in normal birth, it will happen," explains Laraine Guyette, a nurse-midwife and assistant professor of nursing.

Your attitude about your pregnancy may influence the way you experience childbirth, which, may, in turn, influence your labor. However, sometimes labor will be difficult despite the best of attitudes. In such cases, if the nurse-midwife deems it necessary, she can order and administer medications, induce labor, perform episiotomies, and interpret fetal heart monitors. Nurse-midwives are trained to handle a wide range of problems (births can be normal yet still have some problems), although they do not perform cesarean sections, and they rarely deliver multiples or breech babies. Consequently, nurse-midwives work with a backup physician or group of physicians who become your caregivers should any major complication arise during your pregnancy or your baby's birth. If a forceps or vacuum extraction or a cesarean section is required, the midwife will call in her backup physician. You may wish to talk to the backup physician during your pregnancy in order to increase communication in the event that this doctor attends your birth.

A CNM is a registered nurse (RN) with advanced training in childbirth. After she completes an accredited university program and passes an exam given by the American College of Nurse-Midwives' Certification Council (an organization called the ACC), she becomes a certified midwife (CNM). (When I refer to midwives in this book, I refer to either CNMs or "direct-entry" midwives who have had professional training but are not nurses.) Although midwives have been accepted for decades in European countries like the Netherlands, where midwives provide much of the prenatal care and manage a large number of births, their popularity in the United States is relatively recent. It wasn't until the 1960s that hospitals began to allow individual nurse-midwives to practice.

Nowadays, CNMs can deliver babies at your home, in

birthing centers, or in some (though not all) hospitals; they are covered by health insurance, just like doctors. Some have their own practices. Others are members of an obstetrical or family medicine practice. If you want access to both a midwife and doctor, you can have the best of both worlds by finding a medical practice that includes a nurse-midwife. That way you can have a nurse-midwife as your primary caregiver but at the same time become familiar with the physicians who may step in if you have complications in pregnancy or birth.

Empathic Companionship

The term midwife means "with woman." It is the midwife's purpose to give you confidence and empathic companionship during childbirth. "I keep saying, 'I know you can do this. I've seen thousands of women do this, and you're doing just fine,'" says Marion McCartney, a CNM. Many midwives labor-sit, offering you ongoing support during crucial parts of your labor. "Labor-sitting can mean staying with you for the most crucial parts of labor and birth or never leaving your side once you arrive at the hospital or birthing center," says McCartney.

On the other hand, most doctors, especially those with large practices, are rarely able to labor-sit and remain continuously at your side during labor. You will see your doctor on and off during your labor, especially if you are having problems, and your doctor will be present during the birth—that's just how the system is set up. Your physician's role is to manage any possible complications of pregnancy and birth, to utilize high-tech procedures when necessary, to deliver the baby, and to offer you medical advice and some degree of emotional support throughout your pregnancy and birth. However, most doctors simply do not have the time to spend hours and hours labor-sitting.

Although you will be assigned a labor and delivery nurse once you are in the hospital, the nurse may be in and out of your room to take care of another patient, leaving you and your birth partner alone for long periods of time. More continuous nursing support is unlikely due to the current nursing shortage in American hospitals. Consequently, a woman is rarely supported continuously throughout her entire labor. While this system takes care of your immediate medical and surgical needs and provides cutting-edge technology to care for you and your baby, it often is not designed to meet your needs for comfort and reassurance.

A nurse-midwife, on the other hand, attends to both your medical and emotional needs in the hospital setting, at a birth center, or in your own home. Her role is to make childbirth a positive experience for you. She is there to believe in you, to understand you, and to support you in your choices—whether you choose pain medications or a natural birth. She also is there to offer you her medical judgment and experience in order to help you arrive at decisions that are the safest for you and your baby. If you are nervous about hospitals, a nurse-midwife can sometimes make the hospital a friendlier, more human environment and make you feel more at ease—even if you end up needing medical interventions. "Nurse-midwives are a stepping-stone between a home birth and a high-tech, medically managed hospital birth," says Pam Spry, a CNM and Professor of Nursing at the University of Colorado.

Now that nurse-midwives are becoming more popular as care providers, it is possible that your nurse-midwife may be unable to labor-sit because she must attend to her other patients. In this case, you may want a doula to offer you continuous support.

Patience and Support of the Birth Process

Because midwives see labor as "natural" and believe that some labors are longer than others, they may be inclined to let "nature takes it course." For instance, nurse-midwives tend to be more flexible than some physicians in their reaction to a long or difficult labor. Midwives are more likely to suggest changes in your position (to help your baby move more easily through the birth canal) or a relaxing shower before they consider administering Pitocin or calling in a physician to administer pain medication or an epidural.

Midwives tend to see labor as a normal event—even if yours lasts a little longer than the standard times set by the "labor curves" of medical studies. "I don't have a set second stage of labor. Medicine has two and a half to three hours as an upper limit. But if you have a mother who's not exhausted and a baby who's not in distress, you can extend those perimeters as long as necessary," says Pam Spry. Many nurse-midwives think episiotomies can be avoided by slow delivery of the baby's head or by perineal massage and that a woman's perineum often will stretch to adequately accommodate her baby. Some midwives will do episiotomies only in cases of fetal distress when the baby needs to be born quickly.

Some physicians share the midwifery "birth-is-normal" philosophy, have flexible attitudes about length of labor and episiotomy, and are familiar with a variety of birthing positions. If you prefer to be cared for by such a physician, shop for one early in your pregnancy.

Medical Interventions

Although midwives often use natural means to facilitate childbirth, if your labor fails to progress after an adequate period of time, a nurse-midwife may administer Pitocin or other medications to help your labor along. If your labor does not progress or if you develop certain complications, the midwife will refer you to a physician. Most nurse-midwives practicing in American hospitals will call in physicians whenever necessary for the benefit of mother and baby.

Childbirth and Bonding

The midwifery philosophy of birth includes the psychological and spiritual along with the physical components of labor and delivery. From this point of view, childbirth is a profound accomplishment. Most contemporary midwives—whether they are nurse-midwives or "direct-entry" midwives—present childbirth as powerful, difficult, and rewarding work focused on a precious goal: birthing a baby. Even painful contractions are considered constructive in a context where they do the purposeful and valuable work of pushing your baby into the world.

Midwives also believe the time immediately after birth should be used for emotional and physical mother-child bonding. "I think the baby should be delivered and never leave the mother's side," says Pam Spry. Her words are typical of the midwifery philosophy, which holds that babies and mothers should remain together unless it is medically necessary for one of them to receive special care. However, in some American hospitals, examining and weighing the baby, treating it with the appropriate eye drops, and bathing it—a combination of medical requirements and conventional hospital routine—take precedence. In some hospitals, babies are taken to the nursery after birth for anywhere from twenty minutes to several hours.

Midwives are interested in the spiritual ramifications of birth and bonding. Several midwives have written books and articles addressing topics such as the "rapture" or "near-mystical bliss" experienced by some women during or after birth. However, there are also physicians who are sensitive to spiritual issues surrounding birthing and bonding. If you choose a physician as your care provider, and if such spiritual issues are important to you, include questions about the spiritual nature of birth in your initial interview with your doctor.

Alternative Birth Settings

A woman will labor the best where she feels the safest and most secure. For some that will be the home, for some women that will be a hospital, and for some women that will be a birth center.
—Michelle Brill, doula

* * *

Nurse-midwives may practice in a hospital or in an alternative birth setting such as a birth center or your own home, depending on state law and licensing. Most nurse-midwives will offer you a home birth only if you are low risk. But the term "low risk" means different things to different people; some care providers will consider a home birth only for women who have previously had a baby. If you are having a first baby, some nurse-midwives will suggest that you give birth at a hospital or at a birth center.

Direct-entry midwives (CPMs and CMs) are non-nurse midwives who tend to specialize in home births. Sometimes they attend births in birth centers, but they do not have hospital admitting privileges.

Although midwives tend to argue that home and birth centers are safe places to have your baby, they acknowledge that some women—especially older women—may end up being transferred from a birth center to a hospital due to a labor that doesn't progress adequately. Women over forty are more likely than women in their twenties to be transferred for dysfunctional labor. According to a New Zealand study, for all women who plan home birth, one out of four will be transferred to a hospital to give birth. (See Chapter 4.)

Direct-Entry Midwives (CPMs and CMs)

"If your body knows how to conceive this baby and knows how to grow this baby, certainly it knows how to do the other part of the equation: to birth the baby," assures Nancy Wainer Cohen, direct-entry midwife. Wainer Cohen's statement reflects the childbirth-is-normal point of view held by most lay midwives. Like other direct-entry, non-nurse midwives, she believes that birth is so normal that it can be routinely done at home.

The direct-entry midwife has a long history in both the United States and Europe, since most babies in the 1600s and 1700s were delivered by midwives. In the United States, most midwives received no formal training but learned what was then a woman's trade from other, more experienced midwives. In Europe, women attended midwifery schools. It wasn't until the 1800s that male doctors replaced female midwives. The specialty of obstetrics did not appear until the 1900s.

Nowadays, some direct-entry midwives have completed a formal midwifery education program or met midwifery licensing criteria. Although it is sometimes difficult to evaluate the training and skill of a particular midwife, there are national certification programs for direct-entry midwives that provide quality control. One certification program is administered by the North American Registry of Midwives (NARM). Women who complete the certification are called certified professional midwives (CPM). Even though they are not nurses, they are trained midwives, and they have their own professional organizations such as NARM and the Midwives Alliance of North America (MANA). Another national program, administered by the American College of Nurse Midwives, grants certified midwife (CM) certification.

Some direct-entry midwives have no certification. This kind of lay-midwifery is illegal in some states. A lay midwife may be well trained in obstetrics, or she may not—"It depends on the individual person," says Louise Aucott, who was a lay midwife before she became a CNM.

If you are interested in finding a midwife who is licensed as a CNM, CPM, or CM, call the national organizations for referrals. (See appendix for phone numbers.)

Doulas or Birth Companions

A doula can offer labor support, can make things go smoothly, and can decrease the need for pain medication.
—Dr. Susan Porto

* * *

Emotional and physical support significantly shortens labor and decreases the need for cesarean deliveries, forceps and vacuum extraction, oxytocin administration, and analgesia [pain medication]. Doula-supported mothers also rate childbirth as less difficult and painful than do women not supported by a doula. Labor support by fathers does not appear to produce similar obstetrical benefits.
—K. D. Scott, P. H. Klaus, M. H. Klaus. "The Obstetrical and Postpartum Benefits of Continuous Support During Childbirth." *J Womens Health Gend Based Med* 1999 Dec., 8(10)

* * *

When Thelma was in labor with her second child, she felt so isolated that she insisted someone be sent to stay with her. "I kept saying, 'I don't want to be alone! I don't want to be alone in here!'" The nurses sent a cleaning lady in to keep her company. Companionship was all Thelma needed to ease her anxiety during her long labor.

Thelma had this experience in 1946, long before doulas (experienced "female birth companions") were accepted by American hospitals as part of the birthing process. But nowadays, even as doulas become more popular, and as doula-training programs become more available, many women remain unaware of the benefits of a doula. Even if a woman has heard about doulas, she may be unaware of how or where to find one.

Medical studies over the last decade show that "continuous support during labor" by doulas and midwives greatly improves a woman's experience of childbirth and the general well-being of her newborn. Women who have continuous support during childbirth have shorter and less complicated labors, and they need fewer episiotomies, fewer forceps deliveries, and fewer cesarean sections than women who do not have continuous support during labor. Studies show that the continuous presence of a trained support person during labor reduces the need for pain medication and has been associated with lower epidural rates and fewer women describing panic or exhaustion. Studies also show that the presence of a doula may benefit the woman and her newborn by decreasing fetal distress and increasing success in breastfeeding.

The review of medical studies in *A Guide to Effective Care in Pregnancy and Childbirth* (third edition) found that the effects of a labor support person are "remarkably consistent" and beneficial for both mother and baby. Dr. Enkin and his coauthors write: "The continuous presence of an experienced support person who has no prior social bond with the laboring woman reduced the likelihood of: medication for pain relief, cesarean delivery, operative vaginal delivery, and a five minute Apgar score of [less than] 7. Another beneficial effect found in six trials was the decreased likelihood of negative evaluations of the childbirth experience, of feeling very tense during labor, and of finding labor worse than expected."

Both British and American obstetricians now recognize the benefits of doulas. Even standard obstetrics textbooks such as Creasy's *Management of Labor and Delivery* acknowledge that doulas facilitate labor and help reduce pain.

Whether your doula is a trained professional or a trusted friend, she should understand childbirth and function as part of a supportive team that may include your partner, family member, midwife, and/or physician. The doula does not replace your partner, but in helping to support you, she may take some of the pressure off your partner and family, who may be under considerable stress. When Sharlene had her first baby at age forty-eight, a doula supported her through a long labor and massaged her back after Sharlene's husband was exhausted.

"It can be a long time waiting during labor. Husbands are not set up to stay up all night and wait on you hand and foot. They're too emotionally involved. My husband is great—but that's an area he's not good at. Paula [the doula] gave me massages. My husband, Carl, talked to me. We had the lights down low. We had soothing music. It was a really calm environment." Carla, at age thirty-three, was frightened of childbirth, and she needed both her husband and her doula to support her through a long and difficult labor.

Doulas provide emotional encouragement by reinforcing the positive aspects of birth in terms a woman can best understand. A resourceful doula will find encouraging words that appeal to a woman's unique personality. "Sometimes I tell a woman that there are thousands of women doing what you are doing all over the world," says Penny Simkin, doula and childbirth educator. Kathleen Gray Farthing, a Birthworks educator and doula, encourages laboring women to see birth as both a spiritual and physical achievement.

"This is a woman's chance to feel the same exhilaration as a football player," says Farthing. "I tell her, 'Your body did that, and you were stronger than you ever believed.'" Farthing, like many other doulas, believes that within every woman is the knowledge of how to give birth, that every woman is capable of it, and that labor can be made easier if a woman believes in her body and trusts the birth process.

The presence of a doula can complement the medical care

of either a nurse-midwife or an MD. If you are truly high risk or are pregnant with a breech baby or multiple babies, you will need a physician because you may need medical interventions. In any case, the doula can lend support and help you with the baby or babies. If your primary caregiver is a midwife, it still is reasonable—and not excessive—to also have a doula by your side during labor. Kathleen found she needed her doula, her midwife, and her husband to support her through labor with her first child. Each had a different but important role:

"If Svea [the doula] wasn't there I don't know what I would have done. She was really calming. She was there to just support me. The midwife didn't have to do that. My husband couldn't respond that way to support me; neither one of us had done this before. He was rubbing my back the whole time, and I needed him to do that."

Although your midwife may offer emotional support, she must focus her attention on medical matters when necessary. Your doula, on the other hand, is trained to support you, but not to assume a medical role. While the midwife is busy monitoring the baby, checking your contractions, or helping you find advantageous positions in labor, a doula can offer you encouragement, rub your back, and bring you ice chips or hot compresses. If your midwife has another woman in labor and has to go back and forth between the two of you, your doula will stay by your side throughout labor.

A good labor and delivery nurse can make an excellent doula. However, because labor and delivery nurses usually must care for several laboring women at the same time, they are not able to labor-sit.

Choose a doula who will listen to you and support you and represent you fairly. Look for a woman who is sensitive to your needs, mature, experienced, and nonjudgmental about your birth plan. Pick someone who can firmly—but diplomatically—

advocate for you without alienating hospital staff. To find a doula, contact DONA, a national organization of doulas (see appendix). Some hospitals offer low-cost or volunteer doulas. Call your care provider, hospital, and/or local birth center to find a doula in your area.

If you want a doula with you during childbirth, you will need to make arrangements in advance with your care provider and with the hospital or birthing center.

Partners, Friends, and Family

Men can just be there to hold their wife's hand, stay at her side, and give her what she wants. That's the best thing to do. Just show that you're interested and empathic.
—Dr. Susan Porto

❋ ❋ ❋

"You can't control your labor, but you can control your choice of health care provider and whom you invite to your labor," says Mary Sommers, a childbirth educator at the Alivio Clinic in Chicago. In deciding who to invite to your birth, consider who is most likely to be a calming influence and who can be sensitive to your needs rather than absorbed in their own. You may be accustomed to taking care of your partner or other family members—but during labor you will need to free yourself to concentrate on birthing your baby.

You may need to invite several people to cumulatively get the support you need (although your hospital may not allow more than one or two family members or friends). For instance, you may find it emotionally important to you to have your partner, your mother, your sister, or a close friend with you during labor.

Studies show that the presence of a supportive person decreases a laboring woman's experience of pain. There also is evidence that the father's or birth partner's presence during childbirth, the role the partner plays in supporting the use of pain management techniques, and the quality of the couple's relationship may reduce the need for pain medication in labor.

Despite men's fears that they may be too squeamish or useless during childbirth, men often find—sometimes much to their pleasant surprise—that attending the birth of their child is an intense and emotionally satisfying experience that leaves them feeling "high" for hours after the birth and bonds them with their new family in a lasting and positive way.

Many men, lesbian partners, and family members do not realize how soothing their mere presence—their eye contact, touch, smell, voice—can be for a laboring woman.

However, the presence of family or friends is not always reassuring. A problematic relationship can add to your anxiety, fear, and pain and can be counterproductive. If a particular family member or friend tends to cause conflict, you can protect yourself during your most vulnerable moments in labor and birth by either asking the person to visit you after the baby is born or by inviting a protective and diplomatic friend or family member to buffer potential conflict and to support you during childbirth.

Chapter 18

Due Dates: Preterm and Postterm Births

Only about 5 percent of babies arrive on their due date. Seven out of ten babies arrive after their due date. The due date is an estimate, and it is most reliable if you know exactly the first day of your last menstrual period before you became pregnant. If your periods are regular and you know when you ovulate, you will have an easier time calculating your probable date of conception. Often, your real due date is two weeks before or after your predicted due date.

There may be considerable individual variation from baby to baby and not one hard-and-fast date of forty weeks gestational age at which all babies are ready to be born. Some women's pregnancies last only thirty-eight weeks, yet their babies are not born "too soon" since they are already mature and ready to be born. Other women go for forty-two weeks—two weeks past due—without problems. However, there are times when thirty-eight weeks is a bit too soon, and forty-two weeks is a bit too long, in that babies may show signs of distress.

Preterm Labor and Birth
Preterm birth—or birth before thirty-seven completed weeks of

gestation—occurs in approximately 10 percent of all births. If you have high blood pressure, preeclampsia, or severe infection; if your mother took DES during her first trimester of pregnancy; or if you are pregnant with twins or more, you may have an increased risk of going into preterm labor and delivering your baby early.

Preterm delivery may be risky for your baby, especially if the baby is physiologically too immature to breathe well and function on its own. Sometimes preterm labor can be detected early enough to prevent preterm birth, and you will need to go to the hospital immediately to receive treatment to delay labor. Learn to recognize the early signs and symptoms of preterm labor.

Call your caregiver immediately if you experience:

1. Recurrent contractions every fifteen minutes that cause your uterus to tighten and harden, even if they are not painful
2. Cramping in your abdomen
3. A premonition that something is wrong
4. Diarrhea, intestinal discomfort, or pain
5. Vaginal bleeding
6. Gushing or trickling fluid from your vagina
7. Vaginal discharge
8. Backache
9. Pelvic pressure or fullness
10. Abdominal pain

If you experience any of the above symptoms, do not wait for them to go away. Call your doctor. If your doctor is not available, call his or her partners or call the emergency room of the nearest hospital, preferably a hospital with a neonatal care unit. Explain your symptoms, and prepare to go to the hospital to be checked. If you are bleeding or have any of the afore-mentioned symptoms, do not attempt to drive to the hospital. Call 911 if you are bleeding or if you can feel the baby's cord in your vagina (see Part 8).

The sooner you call your care provider, the more effective he or she can be at either preventing the premature birth or managing your labor. If contacted early enough, your caregiver may administer medications to stop your contractions and post-pone labor until your baby is more mature. Sometimes your caregiver can delay labor for only forty-eight hours or more, but that may give you enough time to get to a hospital with a special unit for premature babies—an NICU.

Your doctor may attempt to manage your premature labor without medication. He or she may advise you to drink more fluids, since dehydration can cause premature labor. Your care provider may prescribe limited activity or strict bed rest. Limited activity means that you rest at home, but you are not confined to bed. If you are put on strict bed rest, however, you will be expected to remain in bed—and not putter around the house. Strict bed rest means that you do not subject your baby and cervix to the forces of gravity by being upright: You are not supposed to stand, sit, or kneel. Lie on your side, preferably your left side, since lying on your back for long periods of time can impede the blood flow to your baby. If you are on bed rest, stock up on reading materials, videos, and music and place all these items within easy reach. For extended periods on bed rest, call bed rest support groups (see Chapter 14 and the appendix) since weeks or months on bed rest can be tedious.

Postterm Pregnancy

The basic protocol is when a woman is past her due date you do tests. You do the nonstress test. When the woman is past

forty-one weeks, you schedule her for intervention so she doesn't go beyond forty-two weeks. . . . There are protocols, using prostaglandins, to get a woman to go into labor on her own. The idea is not to have to do a cesarean section. The interventions would hopefully lower the odds of cesarean section. But does intervention lower the instance of cesareans? Done wisely and thoughtfully, it doesn't increase them.
—Dr. Allen Killam

◆ ◆ ◆

The frequency of postterm pregnancy—a pregnancy lasting forty-two weeks or more—varies from 4 to 14 percent of all pregnancies, depending on the medical study and the definition of postterm (whether it is forty-one or forty-two weeks).

A potential problem for postterm babies is that the larger and more mature the baby becomes, the more the baby demands from its placenta. If the placenta is beginning to get old, a condition that may lead to problems with blood flow and nourishment, the baby may be seriously endangered if its birth is delayed by a week or two. Consequently, it is now standard for care providers to induce labor after a baby reaches forty-two weeks gestational age—even in the absence of fetal or maternal problems. Under some circumstances, such as fetal distress, labor may be induced at forty-one weeks of pregnancy.

The management of postterm babies is the subject of medical debate. Some care providers think that routine induction of labor at forty or forty-one weeks gestation is in the best interest of the baby. Others disagree and recommend induction only *after* forty-one weeks. Still others argue that the best approach (as long as both mother and baby are healthy) is to wait and see if labor will occur spontaneously. However, several medical studies show that the baby benefits from an induction of labor in pregnancies lasting *longer than forty-one weeks*, according to

Dr. Enkin and his coauthors in *A Guide to Effective Care in Pregnancy and Childbirth.*

The management of postterm pregnancy is far from cut and dried, according to childbirth expert Henci Goer. Although Goer writes in her book, *Obstetrics Myths Versus Research Realities,* that "routinely inducing [labor] creates more problems than it solves," she adds that no approach to postterm pregnancy is risk-free: "Letting nature take its course is generally best, although that is not risk free either. No course of action (or inaction) guarantees good outcomes. The reality is you pay your money and you take your choice."

Also the subject of debate is whether or not induction of a postterm baby will increase a woman's odds for needing a cesarean delivery. Some care providers believe that inducing labor *before* forty-one weeks with a healthy mother and baby has no advantage for the mother or baby and may increase the likelihood of a cesarean birth. However, there is some evidence that inducing labor *at* forty-one-plus weeks may actually *decrease* the likelihood of a cesarean section.

If your baby is late, discuss your individual circumstances with your care provider to determine what management plan is best for you and your baby. Your care provider may wish to induce labor if your baby has an aging placenta that can no longer effectively provide nourishment or if your baby is in distress. To assess the health of baby and placenta, your care provider may perform some of the following tests: urinary estriol, electronic fetal monitoring, or ultrasound.

If you have preeclampsia or worsening high blood pressure, your care provider may also want to induce labor since your baby could be deprived of adequate blood flow and nutrition within your uterus. In such cases, your baby may be better able to thrive outside your body than inside it. (See Part 8 for a description of induction techniques.)

Chapter 19
What Is Labor?

It was a journey. Now I know what my strength is. If you asked me, "Can you climb Mt. Everest?" I now feel: yeah, I could.
—Carla, thirty-three, was surprised by the extent of her stamina and strength during labor

• • •

Labor is a process initiated by a well-orchestrated, biochemical interaction between you and your unborn child. Your baby triggers a series of events that result in your pituitary gland producing *oxytocin*, a hormone that stimulates labor contractions. Labor is your body's effort to push your baby from your uterus, down through your birth canal, and out into the world. The first stage consists of regular uterine contractions leading to the gradual "ripening" (the softening, thinning, shortening, and opening) of your cervix. The second stage consists of the progressive descent of your baby through your pelvis and birth canal.

The next several chapters are designed to prepare you for childbirth—to explain what your body is doing; what you can physically and emotionally do to cope with labor, minimize discomfort, and facilitate birth; and how you can maintain a positive attitude toward birthing your baby. In the words of the nurse-midwives and physicians whose thoughts contributed greatly to these chapters:

The single most important thing is for a woman to trust her body to know what it needs to do—and then when it's time, her body will function.
—Laraine Guyette, CNM, Assistant Professor of Nursing at the University of Colorado

* * ◆

Women get through labor the same way they get through other hard things in their lives. Every woman's capable of doing it, but she does it in a way that is unique for her.
—Mary Sommers, CNM, Alivio Clinic, Chicago

* * ◆

You have to tell women that labor is unpredictable. They can optimize it by relaxing and understanding what is going on, but they can't control it completely.
—Dr. Edward Quilligan

The 4 P's of Labor: Powers, Passage, Passenger, and Psyche

Obstetric textbooks frequently describe the components of labor in terms of what doctors call "the 3 P's":

1. The powers (the contractions of your uterine muscle),
2. The passage (the architecture of your pelvis), and
3. The passenger (your baby).

Midwives add a fourth "P":

4. The psyche.

The 4 P's explain, in simple terms, four important components involved in labor and birth: the force of your uterine contractions, the shape of your birth canal, the size and position of your baby relative to that of your birth canal, and the state of your mind. These components affect each other during labor. The progressive movement of the baby through the birth canal is affected by the size of the birth canal, the size of the baby, and how well the uterus works as a muscle that pushes the baby. These dynamics are present in every labor, whether you are fifteen or fifty.

The contractions of your uterine muscle, "the powers," cause the cervix to soften and open, and then the contractions push the baby through the birth canal (your pelvis, cervix, and vagina), which adapts to labor by opening up. The powers push the baby through your birth canal, and the baby responds to the shape of the passage by rotating, flexing, and extending as it makes its journey into the world. The relation of your baby's head and body to your pelvis changes as she descends through the pelvic cavity. This process involves a combination of movements working together or in sequence as the baby adapts to different parts of your pelvic passage.

The passage of the baby will be modified by the shape of the pelvis she is moving through. Some caregivers believe that the shape of the mother's pelvis is a "given" that cannot be influenced by maternal positions such as squatting or walking. However, other caregivers believe that birthing positions make birth easier by slightly changing the shape of the passage.

Your baby negotiates your pelvic passage as she moves closer and closer to birth. The size and position of your baby play important roles in determining the ease or difficulty of this journey. However, on the whole, your baby is well designed for birth. Her abdomen is relatively flexible and can adjust to the compression of your uterine contractions. Although birth may appear to be hard on the baby, many doctors believe that labor and birth are actually good for the baby: the contractions of labor force amniotic fluid from the baby's lungs and prepare her for breathing air.

As the baby's head enters the birth passage, her head may change shape by a process called molding. Even though labor may temporarily compress your baby's skull into a kind of temporary "cone head," her skull is designed to move in order to tolerate such pressure. Molding is a beneficial thing, since it allows your child's head to fit the size of your pelvis.

Your *psyche* also may exert an influence on the process of birth. Midwives like Laraine Guyette believe that women who psychologically "let go" and work with the forces of nature—instead of fighting them—are more likely to have easier and shorter labors than women whose fear and anxiety interfere with their contractions and the relaxation necessary for labor to progress. According to this point of view, your mind can influence your contractions and the opening of your cervix and birth canal. Believing in your capacity to give birth may relax you, influence your labor—and become a self-fulfilling prophecy, says Guyette:

"You have to believe in the birth process. Women have been doing this since the beginning of the world. Women need to believe in themselves. If they believe they can birth their child, the birth will happen."

If your labor has slowed or stopped, your care provider may enlist the aid of your psyche by asking you to confront fears that might be hindering you. Sometimes the reasons for a slowing down of labor are physical, but sometimes the reasons may be emotional. For instance, a woman's labor may temporarily stop after she is admitted to the hospital, especially if the hospital environment increases her anxiety level. The anxiety releases stress hormones, and the hormones slow down labor. Anxiety can also come from inner conflicts. Midwife Laraine Guyette believes that some women become fearful of birthing the baby and the labor stops—a phenomenon she refers to as "fetal retention syndrome." When this occurs, Guyette asks the woman to tell her what fears are getting in the way of birthing the baby. Sometimes giving voice to the fear makes labor more manageable, and the labor progresses.

Midwives, doulas, and some physicians will enlist your psyche to increase cervical dilation and the passage of your baby through the birth canal. The care provider may use visualization—a mind-over-matter technique used in healing, relaxation, or meditation—to help you "see" your cervix opening or to imagine a "widening circle" or a flower opening petal by petal. Such images engage your psyche in the task of opening your cervix. Many women find such visualizations useful in coping with labor.

The Mechanisms of Labor

The mechanisms of labor help your baby move through your pelvis during childbirth. These mechanisms are often discussed in terms that seem complex, such as "engagement," "descent," "flexion," "internal rotation," "external rotation," and "extension." However, the movement of the baby is really quite simple.

As the baby moves downward toward your cervix and birth canal, its head engages (if the baby is positioned headfirst) in your pelvis. Thus, the baby no longer floats freely in amniotic fluid and no longer somersaults in your womb, since its head now rests between the pelvic bones near your cervix. If you are having your first baby, 80 percent of the time engagement will occur prior to the clinical diagnosis of labor—sometimes several weeks before labor begins. If you already have had a child, engagement may occur shortly before labor. Engagement positions the baby for birth. It also puts pressure on your cervix, leading to further cervical dilation and opening of the birth canal.

Before your baby can descend through the canal and be born, your cervix must open to nine or ten centimeters. When your cervix is fully open, the baby, pushed by the "powers" of your uterine contractions, descends through your cervical opening during the first stage of labor.

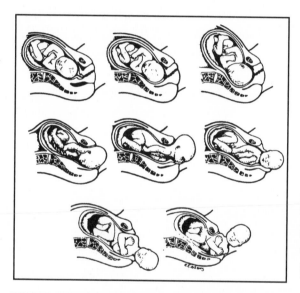

Figure 19-1: The "mechanisms of labor" help the baby descend through the birth canal.

(Creasy, *Management of Labor and Delivery*, p. 66). Reprinted by permission of Blackwell Science, Inc.

As your baby moves through the passage, she accommodates herself to the shape of your pelvis. To facilitate *descent,* she *flexes* her neck and tucks her chin. As she moves through the birth canal, her head and body rotate, and her neck extends as she is delivered.

Nature has ingeniously designed this process so that the top of the baby's head in its smallest diameter comes first, making it small enough to fit through your vagina and perineum during birth (when this position is not achieved, the birth process may become more difficult; see Part 8). After the baby's head crowns, the baby rotates as one shoulder is delivered and then the other.

During the first stage of labor your cervix dilates to allow your baby to descend during the second stage. The baby's descent becomes more rapid at the end of the second stage of labor—the pushing stage. In the pushing stage, uterine contractions become more intense as the uterine muscle pushes the baby through the opening of the birth canal. Your voluntary bearing-down efforts, in conjunction with your involuntary contractions, push your baby through the remaining portion of the birth canal.

Midwives, and some labor and delivery nurses and doctors, believe that by assuming specific birthing positions during childbirth, women can influence the rotation of the baby to "favor descent" and thus aid the mechanisms of labor. (See "Maternal Positions in Labor.")

Signals of Impending Labor

Before the first stage of labor begins, your body may give you signals that soon you will be going into labor. It is important to listen to these signals—and to gauge your activities accordingly. For instance, you may not want to dive into a four-hour executive committee meeting or drive to the beach for a weekend if you are manifesting some of the signs of prelabor (sometimes called *prodromal* labor).

The most commons signals that your body is preparing to give birth are: lightening; bloody show; nesting energy; rupture of the membranes or "bag of waters"; cervical changes; and frequent Braxton-Hicks contractions.

Lightening
The baby drops down and the presenting part (the part that

comes first—usually the head) engages in your pelvis. Consequently, the upper part of your abdomen may feel "lighter." You may feel less pressure against your stomach and diaphragm when you eat and breathe, although the lower part of your abdomen may feel heavy from the pressure of the baby. If you are pregnant with your first baby, lightening most likely will occur one to two weeks before you go into labor. For subsequent babies, lightening may occur shortly before labor begins.

Cervical Changes

Your cervix begins to efface—to soften and shorten. It also begins opening. This may happen days or even weeks before you go into active labor.

Bloody Show

When your cervix begins to soften and stretch due to the hormonal changes of late pregnancy, the mucous plug that covered your cervical opening during pregnancy will become dislodged. Bloody show is the bloodstained mucous from this plug—a discharge that contains pink or bright red streaks. It is not a steady flow of blood. The appearance of bloody show means that your cervix is opening and that the birth of your baby could either be a few days or a few weeks away. You need not dash off to the hospital until other signs of labor are present.

However, if you continue bleeding or spotting or if you bleed heavily, call your doctor or midwife immediately. Profuse or prolonged bleeding may be signs of possible problems such as placenta previa or placenta abruption (see Part 5 and Part 8), conditions that require immediate medical treatment. So do not wait for such bleeding to "go away." Call your caregiver to be safe. Go to the hospital if bleeding persists.

Bloody brown discharge that may appear after vaginal exams can be mistaken for bloody show. Check with your caregiver to determine whether or not your protective mucous plug has indeed dislodged and your cervix is preparing for birth.

Nesting Instinct or Burst of Energy

You may experience a burst of energy shortly before you go into labor. If you find yourself knitting, washing dishes, folding towels and linens with increased gusto, you may be approaching labor. Don't overdo; conserve your energy for birthing your baby.

Diarrhea

Some women experience diarrhea shortly before labor begins. The diarrhea may be accompanied by cramping.

Backache

Some women experience backache just prior to labor. If you are pregnant with twins, triplets, or more, or even with a single baby, a backache could mean that you are going into labor even if you are not experiencing other symptoms. Back pain that comes and goes or any rhythmic back discomfort may be contractions. Call your caregiver for advice.

Rupture of the Membranes (Bag of Waters)

As your baby drops down toward your birth canal, the bag of amniotic fluid surrounding the baby may break as it is pressed between the baby and your pelvis. This is a painless process. Fluid will either gush out or trickle out over time. For some women, this may feel like urination. For others, it is subtle and gradual. Frequently, the bag of waters breaks after true labor has started, but it also may break within twenty-four to forty-eight hours before labor begins.

In approximately 10 to 12 percent of pregnancies, the waters break before labor begins. If you are not in labor when your waters break, expect to be in labor soon thereafter.

According to medical studies, about 70 percent of women whose membranes rupture at term will go into labor within twenty-four hours, and almost 90 percent will go into labor within forty-eight hours. You and the baby are more vulnerable to infection after your waters break, because some care providers recommend that vaginal exams be limited after the waters break to avoid introducing infection into the birth canal.

If your membranes rupture before labor begins, you and your baby may face some risks of infection if labor doesn't begin within twenty-four hours. Your care provider may administer antibiotics to you and later to the baby. Some care providers may wish to induce labor if your labor doesn't begin after a reasonable period of time.

If your membranes are intact at the beginning of your labor, they will usually (but not always) rupture during active labor. Once your waters break, do not have intercourse since your baby is no longer encapsulated in a membrane that protects it—and you—from infection. Make note of the time of rupture; the amount of fluid released; and the color, odor, and clarity of the fluid. Amniotic fluid usually is clear and odorless with white flecks in it.

If your fluid is tinged with green, yellow, or brown, your baby may have passed meconium, which means she has had a bowel movement in utero. This in itself is not a cause for alarm; it means that your baby's gastrointestinal tract is mature. However, meconium should be reported to your caregiver immediately, since you and your baby may require monitoring to determine whether or not your baby is in distress.

Although some women may wait many hours between the rupture of the membranes and the beginning of true labor, the longer the time between the rupture of your membranes and the onset of labor, the greater your risk of infection. If you are not yet in labor when your waters break:

- Notify your caregiver.
- Keep track of the amount of time that has elapsed since your waters broke and note the color, odor, and amount of fluid.
- Save your underwear or sanitary pad in a plastic bag in case your caregiver needs to evaluate the amount or quality of your amniotic fluid.
- Refrain from baths (unless your care provider tells you otherwise).
- Refrain from intercourse.
- Limit the number of vaginal exams, since exams increase your risk of infection.
- Do what you can safely do to stimulate labor by walking, relaxing, using acupressure points, encouraging your own natural oxytocin production by nipple stimulation.
- Stay nourished and hydrated in order to meet the demands of labor.
- Make sure the amniotic fluid has not swept the baby's umbilical cord into the birth canal, resulting in a prolapsed cord.

Upon your arrival at the hospital, tell hospital staff when your waters broke. You may even want to provide "evidence." Anna had to produce her underwear to convince the medical staff that her bag of waters had actually broken en route to the hospital. Call your caregiver when you leak or gush fluid. If your baby is breech or it has not yet engaged, your caregiver will most likely want you to go directly to the hospital.

Occasionally, the baby's umbilical cord may be swept through your cervix and into your vagina with the amniotic fluid. Such cord prolapse is rare, but it is a medical emergency for the baby. If you see or feel the cord at or below the vaginal opening, get on your hands and knees in order to take pressure off the cord and to maintain blood and oxygen flow to the baby. (Wash your hands carefully with strong soap and warm water before manually checking for the cord. *Never* pull on it.) Call 911, and call your doctor.

Things to immediately report to your doctor during prelabor and early labor:

- Prolapsed cord
- Sustained or profuse bleeding
- Intense headache or dizziness
- High blood pressure
- Seizures
- Prolonged vomiting or diarrhea
- Severe abdominal pain
- Repeated fainting
- Visual changes such as seeing shimmering, light flashes, or spots

Braxton-Hicks Contractions and False Labor

In terms of preparation for the older mother, I strongly recommend that once my clients start Braxton-Hicks contractions, they get into a pattern of drinking every hour that they're awake, eating something every two hours, and resting every four hours. That way, when they go into labor, they're not dehydrated, they have enough calories, and they're not exhausted.
—Laraine Guyette, CNM

❋ ❋ ❋

Braxton-Hicks contractions, known as "false labor," help prepare the uterus for birth. Unlike the contractions of true labor that increase in intensity and frequency, Braxton-Hicks contractions are irregular and often painless. However, such contractions are signs that real labor is soon to come.

As your body is preparing for labor and birth, you may experience contractions that come and go or continue in a steady, painless, nonprogressive form instead of increasing in strength, frequency, and duration. Although such intermittent contractions are referred to as "false labor," they have a positive and important role. False labor contributes to the softening and thinning of the cervix that prepares your cervix for full dilation during the first stage of labor.

During false labor, think of your body as readying itself for birth. Don't exhaust yourself timing contractions and micro-managing a labor that is barely beginning. Take care of yourself in preparation for the demands of childbirth. Eat small meals and drink plenty of fluids.

Remain active during the day, but avoid stress and heavy physical exertion. Walk, even if it is only around your office and down the hall. Walking facilitates the birth process by helping the baby attain an optimal position for birth and by stimulating labor. Sleep at night; you'll need to rest in order to have energy for labor and birth. Keep a casual early labor record noting time and nature of bloody show, diarrhea, breaking of waters, and so forth. Time contractions occasionally—every time they seem to increase in frequency or intensity or every hour or two—in order to get a general idea of where you are in the labor process.

Avoid obsessing on your labor at this point, since hyperfocusing during prelabor may increase tension and thus slow your labor. Focus instead on creating a supportive birth environment and decide how you want to spend the hours leading up to the birth of your baby. Set the stage for your labor and birth. The optimal setting will, of course, vary from woman to woman. For some, it will include leisurely walks, warm baths, watching movies, going shopping, or listening to music. For others, the optimal setting may be an absorbing day at work.

Although it is difficult to distinguish between true and false labor, false labor tends to be irregular and to come and go. If your contractions come and go for days, chances are that you're in false labor. However, if your contractions become stronger, longer in duration, more regular, and closer together, you are probably in the first stage of labor.

The Stages of Labor

The process of labor and birth is divided into four stages: dilation; descent and birth; delivery of the placenta; and recovery. The first two stages of labor have several parts or "phases."

The first two stages of labor are what we commonly refer to as labor and are the focus of most childbirth preparation classes.

Stage 1: Dilation of the Cervix

Latent phase (early labor):

The cervix dilates to approximately three to four centimeters; contractions are mild, short, and irregular, although they grow in duration, frequency, and regularity.

Active phase:

The cervix dilates approximately four to seven centimeters; contractions become stronger, more intense, and more regular.

Transition (the last part of the active phase):

The cervix dilates from seven to nine or ten centimeters, and the baby's head begins moving through it; contractions are strong and only about two to three minutes apart.

Stage 2: Descent and Birth

Contractions at three- to five-minute intervals, during

which mother feels urge to push.

Descent:

The baby is pushed down the birth canal.

Crowning and birth:

The top of the baby's head appears, and the baby is born.

Stage 3: Delivery of the Placenta

After the placenta separates from the uterus, the mother pushes the placenta out with several pushes. She is usually assisted by her physician or midwife. Rarely, a placenta may not separate on its own. If this persists for over thirty minutes, or if there is excessive bleeding, the care provider may manually remove the placenta.

Stage 4: Recovery

The uterus continues to contract on its own for several days.

Stage 1: Dilation of the Cervix

I tell my clients not to time their contractions because they'll drive themselves nuts. When the contractions are strong enough, they'll know it because the contractions will be so intense. I had one patient spend much of her labor in a botanical garden. I had another who had a hot tub in her yard (with a temperature below 100 degrees) and sat and zoned out. I had another client who played an enthusiastic game of Trivial Pursuit.
—Laraine Guyette, CNM

The first stage of labor often begins gradually. The cervix slowly softens, thins, and opens to about ten centimeters so that your baby's head can pass through it. During the first stage of labor, you will experience regular contractions that transform the shape and texture of your cervix and that lead to full dilation.

As your body prepares for labor, it produces hormones called prostaglandins that soften your cervix. When your cervix is soft, it can become *effaced* (thinned) and dilated (opened). As the cervix softens and opens, your uterine contractions draw the cervix up into the uterus so that your baby will have a larger passageway through which to make her journey into the world.

Your body also produces *oxytocin*, a hormone that stimulates the muscle of your uterus to contract. As labor progresses and oxytocin continues its influence on your uterine muscle, these contractions will grow in length, strength, and intensity. The contractions will come closer and closer together, although you will always have intervals to rest between the contractions. However, if you have back labor you may feel continuous pain.

The first stage of labor is divided into three phases: the *latent phase*, the *active phase*, and *transition*.

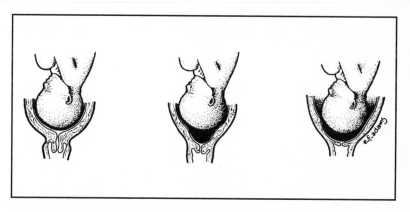

Figure 19-2: Dilation and Effacement of the Cervix

From Creasy, *Management of Labor and Delivery,* p. 72. Reprinted by permission of Blackwell Science, Inc.

The Latent Phase: Strategies for Comfort and Progress

The latent phase can be distressing and painful, and it is very normal for a woman to have a long latent phase thinking she is in labor, but she's really not in active labor.
—Dr. Allen Killam

* * *

Stay home during early labor. Go on walks, take warm baths, get back rubs, and wait to go to the hospital or birth center until the contractions are intolerable and you're not comfortable being home anymore.
—Pam Spry, CNM

* * *

The latent phase is early labor. The biochemistry of your cervix changes, and your cervix is said to *ripen* (become effaced and soft). During the latent phase of labor, your cervix will open to about three to four centimeters. The latent phase often (but not always) begins with contractions that are mild, brief, and erratic. However, as your first stage of labor progresses, your uterine contractions will become more intense, closer together, and longer lasting. As labor progresses, the interval between contractions becomes closer together.

Assigning specific times to your contractions is not necessarily helpful, since every woman experiences labor differently. In general, contractions of the latent phase tend to be fifteen to thirty minutes apart and fifteen to sixty seconds in duration. The latent phase lasts, roughly speaking, anywhere from two to twenty hours. If your contractions are mild enough for you to feel chatty and social and able to easily focus on activities other than labor, you are probably in latent labor.

Do not be alarmed if your latent stage goes on for many

hours, since it is often the longest phase of labor. Because the onset of the latent phase is difficult to determine, the normal limits of this phase are not medically well defined. Signs of the latent phase are subtle and may include bloody show, backache, and frequent bowel movements. As your cervix begins to dilate, you may see a small amount of blood mixed with mucous.

If your waters break during latent labor, call your care provider to determine when you need to come to the hospital— if you should come in right away or if you should stay at home until contractions become regular and strong.

During latent labor, it is important to relax, to be patient with your body, to allow it to do what it needs to do, and to get enough rest and nourishment to prepare yourself for the hard work of active labor that lies ahead.

Use this time to set the stage for your labor. Do things that provide you with pleasant distractions that keep your mind off your discomfort. However, avoid activities that raise your stress and adrenaline levels; early labor is not a good time to work under pressure or race through rush-hour traffic. Some women create a comforting, relaxing environment for their early labor by establishing a pattern of familiar rituals such as running a bath, lathering with fragrant soap, burning candles, listening to music, or watching favorite videos.

As latent labor begins, be prepared to make important decisions that may affect your entire birth experience. Holly made a difficult choice between work and birth priorities when she first went into labor. Instead of taking a walk in the woods with her husband, which is what she had hoped to do, she attended a lengthy meeting in her law firm. "You can still see my fingernail marks on the table," says Holly. "After the meeting I couldn't stand. I was seven centimeters dilated and in transition."

Engaging in activities that you find stressful in early labor may increase your feelings of anxiety, pain, and loss of control as your labor progresses. On the other hand, relaxing activities often decrease your experience of pain and allow your labor to progress.

For Dr. Susan Porto, spending a day at work and taking care of her patients provided a distraction that took her mind off labor pain; she didn't want to stay at home contemplating her contractions and the course of her labor. For Susan, working was an effective form of pain medication. Her labor (with her second child) gradually progressed throughout the course of the day, and her birth experience was quick and uncomplicated.

"My bag of waters broke early in the morning. I kept seeing patients. I figured I'd just keep working until I felt bad . . . I really didn't pay much attention to my discomfort. With that kind of work, you can't really focus on yourself. You can't think of much else except what the person is saying in front of you.

"The patients realized what was going on. I'd have to talk and then stop a minute to catch my breath. It was kind of comical. But I think it was the best way. It was much better than staying home and thinking about the pain. When I finally got to the last patient, my labor started getting active. I left work at 5:00. I went home, changed my clothes, went to the hospital, and had the baby fifteen minutes after I got there."

During your latent phase of labor, do not become obsessed with timing your contractions, since this may only increase your anxiety. Trust that your body knows what to do, and all you need to do is occasionally time your contractions, especially if they seem to be getting stronger and closer together.

If your latent phase of labor comes on during the day, keep walking and changing positions. Assume upright positions, since gravity presses the baby against your cervix and encourages labor. Lying around in bed for hours may slow labor; however, lying down to rest from time to time during the day helps you conserve energy.

If your contractions begin during the night, time them for a few minutes, and if they are still more than five minutes apart and less than a minute in duration, roll over and go back to sleep for a while (if you are pregnant with your first baby). You will need to get some rest, since you may be up late the next night giving birth, and you will need stamina for active labor, transition, and pushing. Do not worry about sleeping though labor and birth; truly active labor will wake you up in time to get to the hospital or birth center. If you are too nervous or excited to sleep, take a warm bath (but NOT if your waters have broken) or stand in a warm shower and then go back to bed.

Take in fluids and calories in early labor. In recent years, some care providers advise women to eat and drink during early labor in order to keep their calorie and fluid levels high enough to prevent exhaustion and dehydration during the demanding second stage of labor. Women who meet their body's energy and fluid requirements will be less prone to exhaustion and thus less inclined to require medical interventions for exhaustion (such as cesarean section, forceps, or vacuum delivery of the baby) later on.

While you are in latent labor, eat small, light, nourishing snacks or meals of bland foods that are high in carbohydrates (crackers, toast with honey or jam, pasta, cereal) and continue to drink juice (diluted with water if you have indigestion), clear fluids, or water. If you are diabetic, you may need to limit your carbohydrate intake or balance carbohydrates and proteins (discuss food for latent labor with your caregiver and dietitian). If you are nauseous, suck on lollipops or other kinds of hard candy to keep your energy level up. You'll need to stay energetic for active labor, just as you would for a marathon race.

Discuss with your care provider his or her food and fluid policy long before your due date in order to determine what kinds of fluids or foods are safe for you in latent and active labor.

The Birth Partner's Role in Latent Labor

We planned to walk around and listen to music and maintain some minimal to moderate level of activity.
—Kevin

* * *

The latent phase of labor is a good time for the birth partner to provide companionship and support (if the laboring woman wants company) and to engage in relaxing, comforting, and distracting activities with the woman in labor. Take a walk, go to the movies, play chess, listen to music—whatever she wants to do. Let her take the lead. Trust that her body knows what it needs in terms of rest and movement. If early labor is going on for a long time, reassure her and trust her instincts about when she needs to go to the hospital or birthing center. Offer her a massage or light stroking of her belly (efflurage) during contractions to distract and relax her. However, some women may not want to be massaged or touched, so don't feel hurt if the laboring woman turns down your offer.

Help your laboring partner to prepare a latent labor chart to keep track of her labor's progress from time to time. Encourage her to focus away from her contractions. Keep track of important events such as the breaking of the bag of waters or the increase in strength and frequency of contractions. This record can give the care provider a good picture of the progress of labor and help the woman and her caregiver decide on the appropriate time for her to go to the birth center or hospital.

Early Labor Chart

Date:_____

Time:_____

Contractions:_____

Duration (how many seconds or minutes the contraction is)

_____

Intensity (how strong, woman's response to contractions)

_____

_____

_____

Frequency (how often)

_____

_____

Bloody Show (when it appears, what it looks like)

_____

_____

Bleeding (report any bleeding to your caregiver immediately)

_____

_____

Breaking of Waters (when it occurs, what it looks/feels/smells like: is it a gush? a trickle? bloody? clear? stained with meconium? odorless? strong odor? [Report odor or meconium staining to your caregiver immediately.])

_____

_____

Loose Stools

_____

Vomiting

___

Backache

___

Temperature

___

Headache or Dizziness (report to your caregiver, especially if you have high blood pressure)

___

___

State of Mind (relaxed, easily distracted from labor contractions, tense, overwhelmed, focused, irritable, etc.)

___

___

___

A Prolonged Latent Phase: What You and Your Care Provider Can Do

It went really slowly. I was walking around the halls of the hospital. The nurse would see me and say, "You're still smiling," and she'd come back and crank up my Pitocin [given intermittently by IV]. I was in early labor from 10 A.M. to 4 P.M. At 7:30 P.M. the contractions started to really hurt, and that's when they stopped cranking up the Pitocin. Paula [the doula] gave me massages. Carl talked to me. We had soothing music. We had massage oil that really smelled good.
—Carla

Your latent stage of labor may be lengthy without being

abnormal. Sometimes it just takes a little longer for your cervix to fully dilate.

If your latent labor is prolonged, you may become exhausted or dehydrated. However, you often can prevent exhaustion and dehydration by:

- Taking in adequate fluid and nourishment during the last weeks of your pregnancy
- Drinking fluid and eating small, bland snacks when mild contractions first begin
- Sucking on ice chips, popsicles, or hard candies to keep up your fluid and blood sugar levels if your care provider wishes you to abstain from food and drink
- Receiving IV fluids to help prevent dehydration and exhaustion during a long latent phase

Your latent phase may be prolonged if you take sedatives or pain medications. However, if you are very anxious during labor, the anxiety may prolong your latent phase and pain medication or sedatives may relax you, help you sleep, and prevent exhaustion, and, in so doing, help your labor progress. Progress may also be enhanced by Pitocin, which can strengthen your contractions, make them more efficient, and shorten your labor. Walking may also help labor progress and help the baby assume a favorable position for birth.

The Active Phase: When to Go to the Hospital or Birth Center

I give women permission to listen to what their body and mind are telling them. When labor gets strong and hard, you'll realize it—and that's a good time to head right in [to the hospital or birthing center].
—Laraine Guyette, CNM

The definition of the beginning of labor is not clear-cut and differs for every woman. However, by the time you reach the *active phase of labor,* your contractions often are uncomfortable, intense, and more frequent and longer lasting than in the latent phase. In active labor, you may find it increasingly difficult to distract yourself from your labor contractions.

Go to the hospital or birth center when you have regular, strong contractions about five minutes apart that last sixty seconds or more—or when you are no longer comfortable laboring at home. If your caregiver thinks your labor is normal and that there is no rush getting to the hospital, and if you feel comfortable at home, stay at home until you no longer feel emotionally or physically comfortable being there, and you would prefer to be in the hospital. If you are birthing your baby at home, call your home birth midwife as you begin active labor (and preferably *before* you begin active labor).

If your doctor wants to monitor you early in labor due to some pre-existing medical condition, or if you are pregnant with a breech baby or twins, it may be best for you to go to the hospital during your latent phase of labor and before your contractions have become regular. However, if your pregnancy and your baby are normal, your labor may progress best if you relax and stay at home during the latent phase. Just make sure you call your care provider when your waters break and that you have timed the drive from your home to the hospital during rush hour, so that you don't miscalculate and end up stuck in traffic while in the midst of your transition stage.

Waiting until you start active labor before you are admitted to the hospital can work to your advantage. Your caregivers may define the onset of your labor based on when you arrive at the hospital, which, in turn, will influence their perception of the length of your labor and whether your labor conforms to the "normal" time limits.

"If you are in a system that is set up to 'do something' to help, it is hard for care providers to sit back and wait," cautions midwife Laraine Guyette. Dr. Allen Killam also expresses concern about women going to the hospital before they are in active labor and thus ending up with medical interventions. He says, "In this country, women sometimes get admitted to labor areas in the hospital before they are really in active labor and that gets them into trouble. They're having contractions that may be painful. So the doctor counts the women in labor even though they are not progressing. Physicians want to get on with it. And patients want to get on with it: 'Do something doctor' is a frequent response because women get tired. This problem leads to a higher c-section rate because people are not patient early in the labor in the latent phase."

When you are admitted to the hospital, the clock starts ticking in terms of the length of your labor, and if you are admitted early in the latent phase, your labor may be defined as "starting" before it actually does. Consequently, the hospital staff may begin to worry that your labor has become "too long," that it is "dysfunctional," and that you need interventions such as Pitocin to strengthen the contractions and speed up your labor.

To avoid a long latent labor in the hospital:

1. Stay at home until you begin active labor. Once you are admitted to the hospital, walk, sit, and engage in relaxing activities. If you must be in bed with a fetal monitor, sit up and change positions from time to time (if it is medically safe for you to do so).
2. If you go to the hospital and are told that you are in prelabor (with dilation less than three centimeters), do not go to bed unless you or the baby have a medical condition that warrants bed rest or continuous fetal

monitoring. Walk the hospital floors if you are admitted to the hospital. If you do not need to be admitted, go home, go shopping, and keep walking, since walking may strengthen contractions and promote labor.

3. Before you go to the hospital, boost your confidence by surrounding yourself with supportive people and positive thinking. Do whatever you need to do to increase your confidence in your ability to give birth: talk to your friends, partner, or doula; talk to yourself and your baby; visualize yourself accomplishing challenging things like skiing, running a marathon, renovating a house, changing a fuel pump—imagine anything in which you succeed at doing something you have never done before. How you perceive yourself and how you present yourself during early labor will influence how your care providers perceive you. If you seem impatient or panicked, your physicians may conclude that something is "wrong" and that they need to intervene in order to "move your labor along."

Prepping Procedures and Hospital Protocols

Prepping procedures in many American hospitals have changed over the past decade, although policies differ from hospital to hospital. Many hospitals no longer routinely shave women, give enemas, start IVs, or strap on continuous fetal monitors, but some do. However, liberal policies about eating and drinking during labor are the exception—not the rule. Discuss your preferences about prepping with your doctor or midwife, your doctor's or midwife's partners, and the hospital staff before you go into labor. Negotiate a birth plan you are comfortable with, and make sure to include a copy of your birth plan with your admission papers and to give additional copies to the nurses on your floor. (See Chapter 16 for details on how to write a birth plan.)

Enemas

Enemas are no longer used routinely at many hospitals, because studies show that they offer no benefits to women in labor unless a woman has impacted stool (a condition that can slow down labor and create discomfort for the laboring mother). However, some care providers believe that enemas, by irritating the bowel, stimulate labor. If you need an enema, ask for a mild kind that will not cause much cramping. Harsh enemas, such as those containing soapy water, may cause painful cramps—something you do not need in the midst of labor contractions. Many women find enemas demoralizing as well as uncomfortable. Since labor is sometimes accompanied by loose stool or diarrhea, an enema may be totally unnecessary.

Pubic Shaving

Shaving was once a common prepping procedure intended to reduce the risk of infection and to make suturing easier in the case of an episiotomy or cesarean surgery, but it is no longer a standard procedure at many hospitals. Not only is shaving uncomfortable; it may cut or scratch the skin and create considerable itching when the hair grows back in the days and weeks following birth.

Nutrition

We have backed off from not letting women drink. . . . Women, within reason, are allowed to drink before labor becomes too hard.
—Dr. Allen Killam

* * *

Withholding food and fluids to women in labor after they are admitted to the hospital is a common hospital procedure. The majority of hospitals withhold solid foods to laboring women, and many hospitals still allow only ice chips or hard candies. Some hospitals allow sips of clear fluids, but only a few hospitals allow women to eat and drink as they wish.

Some care providers prefer that women in active labor avoid solid foods, because they fear that a woman may vomit during childbirth, especially if she receives general anesthesia. If you vomit when you are under a general anesthesia, you could aspirate (inhale the caustic gastric juice and injure your lungs)—a very rare but risky situation. However, general anesthesia is no longer a popular anesthesia choice during birth and often is replaced with epidural anesthesia (which makes aspiration even more unlikely).

On the other hand, some care providers hold that the benefits of eating nourishing food far outweigh the risks (exhaustion and dehydration) of imposed fasting. Talk to your care provider about whether you should eat and/or drink before or after your admission to a hospital or birthing center. Although eating and drinking during active labor is still controversial, taking in fluids and easily digestible foods during early labor is frequently recommended by midwives and by some physicians (as long as a cesarean section isn't imminent) and may help boost your energy and prevent dehydration during labor. If you are allowed to eat, take several small, light meals consisting of fruit juice, cooked eggs, toast, bagels or crackers, clear broth, and cooked fruit. If your care provider is adamant about not eating, try to negotiate for something like popsicles or jello.

If your physician's or hospital's policy strictly forbids food and drink, your care provider may give you intravenous fluids to keep your energy and fluid levels up. Although there is nothing wrong with having an IV, it can limit your movement, prevent you from taking soothing showers and baths, and cause discomfort or irritation. If your caregivers insist on an IV, ask if you can have a cap on the IV so that the IV apparatus can be unhooked from the IV machinery and clamped shut, allowing you to move around as you wish while still giving the medical staff the option of administering IV fluids and medication at a moment's notice.

Monitoring the Baby

There are certain reasons to start monitoring the baby: if you are on oxytocin, if signs of trouble show up, or if you have medical problems. Oftentimes a woman will sit in a reclining chair, or get up and go to the bathroom. The monitor can be off for short periods of time when she can get up and walk around. But the more active her labor becomes, the shorter these periods become. You'll find a lot of flexibility in that.
—Dr. Allen Killam

◦ ◦ ◦

After you are admitted to the hospital, your baby will be monitored by either:

1. Continuous external fetal monitoring
2. Intermittent fetal monitoring or auscultation of the fetal heart rate (this involves listening to the baby's heart with a special stethoscope or a Doppler instrument)
3. Telemetry
4. Internal fetal monitoring
5. Fetal scalp sampling

Many hospitals use continuous fetal monitoring. Because it is continuous, this form of monitoring can be useful in picking up early signs of fetal distress and in reducing the rates of neonatal seizures. However, continuous external monitoring may lead to restriction of your movement during labor, which may, in turn, slow the progress of your labor.

Continuous monitoring may be recommended by care providers if your labor is induced, augmented, or prolonged; if you are pregnant with more than one baby; or if there is meconium in the amniotic fluid. Some health experts argue that external monitors are difficult to interpret and may cause needless alarm (and some unnecessary cesarean sections) unless "unreassuring" results are confirmed with another test—a fetal scalp sampling that involves taking a sample of the baby's blood and examining its acid/base balance for telltale signs of distress.

The internal monitor can be used only after your bag of waters has broken, since the monitor is inserted through your cervix and attached to the baby's head.

Some care providers rely on *intermittent monitoring*—a technique that involves listening to the baby's heartbeat at regular intervals during labor—either by a fetal monitor, a Doppler instrument, or by auscultation with a special stethoscope. However, listening to the baby's heart with a Doppler instrument or stethoscope requires hands-on care, which means that a trained care provider must be available to listen to the baby's heart every fifteen minutes in active labor and every five minutes in second stage labor. In a busy clinical setting, few doctors or nurses are able to spare the amount of time required to carefully monitor the baby by intermittent auscultation. Consequently, some care providers may have you alternate between sitting or lying in bed with the monitor and walking around for fifteen minutes at a time. However, a nurse-midwife who is offering you continuous labor support might have more time to regularly monitor the baby with a stethoscope.

Women who want freedom of movement during labor tend

to like intermittent auscultation best, but some women feel reassured by continuous monitoring and find it worth the physical restrictions.

Coping with the Active Phase

Let the baby press down. Let everything be loose, and open, and soft.
—Louise Aucott, nurse-midwife, advises her patients to relax and "let go" during active labor.

❋ ❋ ❋

A midwife told me, "When you breathe, picture your breath going down to your cervix and opening it up." I did. Amazingly, it just opened up my cervix!
—Claudia

❋ ❋ ❋

The *active phase* of your first stage of labor begins when your cervix is more than four centimeters dilated, and it ends when the cervix is fully dilated at nine to ten centimeters. The last part of active labor, known as *transition,* begins after your cervix has reached about seven to eight centimeters and continues until you are fully dilated at ten centimeters. Most women go to the hospital or birth center during active labor, since labor becomes increasingly more uncomfortable at that time. It is during the active phase that your contractions strengthen, last one minute or more, and come three to five minutes apart.

As you begin active labor, think about the pain as "purposeful" and "productive": The strong contractions of active labor will contribute to the progress of your labor and will bring your baby closer to you. Don't fight the contractions—you'll only get in the way of the natural process. Remember the 4 P's—and that the powers and the psyche can work together to birth your baby. In order to relax, stand in a shower or sit in a Jacuzzi. Many midwives report that simply getting into a warm (not hot), soothing Jacuzzi can further cervical dilation while minimizing the pain. If your waters have broken, some care providers will suggest that you use a shower instead of a bath or Jacuzzi.

You may become quieter and more focused on your contractions during active labor, especially if you are experiencing moderate to strong contractions for sixty to ninety seconds every three to four minutes. Use various techniques from your childbirth preparation "bag of tricks" to comfort and distract you: breathing techniques, hypnosis, massage, aromatherapy, birthing positions, your favorite music. Try some of the following visual images or repeated phrases as part of a mind-over-body strategy to help you cope with labor:

- Visualize your cervix opening
- Visualize concentric circles growing wider and wider
- Imagine that you are riding the waves of each contraction or skiing down a mountain
- Repeat phrases such as: "go with the flow," "my body knows what to do," "the powers are bringing my baby closer to me," "let go"
- Breathe deeply in and out with your birth partner, your doula, your midwife, or the labor and delivery nurse
- Tell yourself that intense contractions are "good contractions"—strong and purposeful as they bring your baby closer to you

Lucy used several powerful images to get herself through active labor and transition. Lucy likened her labor to "riding a wave," training for an athletic event, and a "labor of Hercules" that brought forth surprising strength:

"I was anxious, of course, but I felt I could cope with the pain. It was like very strong menstrual pain. I had suffered from dysmenorrhea [painful menstruation] so that was familiar to me. Labor is not like dental or back pain. It's not continuous. . . . It's like a wave: it goes down. There is always relief. To me, it was like a trial. It was like having to spend a night in training for a prize fight. I had to go through a 'trial of Hercules,' and I didn't want anyone to deprive me of this experience."

As your cervical dilation approaches seven centimeters and you enter *transition,* your contractions may intensify and become more uncomfortable. Some women get tired of being in labor and want the "other mother" to come in and have the baby while they go home and go to sleep. This feeling is normal.

Although you can't totally control contractions, you can influence your experience of labor—and possibly its duration and efficiency—by emotionally and physically preparing yourself for birth and creating a supportive environment for yourself during each phase of labor. To do this, you need to recognize the symptoms of latent and active labor and to make decisions that will put you in the appropriate environment at the appropriate time. For instance, if you are going into active labor, driving several hours to the beach or going to work may put you in the wrong place at the wrong time and set you up for unnecessary stress.

The Duration of the Active Phase

Midwifery data says that cervical dilation at a rate of half a centimeter an hour, in the absence of other problems, is a more appropriate expectation [than the standard one centimeter per hour dilation rate]. It takes longer to have a baby than we previously thought.

—Leah Albers, CNM, Professor of Nursing at the University of New Mexico; author of two studies on the duration of labor

According to the large midwifery study by Leah Albers published in the March 1999 edition of the *Journal of Perinatology,* "normal labor in healthy women lasted longer than many clinicians expect." The study found that the average length of *active labor* was 7.7 hours for first-time mothers and 5.6 hours for women who had previously given birth. However, the length of labor differs from woman to woman and from pregnancy to pregnancy. Furthermore, care providers differ as to what they consider normal progress in labor. The standard measure of progress taught in many American medical schools is that a woman's cervix should dilate about one centimeter per hour during a normal labor. However, some care providers are adopting a more flexible standard of half a centimeter per hour.

Dr. Murry Enkin and his coauthors sum up the debate about the normal rate of cervical dilation in their book, *A Guide to Effective Care in Pregnancy and Childbirth:* "Normal labour can be defined either in terms of the total length of labour or as a rate of progress of cervical dilation often expressed in centimeters per hour. . . . Many doctors use 1 cm/hr as the cut-off between normal and abnormal labour. The validity of this can certainly be challenged. Many women who show slower rates of cervical dilation proceed to normal delivery. A rate of 0.5 cm/hour may be more appropriate as a lower limit for defining normal progress, but this should also be interpreted with discretion in the context of the woman's total well-being."

What the Birth Partner Can Do During Active Labor

It's important to be flexible. Don't go in with any specific ideas of the way things are going to be. I just tried to stay focused and not look ahead. It's sometimes useful to focus on the contraction that's there and not worry about the one that will come in thirty seconds or so.
—Kevin

I ran interference for her. She was very busy! I got the nurse. I got her water.
—Pete, describing the ways he helped his wife, Lucy, through active labor

❋ ❋ ❋

Active labor is often a time when the laboring woman needs her birth partner to support and comfort her, although each woman will have slightly different needs during labor. She may need relaxation or comfort in the form of breathing exercises, back rubs, soft music, a shower, or a Jacuzzi. She may want to walk and may need to stop and lean on you for support during strong contractions.

As a birth partner, you can participate in the progress of labor by assisting the laboring woman (see Chapter 20) and supporting her weight if she wants to try kneeling or other birthing positions during labor. You also can bring her ice chips, rub her back or feet (if she feels like being massaged at this point in her labor), and act as a communications link between the woman and the hospital staff.

Let the laboring woman set the tone, and follow her lead. She may withdraw during active labor as she concentrates on managing intense contractions. However, even if she no longer engages you in conversation, she still needs praise, reassurance, and emotional and physical support. Many birth partners, whether they are men or women, want to "do something" to help ease the pain of labor. But often the best thing you can do is to be supportive. "Recognize from the beginning that childbirth is something you cannot control, and don't try to impose your will upon it," advises Kevin, whose wife had a long active stage of labor.

Some birth partners experience considerable anxiety, especially if they have never supported a woman during childbirth. Even if you feel confident in your ability to offer emotional and physical support, you may worry that your stamina may give out during a long labor. In such cases, you may benefit from employing a doula to provide support for both you and your partner.

The Transition Phase

Open up. The circle of your cervix widens. Let the baby out.
—A midwife's encouraging words during transition

* * *

You can do this. Birth has been happening for years and years and you're just part of that continuum. Your body is designed for this. Millions of women have done this before you. It doesn't last forever.
—Kathleen, remembering the words of Svea, doula and childbirth educator

* * *

Transition means that your labor is progressing, that your cervix is opening up to accommodate the passage of your baby's head into the birth canal, and that nature is working in your favor to push your baby closer to you.

The transition phase of labor is often an intense period in which your cervix dilates from seven to ten centimeters. Some women become irritable and do not want to be touched or distracted. Some women vomit or shake as they begin the transition phase. Many women feel as if they are about to have a huge bowel movement. Even women who have had an epidural may feel rectal pressure or an urge to push.

During transition, you quickly move from one contraction to another and sometimes get only a short break before you need to ride the wave of another contraction. Contractions tend to be strong, last sixty to ninety seconds, and come about every two to three minutes, but every woman is different. The good news is that transition is a relatively short phase of labor (approximately one to two hours).

As you approach full dilation, you may start to feel overwhelmed and out of control. To handle feelings of loss of control, rely on techniques you have used to get through other challenges in your life. Use your childbirth preparation techniques. Make sure your support system is in place, since it is during this phase of labor that you may need the most encouragement from your birth partner, friends, or doula.

Some women find they need to focus on their contractions without outside distractions. Lucy spent her most difficult moments sitting in the bathroom and doing yoga breathing.

What the Birth Partner Can Do During the Transition Phase

When I was dilated to nine centimeters, Kevin was saying, "We can do this." I could hear it in my head: "We can do this."
—Kevin's words became Cathy's affirmation as she progressed slowly through transition.

❋ ❋ ❋

A laboring woman often needs encouragement during transition. Praise her and encourage her using terms that are meaningful to her. Remind her that transition is short, her pain will soon decrease, and her baby will soon be born.

Transition is the time of labor during which she may feel the most out of control, and it is also the time when she may feel intensely irritable and uncomfortable. Don't take her irritability personally. Take your cues from her as to how much physical contact she wants and what form of support she may need. Many women become very absorbed in their labor and are unable to converse during transition. Some women do not want to be massaged at this point, although they may wish to sense your physical presence nearby.

Some birthing women find relief by spending at least part of transition in a warm shower. Others find relief by sitting on a toilet or birthing stool (see Chapter 20). Sometimes just a change of position helps. Encourage the woman to try different positions such as getting on her hands and knees, assuming a knee-chest position, or leaning over the bed and bending at the waist—whatever feels comfortable to her.

Stage 2: Descent and Birth

I liked the pushing. Those contractions were gone.
—Kathleen R.

* * *

I had my own cheering section [husband and doula]—that helped a lot. At one point, I was really exhausted after pushing for one and one half hours. I lost track of time. It became a very internal process. The whole world shrank down to this one little room. For a lot of the time I had my eyes closed.
—Carla

* * *

The second stage—or pushing stage—of labor begins when your cervix reaches full dilation and ends with delivery of your baby. It is often an exciting stage of labor. The intense contractions of transition are over and replaced by pushing—during which you may feel like a powerful, active, and direct participant in your baby's birth. After riding the waves of transition, you can now synchronize your pushing efforts with the urge to bear down. You may find that you enjoy pushing because you feel as though you are finally doing something and are engaged in an athletic event that will achieve a goal: birthing your baby. However, some women find that second stage labor is difficult and painful.

"Push with the urge, relax your jaw, relax your mouth and let it open. Let the baby come down . . . that's good. . . ." are phrases used by midwives and labor and delivery nurses to encourage women during the pushing stage of labor. However, sometimes your caregiver will ask you to refrain from "pushing with the urge," especially if your cervix is not fully dilated or if your baby has not assumed the standard headfirst position.

The pushing stage of labor may last for twenty-five minutes to two hours in a woman having her first baby. It may last as long as three hours if a woman has an epidural and four hours if a woman has an awkwardly positioned baby, or it may be as short as fifteen minutes in a woman who has previously had children. Epidural or spinal anesthesia may increase the length of this stage and may interfere with your urge to push. A "walking epidural," which does not cause complete numbing of the legs, may allow you to push more effectively than a complete epidural (see Chapter 22).

However, sometimes the medication in a walking epidural ends up numbing the nerves that control movement (see Chapter 22), which may make it more difficult for you to push the baby out.

According to nurse-midwife Pam Spry, "some care providers feel that pushing should be delayed for women with epidurals and that the baby should be allowed to 'passively descend;' pushing should begin when the woman feels rectal pressure or when you can see the baby's head."

What the Birth Partner Can Do During the Second Stage

You have to go into it being quite flexible. . . . There is no correct procedure or sequence of events. What matters is the outcome—

a healthy baby—and you can get to that outcome in many ways.
—Kevin, whose wife, Cathy, had a forceps delivery for her first
baby and a cesarean section for her second.

* * *

*I think I'll die with this image: of Kevin's eyes looking at me and
staring at me. I just really felt that he was there for me. He was
solid, and he was concentrating on me, and it was just great. All
he could do was to be there—and that was the most important
thing he could do.*
—Cathy found Kevin's supportive presence and eye-to-eye contact valuable—and unforgettable.

* * *

"I saw my role as being there as a support person, being
there to do what I could do. I never felt shunted aside. I felt
that people with better training stepped in when it was
important to do so," says Kevin, describing the birth of his
daughter. However, many birth partners may start to feel useless or shunted aside during the pushing stage, especially if
the midwife or physician has taken over and is coaching the
laboring woman.

At this point in labor, the birth partner's role may become
less active—but no less important. While the laboring woman is
working to push the baby out, you—as her birth partner—can
support her in the subtle-yet-powerful ways that you have
offered support throughout the course of your relationship: by
the way you look into her eyes, by the sound of your voice and
your words of support, or by being physically present and emotionally tuned in. Cathy saw the look in Kevin's eyes as a connection she will never forget. Lucy found comfort in sensing her
husband's body close to her: "My husband was very important.
He was very supportive. He helped me . . . I had to smell him

and cling to him, feeling his skin. I wanted to touch him. I think human contact is the best. Just presence."

Most birth partners, by staying close by, will give far more than they may realize.

In some births, the birth partner or the family members became active participants during the second stage of labor, says Pam Spry. "I assign jobs and positions—one family member on each side of the bed as needed to help support the legs of the laboring woman as she brings her legs up to push." (See discussion on Stage 3 and Stage 4 in Chapter 21.)

Chapter 20

Maternal Positions for Labor and Birth

The baby is always moving. What the mom needs to do is to try different positions based on what her body is telling her. The pain is giving you a message. If you listen to your body and follow the lead of your body, you will enable the baby to find the best way out.

The pelvis is very mobile. The way you move will give the baby a better angle and more space and will take the pressure off your backbone. As your body moves, the shape of your pelvis changes. . . . By just doing a pelvic tilt, you open the tailbone and create more space around that curve for the baby to move down.

—Michelle Brill, MPH, childbirth educator

• • •

Until relatively recently, most women who gave birth in hospitals in the United States, gave birth lying on their back. The *lithotomy position*—where the woman is lying on her back with her legs raised in stirrups—was preferred by many care providers, since the position easily allowed the monitoring of the baby, viewing of the birth canal, and performing of medical interventions such as episiotomies and vacuum deliveries.

However, according to recent medical studies, women who walk, stand, or sit during part of their labor have shorter labors, on average, than women asked to lie flat. According to the review of several medical studies on maternal position in childbirth by Dr. Murray Enkin and his coauthors in *A Guide to Effective Care in Pregnancy and Childbirth* (third edition), women who assumed upright positions during the second stage of labor had shorter labors and fewer episodes of severe pain. Some care providers say that women who give birth in positions other than the lithotomy position have a decreased risk of vaginal tearing.

Some care providers suggest a variety of birthing positions that may help your cervix dilate and ease your baby into an advantageous position as she passes through your cervix and moves down your birth canal. They believe that if you assume birthing positions that work with gravity, you can facilitate birth and influence the position of the baby. For instance, studies show that by walking during labor, you can use the force of gravity to help bring on contractions and cervical dilation. Similarly, some care providers believe that by sitting, squatting, or standing during the pushing stage, you can make pushing more effective and facilitate the baby's descent through the birth canal.

Your care provider may recommend the positions that follow and suggest that you practice these birthing positions before you go into labor.

Positions for the First Stage: Dilating the Cervix

Going to bed during the latent phase can slow down your labor. At this stage, you want your physical positions to encourage cervical dilation and contractions. Walk and remain upright because gravity will press the baby against your cervix, thereby encouraging cervical dilation. If you need to rest, lie on one side, or sit in a comfortable chair.

If your cervix is dilating very slowly, take a warm bath or Jacuzzi (if your waters have not broken), or sit in a warm shower to relax and encourage dilation.

There are care providers who believe that women whose bag of waters has broken may safely take baths and Jacuzzis, and there are those who believe that bathing is unsafe at this time. Consult your care provider about whether or not you should bathe after your bag of waters has broken.

During your active phase, continue walking between your contractions. Since women who choose their own birth positions during labor require fewer pain medications, moving and changing position might be nature's way of facilitating labor and reducing discomfort. Try whatever positions your body wants to assume; you do not need to adhere to a rigid list.

If you wish to have freedom of movement during labor, make sure you discuss this with your care provider early in your pregnancy. Sometimes your care providers' philosophy—or your medical circumstances—may prevent you from being upright during labor, in which case you may need a backup plan.

During your last weeks of pregnancy, discuss with your caregiver the position of your baby and the positions that may be advantageous for you to assume during labor and birth. Some physicians are familiar with birthing positions and feel comfortable teaching them to pregnant patients. Midwives, on the other hand, frequently recommend birthing positions to facilitate childbirth. It is important that you choose positions that feel comfortable for you and that are appropriate for the position of your baby. Practice the positions, using trial and error to find what feels best.

To prepare for walking during labor, bring sanitary pads with you to the hospital or birthing center. This way, you can walk around after your bag of waters has broken and not worry about leaking amniotic fluid and leaving puddles in your wake.

Positions for the First Stage of Labor (dilation four to seven centimeters)

Walking

Walking is useful during both latent labor and active labor, since your body is working with gravity to bring on contractions, to make your contractions more efficient, and to help your baby assume an advantageous position for its descent through your pelvis. Walking can make labor shorter and less uncomfortable than if you are sitting still or lying down. During strong contractions, you may need to stop walking and to lean against the wall or another person for support (see Figure 20-1).

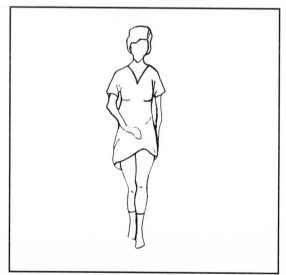

Figure 20-1: Walking

Illustration by Howard Petote.

Standing/Standing and Leaning Forward

Again, you are working with gravity to put pressure on your cervix in order to bring on dilation, make your contractions more effective, and help the baby become well aligned in your pelvis.

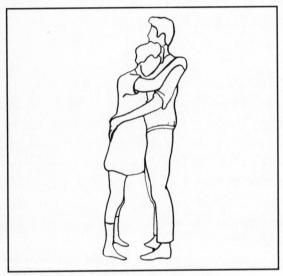

Figure 20-2: Standing and leaning forward

Illustration by Howard Petote.

Sitting Upright/Sitting and Leaning Forward with Support (a Person or Birthing Ball)

In these positions you are working with gravity to get your baby born, but you are also resting. These are good positions for conserving energy and for stabilizing you if you are feeling shaky and for relieving back pain. You often may assume a sitting position during fetal monitoring and thus avoid the slowing of labor associated with lying down. However, sitting for long periods of time without moving may also slow down a labor (see Figure 20-3, 20-4, and 20-5.)

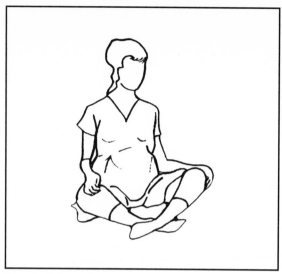

Illustration by Howard Petote.

**Figure 20-3:
Sitting upright**

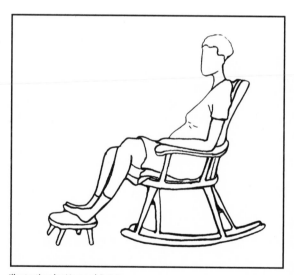

Illustration by Howard Petote.

**Figure 20-4:
Sitting upright/
rocking**

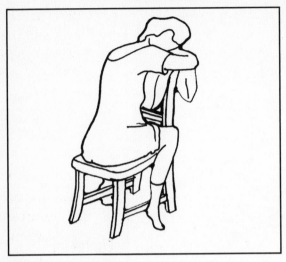

**Figure 20-5:
Supported sitting
while leaning
forward**

Illustration by Howard Petote.

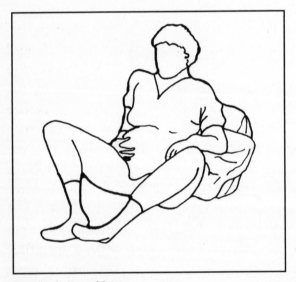

**Figure 20-6:
Semisitting**

Illustration by Howard Petote.

Semisitting

Labor-room beds allow you to assume a semisitting position while still in bed. This is a useful position if you need continuous fetal monitoring and cannot move about freely. The semisitting position allows you to use gravity to help the baby descend and push the baby out. The position also allows you to relax in between contractions and maintain good blood flow to your baby. Ask your birth partner, doula, or labor and delivery nurse to support you from behind (see Figure 20-6).

Sitting on a Birthing Stool, Toilet, or Birthing Chair

Sitting on a birthing stool, chair, or toilet seat may be helpful even if you are in the first stage of labor. This position may help open up your pelvis. Get up and move around from time to time to maintain good blood circulation.

Pelvic Rocking on Hands and Knees

Because this position helps you take the pressure off your back, it is useful for relieving back pain or "back labor" (when your baby is in the "occiput posterior" [OP] position with its spine adjacent to your spine). Try kneeling on the bed or floor, wherever you are most comfortable (but realize that if you labor on the floor, your doctor or midwife may need to get down on the floor with you in order to see the presenting part of the baby). While on your hands and knees you might employ "pelvic rocking" to help your baby move from an OP position (see Figure 20-7). Some care providers believe that by moving your pelvis, you are changing the spatial relationship between your baby and your pelvis and thus giving your baby the opportunity to assume an optimal position for birth. Since an OP baby might create a long and difficult labor, this position is a useful addition to your labor "bag of tricks".

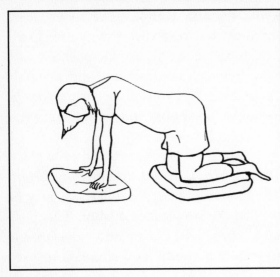

Figure 20-7: Pelvic rocking on hands and knees

Illustration by Howard Petote.

Standing Pelvic Rocking

You may find relief by standing upright, bending slightly at the knees, and rocking your hips back and forth like a hula dancer or a child twirling a hula hoop.

Kneeling, Leaning Forward Supported by Another Person, a Piece of Furniture, or a Birthing Ball

You may want to alternate this with the above-mentioned hands-and-knees position, especially if your wrists get tired or you need to assume a slightly upright posture on your knees and work with gravity to birth your baby. You may find that kneeling hurts your knees but relieves the pressure on your back. In that case, use kneepads, pillows, or pieces of foam to cushion your knees during labor (see Figure 20-8).

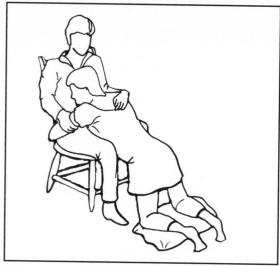

Illustration by Howard Petote.

**Figure 20-8:
Kneeling while
leaning forward
with support**

Squat/Supported Squat

Squatting may improve the alignment of the baby within your pelvis and help you during dilation as well as descent. The position may also relieve backache. Try squatting on the bed or on the floor. If you are on the floor, you might want to stand up occasionally (since most women are not accustomed to squatting for long periods of time). For a more relaxing version, try a supported squat in which your partner, doula, or nurse holds you under your arms from behind. If this position helps you progress in labor, use it. If it doesn't, change positions (see Figure 20-9 and 20-10).

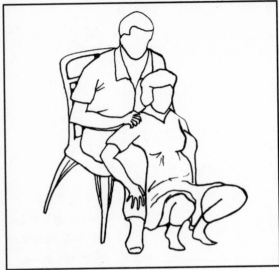

Illustration by Howard Petote.

Figure 20-9: Supported squat

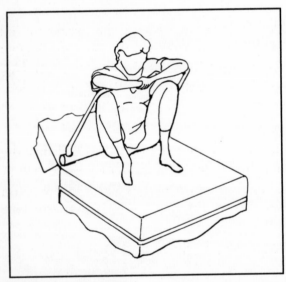

Illustration by Howard Petote.

Figure 20-10: Squat

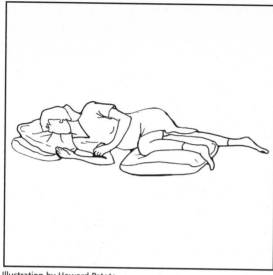

**Figure 20-11:
Side lying**

Illustration by Howard Petote.

Side Lying

This position lessens pressure around the perineum and decreases the risk of tearing and the need for episiotomy, especially if your top leg is held up. The position may promote progress when alternated with walking (see Figure 20-11.)

Lying on Your Back

In this position, you are pushing your baby out against the forces of gravity, which may make your labor more difficult. However, there are some circumstances in which this position is beneficial.

"Back Labor": Maternal Positions and Other Remedies

When the mother changes her position, she alters relationships among gravity, uterine contractions, the fetus, and her pelvis, which may enhance the progress of labor and reduce pain. For example, pressure of the fetal head against the sacroiliac joint [back labor] may be relieved if the mother moves from a semi-recumbent to a "hands and knees" posture. —Murray Enkin et al., "Control of Pain in Labour," *A Guide to Effective Care in Pregnancy and Childbirth* (second edition)

◦ ◦ ◦

When your baby is in an OP position with her spine against yours, you may experience back labor because the back of the baby's head constantly presses against your lower back. This position is also known as the "sunny-side up" position, since the baby's face is looking toward your belly. Childbirth with babies in this position tends to take longer and may include continuous back discomfort.

If you are having back labor, you may find relief in:

- Walking (in early labor)
- Frequently changing position
- Ice packs
- Hot compresses
- Warm showers
- Counterpressure
- Massage
- Hands-and-knees labor position

Changing your position or walking may make you more comfortable and encourage your baby to rotate into the occiput anterior (OA) position. To relieve discomfort and to encourage your baby to turn to the OA position:

- Try a hands-and-knees position to take the pressure off your back and encourage your baby to move from the posterior position.

- Change positions frequently until you find positions that give you comfort.
- Ask your labor and delivery nurses, physician, and/or doula for assistance in finding positions that may help rotate your baby.

Although some women get relief from pain medications or epidural anesthesia (see Part 8), you may find adequate pain relief from ice packs applied to the small of your back, ice massage done with an ice cube on the small of the back, or regular massage. Your partner or birth assistant should massage your back with a circular motion or press firmly against the painful areas on your lower back and sacrum.

You may find that standing in a warm shower with the force of the water massaging your lower back relieves your back labor. Sometimes pressure, in the form of your partner's fist or a tennis ball pressed against your lower back, can ease the discomfort. For do-it-yourself relief, apply pressure by leaning on a tennis ball against the wall. You also may alleviate some of the pressure on your low back by urinating every hour to prevent your bladder from pressing against the uterus and taking up pelvic space that you need for effective labor.

Fortunately, many babies rotate to the occiput anterior (OA) position either during transition or during the second stage of labor, and the mother ultimately achieves a vaginal birth. If the baby doesn't rotate completely, the birth may require instrumental delivery using forceps to rotate the baby (see Part 8).

Positions for the Second Stage: The Pushing Stage

In the second stage of labour, an upright position is associated with fewer episodes of severe pain.

—Murray Enkin et al., *A Guide to Effective Care in Pregnancy and Childbirth* (second edition)

• • •

No matter what position you choose, it helps to have your knees as close together as possible (twelve to eighteen inches apart) to allow the perineum room to stretch as the baby's head emerges . . . Pulling the legs apart or using the lithotomy position puts unnecessary tension on the tissues surrounding the vagina and increases the risk of tearing.
—Pam Spry, CNM/Ph.D.

• • •

During your second stage of labor, you may decrease backache, decrease the length of your labor, and increase your comfort by assuming upright positions at least some of the time. However, there are circumstances when this may not be possible for you. For instance, you may be restricted to bed because of medical procedures such as electronic fetal monitoring, intravenous fluids, and medications that make being out of bed difficult or unsafe. If you are restricted to bed, you may wish to lie on one side and then the other or shift from side lying to semisitting in bed. Discuss the safety and effectiveness of such positions with your care provider.

If you have freedom of movement during your second stage of labor, there is no one "right" position for you to assume; listen to your body and to your care provider to determine the positions that are right for you and your baby. To conserve energy, change your positions from upright ones to resting ones. Since the continuous use of a birthing chair may put stress on your perineum, you may want to use a birthing stool or chair intermittently—rather than constantly—during your labor.

The following positions are useful for pushing and for

delivering your baby. You may already have used some of these positions during your first stage of labor.

Side Lying (on Left Side) with Top Leg Up

This position allows you to relax between pushes. It is helpful during a rapid second stage; some care providers say it may reduce perineal tearing and take the pressure off of hemorrhoids (see Figure 20-11 on page 443).

Lying on Back with Legs Pulled Apart

Although this position may widen your pelvic outlet and help your baby's head slip under your public bone, it may also be tiring since you are working against gravity. Some care providers see this position as an inverted squat that opens the pelvis and shortens the vagina, facilitating the baby's descent (see Figure 20-12). (Lying flat on your back for long periods of time may interfere with blood flow to the baby and placenta. However, some women and care providers prefer this position under certain circumstances.)

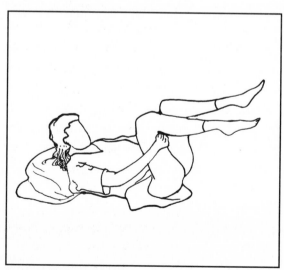

Figure 20-12: Lying on back with legs pulled apart (neck and back supported with pillows)

Illustration by Howard Petote.

Hands and Knees

This position may help the rotation of an OP baby to an easier birth position, reduce backache, take pressure off your perineum and thus prevent tears or aggravation of hemorrhoids, and allow for rocking and tilting movements to promote your comfort. However, you may need to rest from time to time in other positions (see Figure 20-7).

Squat/Supported Squat

You may find that the squatting position is comfortable for pushing. Squatting may facilitate the baby's descent, widen your pelvic outlet, and enhance the proper positioning of the baby. If you use this position, make sure that the floor underneath you is covered with clean paper or towels in case your baby is born. If you begin to deliver this way, also make sure the baby's head is carefully delivered (see Figure 20-9 and 20-10).

Sitting on Birthing Stool, Birthing Chair, or Toilet

This position may help to relax a tense perineum and may enhance descent in some births. If you sit on the toilet, you will need to move for the delivery of your baby. Some women find that sitting on a birthing stool position (see supported squat) reminds them of sitting on the toilet; they associate the birthing stool with bearing down and having a bowel movement—a useful association in the second stage of labor when you are pushing the baby out (see "Maternal Positions for the First Stage of Labor").

Semisitting in Bed

Use this position if you find it comfortable (see Figure 20-6).

What You Can Do to Move Your Labor Along

The normal way a baby descends is with the head flexed so that the baby curls itself into a little bullet—so the smallest diameter of the baby's head can pass through the pelvic cavity. If something happens where there is not enough flexion of the head or there's a little turn here or there that doesn't put the smallest part of the head in the pelvic cavity, you're going to get an obstruction of labor.

Now those things can correct. . . . If the woman doesn't have good contractions, this is where you use augmentation [with Pitocin] or you can use various repositionings. You can put a woman on her hands and knees for a while, depending on what you think the problem is. You can shift her to one side. You can have her stand up. You can have her put one leg up and one leg down—whatever position would seem to maximize the diameter of the pelvis.
—Dr. Susan Porto

* * *

Do not assume that your labor will be long—but prepare for the possibility. You can take both physical and psychological measures that may help you prepare for and, in some cases, prevent or manage a long or difficult labor.

If you have a long labor, try different birthing positions. Sometimes, your labor is prolonged because you stop having contractions or because your baby's position in the pelvis prevents its progressive descent. In either case, try positions that use gravity to bring on contractions or reposition the baby. At other times, your anxiety may interfere with contractions, and you may need to address your psyche in order to keep your labor moving.

Try some of the following physical and psychological measures to manage, and sometimes prevent, a long or difficult labor.

1. During early, active, and second stage labor use positions that promote effective labor contractions and descent of the baby. These positions can help you move forward if you reach a plateau.

2. "Go with" the forces of nature instead of fighting them. Sometime a long intense labor will make you tense up and hold back; it is as if your body is trying to ward off any more discomfort. This is a natural but counterproductive response, since it will not help your labor progress. Instead of trying to control the process or fight it, give in to nature and the forces of labor that will push your baby out of your body and into your arms.

3. Take a warm, relaxing shower, bath, or Jacuzzi. (Shower—but do not bathe—if your waters have already broken unless your care provider gives you *explicit* permission to bathe after the waters have broken.)

4. Accept help from your caregivers. Don't expect yourself to "tough it out alone."

5. Accept support from your birth partner or a trusted friend. You can reduce your anxiety level during childbirth (and thus promote a more relaxed labor) by inviting someone you trust to be at your side during childbirth; this can be your partner, a friend, or a family member.

6. Seek continuous labor support from a midwife or doula. If you do not have female labor support, ask the labor and delivery nurses for support if your labor is prolonged. A good labor nurse makes an excellent doula if she has enough time to labor-sit.

7. Stay hydrated and nourished. During early labor, drink fluids. Eat small, bland, high-calorie snacks if you can. During later labor, stay hydrated with the help of popsicles or ice chips. Suck on hard candies or lollipops for energy.

8. Keep the 4th P—your psyche—confident and well supported. Create rituals that induce comfort and security. Draw on whatever comforts you (music, showers, fragrant massage oils, wrapping yourself in a favorite shawl). Reduce your anxiety by repeating reassuring phrases to yourself, by visualizing relaxing images or events, or by visualizing the natural progression of your cervix widening and your baby moving inch by inch to her birth.

9. Remind yourself that you cannot totally control the birth and to accept variations to your birth plan.

If your labor is long, your care provider may suggest that you take pain medications or medications like Pitocin to help your labor progress. Sometimes narcotic pain medications and "walking epidurals" will help you relax (see Chapter 22), and the relaxation will help your labor progress and allow you enough pain relief to feel more calm and more able to become an active participant in your birth. However, pain medications may lengthen labor or temporarily bring it to a halt.

What the Birth Partner Can Do

The birth partner can help the mother by reminding her of the above strategies for coping with prolonged labor and by protecting her from unnecessary distractions.

If you and the mother have certain relaxing rituals that you have developed during the course of the labor or the childbirth preparation, you may want to implement them.

Encourage the laboring woman. She's like a marathon runner who needs her partner to cheer her on to the finish line—the birth of the baby. Remind her that labor won't last forever—and that she can do it!

Chapter 21
Birth and Bonding

It's a very physical and spiritual thing. . . . I looked into my daughter's eyes and felt this profound love. I carry that with me (the wonder and amazement that I can do this, and I did do this) every time I look at my child.
—Carla

* * *

When I gave birth, I had some kind of metaphysical experience. The only thing I remember distinctly was this feeling of being taken back millions of years. It was like being brought to a primitive time, to my first relative who gave birth.
—Miriam, thirty-eight, had an easy labor and delivery

* * *

I was so high after the baby was born, I didn't sleep from Friday morning until Tuesday at 3 A.M.
—Kathleen R. had wanted to have a baby for many years and was thrilled by the birth of her son, Austin

* * *

The actual birth of your baby is the exciting culmination of many months of anticipation. It is an emotional, a physical, and, for some, a spiritual achievement marking the end of pregnancy—and the beginning of motherhood.

The excitement often sets in just before the baby is born, as its head crowns and you can see—and feel—the top of your baby's head at the opening of your vagina. The head will "crown" in between contractions. You may want to reach down and touch your baby's head for the first time. This will distract you from the stretching, burning sensation (the "rim of fire") you may be feeling in your perineum.

To relax your perineum and help prevent vaginal tears, midwives recommend perineal massage in the weeks preceding birth or hot compresses on your perineum during delivery. Sometimes your caregiver will deliver the baby's head slowly by supporting your perineum and gently controlling the baby's head as it emerges. Some caregivers may ask you to stop pushing hard and instead try to ease the baby out when you feel the burning sensation of the "rim of fire." A slow delivery of your baby's head helps prevent vaginal tears and may make your experience a more comfortable one. However, if your baby is in distress, the baby may need to be born as quickly as possible.

Some women are exhilarated during delivery; others are exhausted. For most women, the actual birth and the hours immediately afterward will be forever etched in their minds. Consequently, it is a good idea to plan for these moments and to have your wishes clearly spelled out in your birth plan.

It is also wise to realize that your birth may not go according to plan. Rhonda had wanted a natural birth and a home birth, but neither was in the cards for her. However, she had decided not to set herself up for regrets by having rigid expectations. Consequently, her birth experience was a positive one even though she ended up with a cesarean section.

If you are accustomed to your life going according to plan, make an exception for birth. Childbirth is full of surprises—all you can do is to be prepared for some of them. Lay the groundwork for the birth you want, but don't expect to control birth or bonding with your baby. For some women, the bonding is immediate; for others, bonding may take weeks or months.

Birth: What the Birth Partner Can Do

Being there when your child is born is one of life's natural highs. It's like you're present for a miracle. It moves me just to think about it . . . to see this little person emerge. I can't imagine missing it.
—Reyn, a father at age forty-nine

• • •

During the birth, the doctor or midwife will be present, which may make you feel less necessary than you were during the earlier parts of labor. However, the laboring woman may still rely on your presence and support. Just knowing that you are "there" with words of encouragement and praise may be very important to her, even though a midwife or doctor may also be encouraging or directing her efforts.

While the baby is being born, you can draw the mother's attention to the emerging baby, so that you both can experience the birth of the child. If you feel squeamish about watching the birth itself, focus on the mother's face. However, don't be surprised if you get caught up in the mounting excitement as the baby is born. Peter was astonished at the way his children seemed to leap into the world: "The baby looked like a seal sliding up out of the sea onto a rock. It looked like it was her act to be born."

After the birth, you may cut the cord (if you wish), hold the baby, place the baby gently on the mother's chest, and cover the baby's body (but not its head) with a blanket. If the baby must be taken to the nursery for treatment, you may either accompany the baby or stay with the mother.

If you are present during a cesarean birth, you can support the mother and experience the excitement of the baby's birth without viewing the actual surgery. Often, the doctors place a screen over the mother's chest to keep the surgery comfortably out of sight. To stay focused on your partner rather than the medical procedure, look at her face and keep your gaze there. After the baby emerges, the screen may be lowered or the baby lifted above the screen and presented to you and your partner.

Discuss with your partner what your role might be in the case of a cesarean birth. Keep in mind that a cesarean birth can still be a beautiful birth.

Stage 3: Delivering the Placenta

The third stage of labor begins with the delivery of baby and ends with separation and delivery of the placenta. During this time, you probably will be absorbed in getting acquainted with your baby.

Delivery of the placenta is relatively easy and painless. You will be asked to push the placenta out, and it usually slips out with little effort on your part. In order to minimize blood loss and to help your uterus recover from the birth, your care provider may massage your abdomen in order to encourage your uterus to contract. If you want to learn how to do this, ask your care provider to show you during the course of your pregnancy. However, you may literally have your hands full with your new baby during the time when massage is needed.

Nursing facilitates the delivery of the placenta, since nursing your baby is nature's way of preventing postpartum bleeding and helping your uterus contract after birth. The oxytocin that your body produces in response to your baby's suckling causes the uterus to contract and to stop bleeding.

Bonding with Your Baby

Some of the things that have been identified as strengthening the bonding process in the early hours after birth are closeness between the baby and the parents in the first few moments following birth, skin-to-skin contact between baby and mother, stroking movements on the part of the mother, warmth and relatively dim lighting with a reduced amount of noise, early nursing, and the irreducible minimum of interruptions for such things as footprinting.
—Dr. Alan Guttmacher and Dr. Irwin Kaiser, *Pregnancy, Birth, and Family Planning*

◆ ◆ ◆

"She was very alert and had this very adult look. It was amazing having this alert human being there," marveled Pete, who was surprised that his newborn daughter responded to him and his wife, Lucy, immediately after the birth. Many parents do not realize that newborns can be very responsive. If you have not received drugs during childbirth (and in some cases even if you have), your baby may be awake and extremely alert for the first hour or two after birth. Your newborn may grip your fingers, root around for your nipple, or gaze into your eyes. Many mothers automatically caress their newborns, an activity that some believe provides both stimulus and comfort for the baby.

As you and your baby become acquainted after birth, the baby may instinctively begin to search for your breast. Similarly, you may instinctively put the baby on your chest—which feels cozy and also places the baby near the breast.

Medical studies show that women who have unrestricted contact with their baby directly after birth tend to bond more easily and quickly with their baby. According to Drs. Klaus and Kennell, mothers who hold their babies immediately after birth, maintain skin-to-skin contact with the baby, are given uninterrupted time to become acquainted with the baby, and care for the newborn at least five hours a day, develop a stronger bond than if their early contact was not permitted.

Consequently, many doulas and midwives advocate close contact between mother and child immediately after birth and recommend that mother and child remain together, with a blanket over them (but not over the baby's head), for an hour or two. Breastfeeding experts believe that this sustained contact also promotes successful breastfeeding as well as the mother-child bond.

Some women bond with their babies immediately after birth. For others, it takes longer—weeks or even months. Be patient with yourself. If you are concerned that you are not bonding quickly enough, remember that new motherhood can be an overwhelming experience, and you may simply need time to grow accustomed to your new life and the demands of your new family member. Leslie advises new mothers that bonding will come, even if it doesn't happen right away: "I feel that my daughter has been the most important event of my life, but that wasn't immediately clear. You shouldn't assume that some epiphany will come to you one hour after the baby is born. . . . Allow yourself time to bond. Magic happens—but you can't push it. We're going on nine years—and it gets better every year."

Ask your family, friends, and partner for support (from moral support to cooking and performing household tasks) in order to give you time to relax and connect with your baby.

However, if you experience persistent problems with

bonding, you may be experiencing a version of postpartum depression. Speak to your care provider and seek counseling.

Breastfeeding after Birth

It was a peak experience. I think you experience a level of bonding with your baby that would not happen otherwise. Nursing forms a deep attachment.
—Linda-Carol

❖ ❖ ❖

A baby is guided by instinct to its mother's breast after birth. If you wish to breastfeed, it is helpful to work with nature and to begin nursing your baby following birth. Be patient, and allow time for you and your baby to become acquainted. Although breastfeeding is natural for babies, and babies practice their sucking response while still in the womb, you and your baby may need some coaching.

Some experts advise that breastmilk become the baby's sole source of nourishment—and not be supplemented with sugar water or formula—in order for successful nursing to be established, since the baby will see nursing as her primary source of nourishment and will be hungry when she begins to nurse. The more often your baby nurses, the more milk you will have—one of nature's convenient feedback loops. Demand increases supply.

If your baby is given a bottle in the nursery, she may not be as interested in breastfeeding. Discuss breastfeeding options with your care provider, and state your preferences in your birth plan. Also discuss with your caregiver possible circumstances in which your baby may need formula, sugar water, or breastmilk from the hospital's milk bank to supplement your breastmilk. If you are having multiples or if your baby is premature, discuss with your care provider how you can breastfeed your baby (or babies) in the NICU, where most preemies spend their first days or weeks.

Breastfeeding provides excellent nourishment for your baby, since the rich *colostrum*—the first milk that comes into your breasts—protects the baby's stomach from infection and provides the baby with all of your antibodies to disease. Your breastmilk also has the unique capacity to adjust its contents to meet the needs of your infant. For instance, colostrum is nutritionally well designed for newborns since it is higher in protein and lower in fat than the milk you produce as the baby matures.

Although infant formula has been in vogue from time to time, most midwives and doctors now agree that "the breast is best." According to John Riggs and Jorge D. Blanco in *Management of Labor and Delivery,* a standard medical school obstetrics textbook:

"Although infant formula is commercially prepared to meet the nutritional needs of infants, at best it can only approximate what is known about the composition of human milk. . . ."

You may fear that breastfeeding will prolong your state of feeling large and pregnant, but the opposite is the case. Breastfeeding stimulates the release of oxytocin—the hormone that makes your uterus contract.

If you have a cesarean birth, you may need help positioning the baby and finding a comfortable breastfeeding position. Rhonda's nurse and her husband helped her prop her son up on a pillow beside her so she wouldn't put strain on her cesarean incision as she nursed.

Should you encounter problems breastfeeding your baby, seek the assistance of a lactation consultant or La Leche League before you give up. You may find that the problems are easily solved. If you have nursing problems in the hospital, ask for a lactation consultant or call the La Leche League twenty-four-hour support (see appendix).

Episiotomy: Changing Philosophies

Perineal massage is beneficial if done prior to labor or the last few weeks before delivery. You can use vitamin E oil. Women who do this daily have less need for repair.
—Pam Spry, CNM

• • •

An episiotomy is a surgical cut in your perineum, the area just behind your vagina. The rationale behind doing episiotomies is that, by widening the vaginal opening before the baby's head comes out, the care provider can prevent perineal tearing and other injuries to the mother as the baby is born. Episiotomies are also performed to protect the baby; in the case of fetal distress, an episiotomy can speed the delivery of the baby.

Physicians who routinely perform episiotomies, especially at a first birth, believe that surgical cuts heal better than spontaneous tears and that the intentional cut performed during episiotomy prevents "uncontrolled tearing" that could cause future incontinence or pain. However, medical studies have called into question the routine use of episiotomy by showing the procedure may not decrease rates of incontinence due to bladder injury during birth and may actually increase risk of pain and tears extending to the anus.

Like any other surgical procedure, episiotomy has benefits and risks. The procedure may be beneficial when the baby is distressed. However, episiotomy carries the risks of bleeding and infection, and it may create additional injury and pain. This procedure may cause considerable discomfort during early motherhood and, in some women, problems in the months or years after childbirth.

Some care providers have a policy of "selective" episiotomy: If the baby's head will deliver without a serious tear, they refrain from episiotomy. Other care providers argue that small tears do not pose a problem for the mother and that they heal faster and hurt less than the surgical incision of episiotomy. Ask your caregiver if he or she performs routine episiotomies. If not, ask under what conditions episiotomies are performed and what percentage of his or her patients receive episiotomies.

Midwives tend to avoid episiotomies and frequently recommend perineal massage—massaging the perineum with olive oil, vitamin E oil, or other oils—weeks before labor begins in order to stretch the tissues, reduce perineal tearing, and avoid episiotomy. However, not all care providers agree that perineal massage prevents injury. Some argue that massage increases blood flow and swelling, which may increase the risk of bleeding during birth (especially if the perineum is massaged during childbirth).

Dr. Donna Kirz and nurse-midwife Pam Spry represent two different philosophies on performing episiotomies. Spry is antiepisiotomy unless the baby is in distress. Like other midwives, she attempts to solve the tearing problem with natural means such as birth positions that protect the perineum. "Lying on your side with your knees close together gives more stretch to the perineum," advises Spry.

Dr. Kirz, on the other hand, takes the selective episiotomy approach. "If I really think it [birth without tearing] is not going to work, my tendency is to cut a controlled episiotomy rather than let somebody tear. I think midwives tend to let people tear. It's just two different perspectives," explains Kirz.

If your baby's head is large and your perineum is inflexible, you may need an episiotomy. If you require a forceps-assisted delivery you may or may not need an episiotomy, depending on the kind of forceps delivery, the response of your body, and the philosophy of your care provider.

If you have tears or an episiotomy that need stitching, ask for an ice pack to reduce pain and swelling.

Stage 4: Recovery

During the week or two following your birth, you will regain your strength and your body will gradually return to its prepregnancy state. Expect some kind of vaginal bleeding or bloody discharge in the days or weeks after the birth. Always report bleeding or vaginal discharge to your care provider and keep track of how many sanitary pads you use a day in order to monitor the extent of your bleeding.

Chapter 22
Pain Relief in Childbirth

I don't offer pain medication to every woman routinely. However, if somebody asks for it, or if somebody really would benefit from it, I certainly think there is a place for it. Childbirth is supposed to be a happy experience, and I don't want a patient looking back and being angry about a bad experience.

—Dr. Susan Porto believes that women should have realistic expectations about childbirth: that it should be a positive experience—but not without discomfort. She says, "That's why we call it labor."

• • •

Women who are in control and confident do so much better than women who are out of control and anxious. This is why epidural or narcotics will often turn a labor around. The woman relaxes; labor develops a good pattern. It is better to do pain management with suggestions, helpful hints, being there, and supporting a person emotionally. But when that's not doing the trick, then the narcotics and the epidural really are helpful.

—Dr. Allen Killam

• • •

Labor is often painful, but the nature of the pain varies greatly from woman to woman. Some women experience manageable pain. Other women find the pain overwhelming and request medications for pain relief or some form of local or regional anesthesia.

In this chapter, I will focus on medical approaches to pain management such as epidural and spinal anesthesia, as well as medications such as analgesics and sedatives. I will also briefly discuss alternative methods of pain management such as hypnosis, acupuncture, and continuous support in labor.

Taking medications to relieve pain is a choice, not a sign of your failure to have a "natural birth." In some cases, pain medication may have significant benefits: the medications may give you enough pain relief to allow you to rest or sleep during a long labor, enabling you to regain your energy and concentration and helping you achieve a vaginal birth. However, there are also distinct disadvantages to taking drugs during childbirth. Many medications that you take can pass from your bloodstream through the placenta and into your baby's system. The amount of drug that crosses the placenta and finds its way to the baby may be minimal. However, some drugs are potent enough to make you or your baby groggy or unresponsive and may thus interfere with breathing, breastfeeding, or the precious moments of getting to know your newborn.

Because the choice of taking medications or not taking them has both emotional and medical consequences, it is important for you to become well informed about the medications you might be offered and the advantages and disadvantages that they create for you and your baby. Talk to an anesthesiologist who does labor and delivery pain management during the last month or two of your pregnancy, so that your questions are answered *before* you go into labor.

Regional Anesthesia: Epidurals and Spinals

Epidural Anesthesia

I'm not going to stand up and say, "Epidural anesthesia is for everyone," because I really don't think that. When a woman comes to me and she's eight months pregnant and wants to talk about anesthesia choices, I tell her: "Don't make a decision now. Don't even make a decision when you go into the hospital. Just get as much information as you can, and then when the time comes you can make a decision. You don't really know what your labor is going to be like until you actually experience it." So don't say, "I absolutely want an epidural," and don't say, "I absolutely won't have an epidural."

I think that's the bottom line. I think that's the best advice I can give any pregnant woman. Because she just doesn't know. Even if in her last labor she breezed through and didn't need an epidural, or in her last labor she did need an epidural—every labor is different. Two different babies are going to be different; the presentation is going to be different. Things change.

You shouldn't go in with a hard-and-fast plan. That's the anesthesiologist's view of birth plans. Be mega-flexible, and don't be disappointed if your plans don't work out.

—Dr. Louise Kirz, an anesthesiologist at the University of Oregon and mother of two

❀ ❀ ❀

The standard type of epidural anesthesia works by blocking the nerve pathways that transmit pain messages as well as the nerves that give you motor control (the ability to move), resulting in a loss of most sensation and movement below the waist. A "walking epidural," on the other hand, allows you to maintain movement and some control over the muscles used for bearing down and pushing the baby out during your second stage of labor, because this type of epidural is designed to block the small nerve fibers that carry pain sensations but not the bigger fibers that control the movement and pressure sensations that make you push during the second stage of labor. Thus, the walking epidural may give you several advantages, allowing you to actively participate in birthing your baby while relieving the pain of childbirth. It also allows you to change labor positions, although it does not always give you enough control to literally "walk." In most cases, at least, the walking epidural (which has become a popular form of epidural anesthesia) will allow you some control over pushing, although it is difficult to predict how each individual woman will respond to an epidural.

Both the standard epidural and the walking epidural will usually contain anesthetic medications to block pain and analgesic medications (such as morphine or other narcotics) to dull pain. Walking epidurals tend to have more narcotic than anesthesia, and it is this decreased amount of anesthesia that allows you to move to push.

An epidural is administered by an anesthesiologist who inserts a hollow needle into your back just above your waistline. The object of this procedure is to numb the nerves in your back that are connected to your lower abdomen—where the contractions are taking place. These nerves (as well as your brain and your spinal cord) are floating in cerebral spinal fluid and are enclosed in a thick membrane called the *dura*. An epidural is an injection of local anesthesia that reaches just outside or above (epi) the membrane (dura), and does not puncture the membrane. After the needle is inserted, the doctor threads a tiny plastic tube through the needle and leaves the tube in place throughout your labor so that epidural solution can be pumped through the tube as needed. The solution seeps across the dura and numbs the nerves leading from your spine to your abdomen. The specific kinds and amounts of solution and the anesthetic-to-narcotic ratio vary from hospital to hospital. At some hospitals, the dose of anesthesia is relatively light, resulting in a true "walking epidural." At others, the dose may contain more anesthesia and thus lead to more numbing of the motor nerves, resulting in less mobility.

The epidural catheter allows the doctor to administer additional anesthetic or analgesic (morphinelike pain medication) during the course of your labor. If you need a cesarean section, more anesthetic can be given to you through the narrow catheter in your back, and pain medication may be given to you at intervals during the twenty-four hours following your surgery.

When an epidural is administered, you will be asked to lie curled on your side or to curve your back forward in order to give the doctor easier access to the epidural space. Before the doctor inserts the hollow epidural needle, she will inject some local anesthetic, like the Novocain used by your dentist, to numb the area of the injection site. This will sting a little. Then, the epidural needle will be inserted in the lower portion of your lumbar spine—just below the part of your back that contains the spinal cord. You will feel pressure. When the medication is injected into your epidural space, you may feel a tingling or achy nerve feeling down your leg(s). Within approximately thirty minutes, you should feel little or no pain from the labor contractions. Although you may be aware that the contractions exist, they should not be painful. Most of the time, the epidural will be effective, although occasionally it may be uneven—numbing one side but not the other.

Because you will not be able to control urination if you have an epidural, a nurse or doctor will insert a catheter up your urethra and into your bladder. Since this procedure may burn a little at first, you may wish to ask your caregivers to insert the urinary catheter after the epidural takes effect.

It is always best if your anesthesiologist is experienced in administering epidurals to obstetrics patients.

When to Choose Regional Anesthesia

If the problem is that a woman is very tense, there are some strong therapeutic arguments for a labor epidural. I don't use labor epidurals routinely, but there are some cases where they are well utilized. If the woman just needs a little relaxation, I'd go with a narcotic. But narcotics are not really good at relaxing the pelvic floor. If I have a woman having her first baby, and she's been up for twenty-four hours straight with contractions, and she really needs something that's going to let her sleep, sometimes a labor epidural will do it. A lot of times the woman will wake up with her baby's head starting to come down.
—Dr. Susan Porto

* * *

Dr. Susan Porto decided not to have an epidural for childbirth. She felt confident that the natural birth process works well most of the time, and she didn't want to interfere with her body's instinctual way of handling childbirth, at least not unless absolutely necessary. "I went in hoping I would not need any pain medications, because my preference was not to accept anything." Luckily, both her labors (at age thirty-nine and forty-one) were fast, uncomplicated, and easily managed without pain medication. Nature worked as well for her as she expected it would.

Nature didn't work as well for Cathy. Cathy's labor was difficult, and she became too distracted by intense back labor to concentrate on her pushing—that is, until she received an epidural. "I pushed and I pushed and I pushed. Susan was turned 'sunny-side up'—in the OP position. She turned out to have a very large head—the 100th percentile. We finally decided to have an epidural. It made an amazing difference! Once the pain was gone, I was more aware of what was happening. I could participate more in the pushing. The epidural was great! Yes, I vote for it. Thank God for modern medicine; it was magic."

After the medication took effect, Cathy felt more clear-headed and able to work with the forces of nature. However, even her best pushing efforts couldn't compensate for cephalopelvic disproportion: Cathy's pelvis was not large enough to accommodate her baby, and the baby was born by cesarean section. Since her epidural was already in place, Cathy's doctor simply administered more anesthetic through the epidural tube to prepare her for cesarean birth.

Epidural medication, known as the "Cadillac" of anesthesia, has many potential benefits. It can help you rest and thus regain the stamina and presence of mind necessary to complete a painful or strenuous labor. But an epidural is not the best choice for every woman, since epidurals can slow down your labor. The choice will depend on the circumstances of your labor, your baby, and your medical and emotional condition.

Before signing up for an epidural, do some research. Discuss your individual circumstances with your caregiver to decide whether or not an epidural would benefit you during childbirth. Ask your caregiver at what point during labor and under what circumstances he or she recommends epidurals. Do not forget to ask your caregiver about risks, since every medication has risks as well as benefits. Talk to women who have experienced births with epidurals and women who have experienced births without them. Women who have had both kinds of birth experiences may offer you a particularly useful perspective. However, do not assume that your birth experience will resemble theirs, since every birth is different.

If possible, ask your doctor to recommend particular

anesthesiologists that he or she likes to work with and who might be available when you go into labor. Because you can't be sure when you will have the baby (unless you are having a scheduled cesarean), and because you cannot be certain which anesthesiologist will be working when you are in labor, you probably will have to take potluck once you arrive at the hospital. However, by talking to one of the anesthesiologists at your hospital you will be able to get information about the kind of anesthesia available at that hospital and about the anesthesia team's attitude toward epidural, spinal, and general anesthesia. Have this discussion by your eighth month of pregnancy (or earlier if you are pregnant with multiples) because you may need a month or more to mull things over before the birth.

If you are having a scheduled cesarean section you may be able to choose your anesthesiologist in advance.

If you are planning on having an epidural, make sure your anesthesiologist or nurse-anesthetist is experienced in doing epidurals for obstetrical anesthesia. If your anesthesiologist only does general anesthesia and if general anesthesia is all your hospital ordinarily offers for childbirth, do not press the doctor to do a procedure he or she is uncomfortable with. If you are not happy with the options presented to you, find a hospital that offers the kind of obstetrical anesthesia that you want. Usually, large hospitals or university hospitals offer a wider ranger of anesthesia options than small community hospitals. But you won't know for sure unless you ask.

Discuss your medical history and allergies with your anesthesiologist to determine which kind of anesthesia might be safest for you. For instance, if you have ruptured disks, or have had spinal surgery, or have rods in your lumbar spine, you may not be able to have an epidural. If you have had extensive surgery in the part of the back where epidurals are ordinarily placed, starting an epidural may be difficult.

If you have had no surgery and have a limited injury confined to one or two vertebrae, there may be no problem if the anesthesiologist can insert the epidural needle in an uninjured portion of your back. Discuss with your obstetrician and anesthesiologist whether or not an epidural is advisable for you.

Although many doctors agree that the timing of an epidural and/or the kind of epidural solution used are important if you want to avoid prolonged labor or an instrumental (forceps or vacuum) delivery, care providers disagree as to *the best time* to insert an epidural. "Early and late epidural: again, there's a real controversy," notes Dr. Allen Killam, who believes "that too, too early is not good." However, Killam thinks that "timed appropriately and given in the modern way, the 'walking epidural' is very useful and doesn't delay labor significantly."

Some doctors determine "good timing" by the degree of a woman's cervical dilation, and these doctors will begin an epidural only after a woman's cervix is dilated five centimeters. Other doctors, like Susan Porto, use the position of the baby, the regularity of effective uterine contractions, and the degree of softening of the cervix to ascertain when a woman can receive an epidural without jeopardizing her progress in labor. Dr. Porto says, "The timing of an epidural is important. I think the baby's head should be low in the pelvis, the cervix at least 80 percent effaced [softened], and the contractions regular and adequate. Those are my criteria. . . . If you place the epidural in a timely manner, it won't interfere with pushing because the baby's head will be far down in the pelvis, so the woman won't be able to resist the urge to push."

However, contrary to many doctors' clinical experience, the findings of a 1994 medical study by Dr. Chestnut et al. showed that the timing of epidurals did not adversely affect the progress of labor or the outcome of delivery.

Discuss the timing of your epidural with your physicians.

Before choosing an epidural, you may wish to consider the psychological effects that an epidural may have on your birth experience. An epidural may further "medicalize" your birth and make you feel more like a passive patient, especially if you are hooked up to an IV and a urinary catheter, medicated with Pitocin, and attached to a fetal monitor. On the other hand, you may feel, like Cathy did, freed from pain and more able to focus and actively participate in the birth of your baby.

Ask your care providers about the benefits and risks (to you and your baby) of the different kinds of anesthesia. Ask about the frequency of spinal headaches or other possible side effects. Find out whether or not epidural and spinal anesthesia are frequently offered to women at that hospital, and if you will have the option of a "walking epidural."

Possible Effects on the Baby

Care providers disagree as to whether or not epidurals may cause problems for the baby. Most American obstetricians and anesthesiologists think that epidurals are safe for the baby. Even if a tiny amount of the narcotic in the epidural solution should enter your bloodstream and pass to your baby, many doctors say the small dose of medication is not problematic for the baby. However, some care providers believe that epidurals may temporarily affect the baby's behavior just after birth, resulting in delayed rooting or nursing responses. So far, much of the concern about nursing and infant behavior is based on "anecdotal evidence" (the least reliable kind of medical evidence) and not medical studies. However, because few well-designed studies have been conducted to investigate the effects of epidural anesthesia on infant behavior, we do not know for sure whether or not epidurals adversely affect the infant's nursing instincts or other behaviors.

However, we do know that a baby may develop an

epidural-induced fever after birth, especially if the mother has developed a fever from her epidural during labor. A 1997 study of 1,650 women found that 15 percent of women with epidurals ran fevers of 100.4 degrees, whereas only 1 percent of women without epidurals ran fevers during childbirth. In another study, researchers found that epidural anesthesia increased the odds by 25 percent that the newborn would have a fever after birth.

A baby with an epidural-induced fever must be carefully watched, tested, and sometimes taken from its mother's side to the nursery or NICU for observation, to make sure the fever is merely a passing thing that is due to medication—and not a more serious problem caused by infection. Babies with fevers may receive a "septic workup," which may include blood tests, a spinal tap, and antibiotic treatment.

Possible Effects on the Mother

Although epidurals are generally quite safe, no anesthetic is without risks. Some problems caused by epidural anesthesia include spinal headache, decreased maternal blood pressure, prolonged or dysfunctional labor resulting in forceps or vacuum deliveries, itching, bladder dysfunction, and back pain. Sometimes a "walking epidural" results in more numbing and loss of motor control than anticipated.

Spinal Headache

The biggest side effect that women need to be aware of from an epidural is spinal headache. A spinal headache is probably the worst headache you can imagine—it's on par with a bad migraine. When you puncture the membrane [the dura] with a very small needle, there's not a problem. If you puncture that membrane with a big needle, the needle leaves a hole, and fluid leaks out through that hole: and that's what causes a spinal

headache. Now an epidural is not supposed to puncture that membrane, but between 1 and 2 percent of the time it does. . . . That's one or two out of one hundred.
—Dr. Louise Kirz

* * *

Spinal headache is one of the most common side effects of epidural anesthesia. This kind of headache typically worsens when you sit or stand up and is a symptom of a "misplaced" epidural needle that goes just a little bit too far and punctures the dura. As a result, spinal fluid seeps through the hole in the dura and, if the hole is large enough, creates a spinal headache. The headache may last five to ten days. Often the headache is at its most intense on Day 2, which is the day you are going home with your new baby. It starts to get better by about Day 4 or 5, and within a week it is usually gone.

Spinal headaches can be treated with analgesics, bed rest, and fluids. Although these treatments may help you feel better, they may not make the headache go away. Sometimes you can partially relieve the pain by lying flat.

When the pain continues for longer than normal or is unbearable, your care provider may suggest a procedure called a "blood patch." This procedure involves the doctor taking blood from your arm and injecting it in the place in the epidural space where the initial puncture took place.

Drop in Blood Pressure

Although epidural anesthesia may cause your blood pressure to fall, this drop in blood pressure may be prevented by keeping your blood volume (and thus your blood pressure) up with IV fluids. Usually, the IV is started before you are given the epidural to prevent a sustained drop in your blood pressure that could diminish the blood flow to your uterus and your baby.

Problems with Labor
Eleven studies of 3,157 were included [in this review of the med-
ical literature on epidurals]. Epidural analgesia was associated
with greater pain relief than nonepidural methods, but also with
longer first and second stages of labour, an increased incidence of
fetal malposition, and increased use of oxytocin and instrumental
vaginal deliveries [forceps, vacuum extractions]. With new trial
data [research information] included, no statistically significant
effect on caesarean section could be identified.
—C. J. Howell, "Epidural Versus Non-Epidural Analgesia for
Pain Relief in Labour," *The Cochrane Library*, Issue 3, 1999.
Oxford: Update Software

* * *

Because women are a little more aware of their contractions [with
a walking epidural], their pushing is a little more coordinated—
but it's still not as good as someone who doesn't have an epidural.
. . . I think with proper coaching with a good labor nurse, or mid-
wife, or both, or a good OB, a woman can push effectively with
an epidural, but it seems that the reflex to push is blocked.
—Dr. Louise Kirz

* * *

Whether or not epidural anesthesia—especially an epidural
used early in labor—causes problems in labor is the subject of
debate. Some caregivers think that epidurals may slow both first
and second stage labor. According to several medical studies,
women who have epidurals need Pitocin to enhance the contractions of first stage labor more often than women who do
not have epidurals. In addition, women with epidural anesthesia may tend to experience a lengthened pushing stage of
labor as well as problems with the baby's descent and rotation,
leading to an increase in forceps and vacuum deliveries.

Consequently, many physicians allot more time for labor in a woman who has had an epidural than for a woman who has not been so medicated.

Does epidural anesthesia increase the incidence of cesarean sections? Some doctors say it does; others say it does not. According to Dr. David Chestnut, an expert in epidural anesthesia, a "light" or "dilute" solution of local anesthetic may be "less likely to increase the risk of cesarean than administration of a more concentrated solution."

However, Dr. Chestnut writes in "Epidural Analgesia and the Incidence of Cesarean Section: Time for Another Close Look" (*Anesthesiology*, September 1997) that this distinction between light and heavy epidural solutions is supported by some studies but not by others. It is also possible that factors other than the use of epidural anesthesia may contribute to an increased cesarean rate: The medical circumstances of the mother and baby and the obstetric management may influence the cesarean rate.

Back Pain

Some women experience short-term back pain after an epidural. Most often, they experience pain only briefly at the site of the injection, but occasionally the discomfort remains for weeks or months.

Bladder Dysfunction

Occasionally, women have temporary trouble urinating after receiving an epidural. This problem may last from a few hours to one to two days.

Itching

The narcotic in an epidural may cause intense itching all over your body. Fortunately, this itching is easily treated.

Other Possible Side Effects

Another possible effect on the mother includes accidental total spinal anesthesia. Rare complications include neurological effects, respiratory insufficiency, and, very, very rarely, death.

Spinal Anesthesia

You put your medicine in. The patient lies down. She gets numb.
—Dr. Louise Kirz

* * *

One should not persuade an anesthesiologist to give a spinal unless he or she is trained in its administration and management in the obstetric field.
—Robin Russell and Felicity Reynolds, "Pain Relief and Anesthesia During Labor," in *Management of Labor and Delivery*

* * *

Spinal anesthesia is often done to provide regional anesthesia for cesarean sections, but not for labor, since a spinal is time limited and there is no telling how long a labor will last. A spinal is administered by a very small needle that is inserted into your lower back. It is "deeper" than an epidural in that the needle punctures the dura, injects anesthetic directly into your spinal fluid, and quickly results in the numbing of the nerves leading to your abdomen and legs. After a dose of anesthetic is given, the needle is withdrawn. No plastic tube is left behind to administer continuous doses. Consequently, the spinal lasts about two and a half hours—long enough to numb you from the waist down for a cesarean birth but not long enough to cover hours of labor.

Spinal anesthesia is used for emergency cesareans since it takes effect much faster than an epidural—in about five minutes as opposed to thirty minutes. However, epidurals are often used for cesareans that are not emergencies and for some abdominal surgery, like fibroid surgery, in which waiting thirty minutes for the anesthetic to take effect presents no problem.

The possible side effects of spinal anesthesia are similar to those with an epidural: headache, drop in blood pressure, difficulty with urination, respiratory depression.

Analgesics (e.g., meriperidine [Demerol], nalbuphine [Nubain], and butorphanol [Stadol])

If a woman's contracting painfully and not progressing, and if she's getting tired and upset, if you give her a narcotic, the drug may let her sleep and then wake up in active labor, rested and ready to go. This approach is probably underutilized now. It was utilized in the old days when we had below 5 percent cesarean rates. It's a thing that works very well, but it's become a lost procedure.
—Dr. Allen Killam

* * *

Narcotic pain medications may offer temporary reduction in labor pain for two to four hours. For some women, this much-needed break from pain allows them to relax, to rest or sleep through their contractions, and to regain the energy and calm necessary to tolerate labor and go on to have a vaginal birth.

When anxiety is getting in the way of your progress in labor, narcotics can speed your labor by reducing your anxiety. This temporary break from pain and stress may ultimately turn a difficult labor around. Because you are no longer fighting against the strong contractions that dilate the cervix and open up the birth canal, your labor can proceed more easily.

If you are having back labor, you may benefit from narcotic assistance, since the pain relief may help you relax enough for labor to progress and for the baby to rotate to a more advantageous position for birth.

Some caregivers think the benefits of narcotic pain medications outweigh risks to the mother insofar as the medications may help the mother tolerate labor and proceed to a vaginal delivery of her baby. Some caregivers argue that narcotic pain medications, by helping the mother, may *indirectly* benefit the baby—if the medications ease a woman into a less stressful, less complicated labor than she would have had without them and help her achieve a normal vaginal birth. In such a case the baby is spared a long, difficult labor and the risks of instrumental deliveries.

However, narcotics *do not directly benefit the baby,* since the drugs cross the placenta and may cause short-term problems and respiratory depression in the baby immediately after birth. Some experts argue that narcotic pain relief, if it is given at all in childbirth, should be given only in moderate dosages and while the placenta can still help the baby get rid of the narcotic in its system.

Narcotic pain medications may be given to you intravenously, though an IV, or in a muscle. The IV medication takes effect quickly and it also leaves your system more quickly (which may be safer for your baby, especially if your labor is shorter than expected). The intramuscular injection affords longer-lasting pain relief.

Possible Side Effects on the Baby
Narcotics cross the placenta, and this may cause respiratory depression in the baby. . . ."
—Dr. Murray Enkin et al., *The Guide to Effective Care in Pregnancy and Childbirth* (second edition)

If you take a narcotic during childbirth, so does your baby. Narcotic pain medications in childbirth may depress the baby's breathing. However, often this effect can be immediately reversed when your doctor gives the baby Narcon or similar drugs to counteract the narcotic effects (unless the baby is premature or has other respiratory problems). Some experts warn that babies exposed to narcotics in utero are more likely to be sleepy at birth and consequently less responsive, slower to nurse, and more likely to have behavioral side effects than babies not exposed to narcotics.

The degree of side effects experienced by the baby depends upon at what point in your labor you took the drug, the dose of the drug, and the overall health of your baby. The new shorter-acting drugs (such as Nubain, Stadol, Sublimaze) are safer for the baby since they will be excreted from the baby's system sooner than the longer-acting drugs like Demerol. High or frequently administered doses of narcotic are more likely to affect the baby than low doses.

Premature infants are more susceptible to narcotic-induced respiratory depression, since preemies are more likely to experience respiratory distress in the first place, and the combination of narcotic medication and prematurity can create additional problems for them.

Possible Side Effects on the Mother

Demerol may cause nausea or vomiting, although it can be given with medications to reduce nausea. Many of the narcotic pain medications may also cause dizziness, euphoria, hallucinations, respiratory depression, itching, and difficulty with urination. You may feel zoned out, detached, or drunk after a narcotic is administered. Cathy felt that the narcotics made her feel too drugged to fully participate in the birth of her first child. According to Dr. Porto, the drugged feeling can take on numerous forms:

"With the narcotics, the worst effect on the mothers I see is that they can get really stuperous. Sometimes they don't remember anything, or they lose their ability to follow their own instincts. They may be getting ready to deliver, and they can't push. It's like being extremely drunk and trying to do heavy work. They can't do it because they are too sleepy from the medication to be able to help their bodies out. They end up losing a lot of nature's cues. Some women end up having problems with nausea, headache, or vomiting. Narcotics give some people a hangover side effect."

However, some women feel more relaxed and in control after taking narcotics for labor pain.

Tranquilizers and Sedatives

Although barbiturates are sometimes used to sedate women during early latent labor, they are not popular because they do not effectively control pain, and they have "a profound depressant effect" on the baby. Tranquilizers may occasionally be given in childbirth, sometimes in combination with narcotics, because they may reduce narcotic-induced nausea or vomiting. However, some childbirth experts say that the effects of tranquilizers such as diazepam (Valium) may have potentially harmful effects on the baby. Tranquilizers, if taken during birth, may make the baby limp, "floppy," and slow to suckle. The drugs also may lower the baby's body temperature.

General Anesthesia

If you require an emergency cesarean section, your anesthesiologist may use general anesthesia, since these anesthetics act very quickly. General anesthesia may also be used if, for some reason, you are unable to have epidural or spinal anesthesia—either because you have medical contraindications, such as previous spinal surgery, or because your hospital does not regularly offer epidural or spinal anesthesia. Occasionally a spinal or epidural will only partially numb your abdomen prior to cesarean section—in which case you may require general anesthesia for the surgery.

General anesthesia involves a loss of consciousness and sensation. First, you are given intravenous medications to relax you. Next, you inhale gas and quickly "go to sleep." Once you are asleep, you will be intubated: A tube will be put down your windpipe to ensure that your airway remains open and that you receive sufficient oxygen while you are unconscious. Sometimes this tube will irritate your throat and make it sore after you awaken.

The benefits of a general anesthesia are (1) you will be unaware of the surgery, (2) the surgery can begin very quickly, and (3) most anesthesiologists are accustomed to administering it. However, general anesthesia is not without risks.

Possible Side Effects on the Mother

General anesthesia may give you a hangover that makes you feel nauseous and sluggish. On rare occasions, it can cause vomiting while you are asleep—which is why some care providers restrict eating and drinking in laboring women, especially in those who may need an emergency cesarean. An unconscious patient may, while vomiting, inhale gastric juices or other stomach contents. In the *extremely unlikely event* that this happens, the patient may develop aspiration pneumonia, which may result in death. However, given the careful monitoring of surgical patients and the protection afforded your lungs by intubation, aspiration is very rare. Certain drugs, especially opiates and muscle relaxants, when administered in large or frequent doses prior to general anesthesia, may contribute to the risk of anesthesia-related mortality. If you have been given systemic opiates during labor and then again during and after surgery, you will need to be carefully monitored in the recovery room after your surgery.

The intubation procedure involved in general anesthesia makes the anesthesia safer because the anesthesiologist can "secure an airway," making it easier for you to breathe during the surgery. Although intubation usually proceeds smoothly, occasionally the intubation process is problematic.

Possible Side Effects on the Baby

Other drawbacks of general anesthesia include the possibility of respiratory depression and poor muscle tone in the baby and the possibility that the mother and birth partner will miss the birth and the first hours of bonding with the baby.

Discuss your individual benefits and risks with your doctor.

Natural and Alternative Choices: Strategies for Managing Pain

Some choices for labor are "natural choices" like breathing and relaxation techniques . . . if you can get your body to relax, the pain is there but the labor tends to go more quickly.
—Dr. Lousie Kirz

＊ ＊ ◆

You have many pain management options for labor that do not involve drugs. Helpful nonpharmaceutical approaches to pain control include relaxation and breathing techniques; self-hypnosis and visualization; continuous support from a doula, midwife, or labor and delivery nurse; birthing positions; warm showers; and acupuncture or acupressure. Many of these pain management approaches involve positive thinking techniques that help you view contractions as "productive," "strong," and "good" (rather than "painful") because they do the work of labor and bring your baby closer to you.

Many childbirth education classes include pain management in the form of the previously mentioned techniques. In most pain management techniques, relaxation is key. To increase your relaxation during labor and birth, include people, rituals, activities (warm showers, Jacuzzis, back rubs), and objects in your environment that bring you comfort.

To supplement your nonpharmaceutical "bag of tricks" for pain control, you might want to use acupuncture or acupressure. Since some acupressure points may increase your contractions or induce labor, consult an experienced, licensed acupuncturist. Call a local or regional acupuncture college for referrals. The accupuncture point called Large Intestine 4 (on the back of your hand in the soft webbed area next to your thumb) is an all-purpose point for pain and stress. If the point is sensitive or hurts when you press it, you have probably found the right spot. (See appendix for references.)

If you have emotional issues resulting from bad experiences with previous births, medical staff, or hospitalizations (e.g., previous surgeries or serious illnesses) that may add to your tension and pain during labor, try to acknowledge these experiences and work through them before you give birth. Traumatic memories concerning sexual assault or physical abuse may be ignited by the emotions and sensations of childbirth, and you may wish to seek support from a counselor or other health professional in order to prevent past associations from adversely affecting your birth experience.

Part Eight

Childbirth Interventions, Variations, and Complications

In each case my wife just tried and tried. When it came time to make decisions, there weren't any other reasonable alternatives. . . . We didn't feel stampeded into it [forceps delivery for the first baby and cesarean delivery for the next baby]. Natural childbirth is terrific if you can pull it off. If you can't, it doesn't mean that the end result is diminished.
—Kevin

* * *

Plan for a normal birth, but prepare yourself for possible *variations* or *complications* in your childbirth experience, some of which may call for medical or surgical *interventions*.

A labor *variation* falls within "the wide range of normal," writes Penny Simkin and her coauthors in *Pregnancy, Childbirth, and the Newborn*. Such variations, however, may present you and your care providers with additional challenges during labor and birth. This section will discuss such variations as breech babies, big babies, postdate babies, and long labors. Some of these variations may require that your care provider intervene by administering medications to stimulate labor or by using forceps or vacuum instruments to facilitate your baby's birth. Sometimes the birth will require patience and stamina rather than any direct intervention. At other times, the birth may require a cesarean section. In any case, it is best if you have a "bag of tricks" for each scenario and the necessary information to help you make reasonable decisions despite possible interference from labor contractions and fatigue.

This section will also discuss a range of *complications* of childbirth that pose potential risks to you and your child and thus require your care provider to medically intervene or to carefully monitor you and the baby. Fortunately, true childbirth emergencies are rare, but it is important that you learn to recognize potential problems in order to know when to seek and accept medical care.

My intention in Part 8 is to provide you with information that you can use to think through your options, make informed choices before and during labor, and actively participate in important decisions affecting you and your baby. By informing yourself about potential problems early on, you will be better able to make good decisions during labor and birth.

I begin this section with the most common decisions that you may have to make during childbirth and end with the least common. If you think that reading about rare problems, no matter what the context, may unnerve you, skip Chapter 27. However, if you want to be reassured that rare things probably won't happen to you—and to be prepared just in case they do—read that chapter.

Chapter 23

Inducing Labor, Suppressing Labor, and Other Medical Interventions in Childbirth

One worldview is that you do not know that pregnancy and birth are normal until after the fact, and we must do everything we are capable of doing to ensure a healthy outcome. The other worldview is one in which birth is a normal process, and if you are patient with it, nature will work. Providers inherently favor one view over the other but may be anywhere on the continuum, and they may move in one direction or the other as a situation changes. Midwives tend to be closer to the position of being patient with the birthing process, and physicians tend to be closer to the "do what you can do to help the process" end of the continuum. But either provider can be at any point depending on the situation.
—Laraine Guyette, CNM, Ph.D.

◆ ◆ ◆

Among care providers, there is, as nurse-midwife Laraine Guyette puts it, "a continuum of belief in the normal birth process." Individual care providers (whether they are midwives or physicians) may fall anywhere along that continuum, depending on their general birth philosophy and the particular circumstances of the laboring mother and her baby.

For instance, some care providers take what is called a non-interventionist or *expectant* "wait and see" approach. Such care providers tend to believe that birth is a normal event and have confidence that the process will usually proceed normally. They believe that some births take longer than other births and that both woman and care provider will often do best by simply working with nature and supporting the natural course of a woman's labor—even if it is a little longer than "average." Thus, they tend to let nature take its course and suggest that the laboring woman engage in activities that facilitate her progress in labor, such as walking or assuming different positions.

Because expectant management is a wait-and-see philosophy, it requires patience on the part of both laboring woman and care provider. For instance, if your waters break, expectant management might mean that your care provider will wait and see if your labor starts on its own in a reasonable period of time—usually anywhere from twelve to forty-eight hours—before intervening and inducing labor.

Other care providers, however, may take a more active, *interventionist* role in promoting the progress of your labor. In this case, your care provider may induce labor.

Generally speaking, the expectant and interventionist philosophies are equally valid, although you may find that you are more comfortable with one philosophy than the other. Consequently, it is useful for you to be aware of your provider's views since they will influence his or her obstetrical practice and your birth experience. Discuss with your care provider how his or her childbirth philosophy may apply to you and your baby.

Preterm Labor and Birth

About 10 percent of all babies are born prematurely—before the thirty-seventh week of gestation. Babies born before thirty-two completed weeks of gestation are considered to be "very preterm," and those born at a gestational age of less than twenty-eight completed weeks are considered "extremely preterm." If you start going into labor prematurely, this is not the time to adopt an expectant wait-and-see philosophy. Call your care provider immediately, since premature labor can sometimes be treated and stopped if caught early enough.

If you are in premature labor, your care provider may suggest one or more of the following interventions to prevent your baby from being born right away:

- Bed rest (although bed rest is no longer as frequently recommended as it once was)
- Increased fluid intake
- Treatment with drugs that relax the uterine muscle and stop labor contractions
- Corticosteroid treatment to enhance your baby's lung maturity
- Antibiotic treatment if it has been twenty-four to forty-eight hours since your waters broke

You are more likely to have premature labor if you are pregnant with multiples (see Part 6) or you have a uterus or cervix with structural abnormalities (a T-shaped uterus, a weakened or incompetent cervix, a very large fibroid within or abutting the uterine cavity); uncontrolled high blood pressure or preeclampsia; placental problems; premature rupture of your membranes; or if you or your baby is ill.

If you are having premature labor, your care providers may recommend that you drink fluids (unless you have a medical condition that would prohibit this for some reason), since dehydration may cause premature labor. Your caregiver may recommend bed rest and suggest that you lie on your left side to ensure maximum blood flow to your baby. Instead of bed rest, your care provider may suggest that you take time off from work, stay home, and limit your activity. To treat preterm labor, your care provider may also recommend treatment with one of several medications that can relax your uterus and stop the contractions for a while, to give your baby more time to mature.

Drinking fluid is perhaps one of the safest treatments for suppressing preterm uterine contractions. Drug therapies have both benefits and risks that you should consider with the help of your caregiver and pharmacist. For instance, betamimetic drugs are used to suppress contractions, and these drugs have been shown to reduce the number of deliveries that occur within the first twenty-four to forty-eight hours after treatment begins. However, these drugs may pose risks to both mother and baby. Corticosteroid therapy, a treatment for the baby, has had beneficial effects in successfully treating very premature babies whose lungs are not mature; these drugs accelerate the maturation of the baby's lungs so the baby can breathe adequately outside the womb.

Other important treatments for your baby occur immediately after birth. If your baby is very premature and must spend time in an NICU, you may take heart in the fact that over the last thirty years, modern medicine is responsible for impressive survival rates in very premature babies. At twenty-nine to thirty weeks of gestation, or at birth weights over 1,500 grams, the survival rate for preemies is almost 90 percent.

Fortunately, the neonatal survival rates of extremely premature babies between twenty-three and twenty-six weeks of gestation have also dramatically improved over the last ten to fifteen years (for babies cared for in NICUs). Babies at twenty-five weeks gestational age now have survival rates of around 80 percent.

When Your Baby Won't Wait

Sometimes birth occurs unexpectedly, although not necessarily prematurely, when you are at home, at work, in the car—or even in a taxi en route to the hospital.

If you feel the urge to push, feel your baby coming, or see your baby's head or feet pushing out of your vagina, you are giving birth. If this happens, try not to panic. Remind yourself that women have been giving birth outside of hospitals for thousands of years. Trust your instincts and the birth process but also call for assistance.

First call 911 and tell them you are having your baby (*now!*) and that this is an emergency. (Paramedics and emergency medical technicians on ambulances are trained in the basics of childbirth.) Either you or your partner or a friend should then call your caregiver to ask for instructions. At that point, your doctor may arrange to meet you at the hospital. Next, call the emergency department or labor and delivery ward of a hospital close to you and ask for emergency advice while you wait for the paramedics to arrive. Call someone you know—friend, partner, neighbor—who is likely to answer the phone and ask him or her to help you.

If the baby is about to emerge, spread clean towels or sheets down on the floor or bed. If you are in the car, spread clean towels or a robe on the seat or floor of the car. You will need a clean and relatively padded spot for your baby, especially if you are kneeling or squatting and the baby could land on a hard floor. Remember that newborns are slippery and may emerge quickly.

Carefully reach over and guide the baby's head as the baby is born.

Once the baby is born, wipe mucous from her mouth and nose so she can breathe well; put the baby on her side on your bare abdomen; dry the baby's head and body off with a clean cloth or, if you are en route to the hospital, with any clean piece of clothing; cover the top of the baby's head with a make-shift hat; and cover her body (but not her face) with a warm blanket. Stroke the baby gently—and try to relax.

Do not cut the cord. If your placenta emerges, leave it intact and put it and the baby on the same level so blood in the placenta does not drain excessively into or from the baby.

If the baby does not breathe immediately, rub the baby's chest gently with your knuckles—this may stimulate the baby to breathe. If she doesn't breathe, do this again. You may also stimulate the baby's breathing by slapping the soles of her feet. If neither method works, attempt extremely gentle and extremely careful rescue breathing. Do *not* attempt to use the CPR routine designed for adults! A baby is not a little adult; its neck and lungs are very delicate. To attempt rescue breathing, cradle the baby in your arms, place your mouth over its little nose and mouth, and blow very, very gently. Do not inhale and blow from your lungs into the baby's nose and mouth. Instead, partially fill your cheeks with air and very very gently puff into the baby's nose and mouth. Blowing too hard or bending your baby's neck back too far can cause serious and permanent damage! If you see the baby's chest rise, the air has reached its destination. Blow once every three seconds until the baby responds. Once the baby starts breathing on its own, stop the rescue breathing. You do not need to force air into the baby once she is breathing on her own. Consider taking infant CPR as part of your preparation for parenthood (see appendix). If your baby needs help breathing, call 911 immediately for a paramedic ambulance, and ask for assistance while you are beginning the rescue breathing. Explicitly tell the 911 operator that the baby is not breathing.

If you find that you are bleeding profusely, firmly knead

your abdomen to help your uterus contract, encourage the baby to nurse, and/or stimulate your nipples (since any stimulation of the nipples causes your body to produce oxytocin, which reduces bleeding by making your uterus contract). If the bleeding continues, lie down with your knees bent or put your feet up on a chair or pillow so that your legs and feet are higher than your head and torso. This position may reduce your chance of going into shock from blood loss.

Postterm Birth

. . . An abundance of older as well as more recent data has firmly established that although the fetal risk associated with a prolonged pregnancy is small, it is real. Consequently, the pregnancy that continues beyond 42 weeks requires careful surveillance.
—Dr. Robert Resnick and Dr. Andrew Calder, "Post-Term Pregnancy," *Maternal-Fetal Medicine* (fourth edition)

* * *

In light of the available evidence, the best policy is to offer women a choice of induction of labour by the best method available once the duration of pregnancy has with certainty attained 41 weeks or more.
—Dr. Murray Enkin et al., "Post-term Pregnancy," *A Guide to Effective Care in Pregnancy and Childbirth* (second edition).

* * *

A term pregnancy is completed in thirty-eight to forty-two weeks, and pregnancy is considered prolonged when it exceeds forty-two weeks, according to *Maternal-Fetal Medicine,* a standard obstetrics textbook. The World Health Organization (WHO) also defines postterm pregnancy as a pregnancy that *exceeds* forty-two weeks of no menstrual period. However, some caregivers define a pregnancy as postdue after forty weeks, others after forty-one weeks, and still others after forty-two weeks. Consequently, there is disagreement among care providers as to when after forty weeks of pregnancy labor should be induced.

Many care providers consider inducing labor after forty-one weeks. Medical studies indicate that after forty-one weeks of pregnancy certain risks for the baby may begin to increase. If labor is induced at forty-one weeks or more, studies show a decrease in infant mortality. However, there is no change in infant mortality if labor is induced at thirty-nine to forty weeks.

Care providers who argue for inducing labor at forty weeks (instead of forty-one) say that the earlier induction gets the baby born before it suffers from fetal distress and *uteroplacental insufficiency* (the failure of an aging placenta to provide adequate nourishment to the baby) and before the baby can become *macrosomic* (too large).

Those who argue against inducing labor at forty weeks say that such early induction may result in an increased rate of operative delivery and may not benefit the baby.

Inducing labor at less than forty-one weeks "is not associated with any advantage apart from a small reduction in meconium staining of the amniotic fluid" and "the reduction in perinatal death appears to be confined to pregnancies of 41 plus weeks duration," writes Dr. Murray Enkin in his review of the medical literature in, *A Guide to Effective Care in Pregnancy and Childbirth* (third edition). However, Enkin and his coauthors argue that induction *after forty-one-plus* weeks may offer benefits to both baby and mother. After reviewing the medical literature, the authors conclude that inducing labor after forty-one-plus weeks "is not associated with any disadvantage" and "reduces the risk of perinatal death and early neonatal convulsions." They conclude that when appropriate induction methods are used, inducing labor at forty-one-plus weeks may reduce the risk of cesarean section for postterm mothers.

Keep careful track of your ovulation and your date of conception to help avoid confusion as to whether or not your baby is postdate.

Inducing Labor

Let's say you decide to induce labor. Before you induce labor, be sure the cervix is as favorable as possible—that it is effaced or ripe [thinned, soft, dilating]. The baby's head needs to be in the birth canal and relatively well engaged. If those circumstances aren't fulfilled, you first use cervical ripening agents [such as prostaglandins].
—Dr. Watson Bowes Jr.

*   *   *

Elective inductions solely for convenience are not encouraged.
—Julia E. Solomon and Mary E. D'Alton, "Induction of Labor."
Management of Labor and Delivery

*   *   *

Older women tend to have higher rates of induced labor than younger women, particularly among first births, says Dr. Gertrude Berkowitz, an epidemiologist at Mt. Sinai Hospital in New York City. Older women are also more likely to have preeclampsia and diabetes and other medical conditions that may necessitate induction of labor.

"Before you induce, you need to decide if birthing should begin in order to benefit the mother or the baby. You make that decision first," says Dr. Watson Bowes Jr., explaining how doctors decide whether to induce labor. Then, says Bowes, doctors decide on the safest method of induction for the mother and baby. Deciding whether or not to induce labor is an important decision, not a trivial one, and many doctors believe that labor should be induced only for very good reasons.

Labor may be induced by pharmaceutical or mechanical means or by "natural" remedies such as nipple stimulation (some midwives swear by this). Induction is most successful if your cervix is ripe, which means that it is soft, thin, and dilated. If your cervix is not ripe, it can be softened by prostaglandins, hormonal drugs inserted into your vagina in suppository form. When used in small doses, prostaglandins can change the cervical tissue enough to soften it and ready it for labor. Primrose oil, an herbal remedy used by some midwives, may also ripen the cervix and precede further methods of induction. (However, primrose oil has not been thoroughly studied.)

Mechanical means of inducing labor may include any of the following interventions: stripping or sweeping the membranes (the bag of waters); rupturing the membranes; or inserting a Foley catheter or laminaria japonicum (a type of expandable seaweed) into the cervix.

Nipple Stimulation

Nipple stimulation increases your production of oxytocin—the hormone that causes your uterus to contract. Theoretically, nipple stimulation may induce labor in the same way that oxytocin can. Intercourse and orgasm can also stimulate oxytocin production and may also induce labor. Although nipple stimulation is safe, intercourse at the end of pregnancy is not always safe, especially if you have a weakened cervix or a placental problem. Discuss such induction remedies with your care provider before deciding to try them on your own.

Stripping the Membranes

If your cervix is already ripe and your labor has not yet started, your caregiver may wish to induce labor by "stripping" your membranes. The procedure sounds more invasive than it really is. Your care provider stretches your cervix to loosen the membranes around your bag of waters without breaking them. The stretching of your cervix is probably the most uncomfortable aspect of the mechanical procedures.

The procedure frequently stimulates labor, especially if you walk around so that gravity will press the baby up against your cervix; your waters usually will break spontaneously as labor progresses. This method offers a relatively natural way to induce labor, since your body is allowed to function on its own time clock. One of the major benefits of stripping the membranes away from the cervical opening is that your membranes remain intact, thus protecting you and your baby from infection. Because stripping the membranes is a relatively low-risk procedure, it can be done in your care provider's office and afterward you may return home.

Rupturing the Membranes

Rupturing the membranes is usually painless, although it is actually more invasive than stripping your membranes since your uterus and baby are no longer protected by the membranes. Rupturing the membranes usually produces labor contractions within twenty-four to forty-eight hours.

Your care provider may suggest artificial rupture of the membranes (known as ARM or amniotomy) to induce labor. Amniotomy is a painless procedure (the membranes that are being ruptured have no feeling) that may reduce the length of your labor. After an amniotomy is performed, your amniotic fluid may gush out or trickle out as it would if your membranes had ruptured spontaneously.

Along with speeding up your labor, amniotomy gives your care provider valuable information about your baby, since the amniotic fluid may help the care provider assess how mature your baby is and how well he is responding to labor. Many women fear that meconium in the amniotic fluid indicates fetal distress, but this is not necessarily the case. The mere presence of meconium does not in itself mean that your baby is in distress; it may simply mean that your baby's intestines are mature enough to have a bowel movement (see "Demystifying Meconium" later in this chapter).

If your baby does appear to be in distress, your care provider has better access to the baby once the membranes have been broken. To further assess the condition of your baby, your caregiver may either use a scratch test of the baby's scalp to make sure it is getting enough oxygen or monitor your baby's heart rate through an electrode attached to its head. Many care providers use this test to assess the extent of a baby's distress before performing a cesarean section.

A downside of amniotomy is that, because your membranes are ruptured, you and your baby are more susceptible to infection. For this reason, some care providers limit the number of vaginal exams after a woman's membranes rupture. Infection is relatively rare, but since the risk of infection increases with time, many care providers will want you in active labor within twenty-four hours of breaking your waters. Others will wait forty-eight before deciding to administer Pitocin or other labor-inducing drugs to move your labor along.

Acupuncture

Acupuncture has been used to induce labor with varying degrees of success, depending on the study, the practitioner, and the acupuncture points used. If you are interested in trying acupuncture, discuss this option with your care provider first and then, if your care provider deems acupuncture appropriate, seek an experienced, licensed acupuncturist.

Medications

If labor is not effectively induced by the mechanical methods described above, and if your cervix is not yet ripe enough for labor to safely begin, your care provider may use medications to ripen your cervix and thus facilitate the induction of labor. Your care provider may administer prostaglandin drugs to ripen your cervix. After your cervix is ripe, your care provider may use either oxytocin or a prostaglandin medication to induce labor contractions and cervical dilation. Some prostaglandins are administered vaginally, although one has been used orally for inducing labor. Oxytocin is administered intravenously. Both kinds of labor-inducing drugs have their particular risks, and your care provider will need to closely monitor you if you have a drug-induced labor to make sure that the drug does not overstimulate your uterus and make your contractions too intense for both you and your baby. Discuss the pros and cons of various induction methods with your care provider.

If Labor Does Not Begin

If you do not go into labor after what your care provider considers a reasonable time, or if your cervix remains hard or your baby is in an unfavorable position for birth, your caregiver may consider delivering the baby by cesarean section.

Although induction of labor and cesarean section are interventions that offer potentially lifesaving benefits for the baby, these interventions are not without risk. "One of the downsides of inducing labor is that the natural onset of labor begins in the baby," explains Dr. Bowes, referring to the physiological changes that happen in a baby when it is ready for birth. During the days just before birth, fluid is pumped out of the baby's lungs, allowing the baby's lungs to expand when it is born. Problems may arise, however, if labor is induced before the changes occur in the baby. "The danger of induction or cesarean section is getting a baby that isn't ready to be born and can't make the transition," says Dr. Bowes.

Such potential problems contribute to the debate over when to induce labor.

Demystifying Meconium

Meconium-stained amniotic fluid occurs in approximately 12% of live births. In approximately one third of these infants meconium is present below the vocal cords. However, meconium aspiration syndrome develops in only 2 out of every 1,000 live-born infants. Ninety-five percent of infants with inhaled meconium clear the lungs spontaneously.
—Vern L. Katz and Watson A. Bowes Jr., "Meconium Aspiration Syndrome: Reflections on a Murky Subject," *American Journal of Obstetrics and Gynecology* (1992; 166: 171)

❀ ❀ ❀

Meconium is the baby's first bowel movement. If the baby passes meconium after birth, there is no medical fuss—just a little cleanup. However, sometimes the baby passes meconium while she is still in the uterus, which results in meconium-stained amniotic fluid. This is a relatively common event, occurring in about 12 percent of all live births.

"Meconium can be benign or it can be a warning," says Dr. Donna Kirz. Contrary to popular myth, the presence of meconium-stained amniotic fluid does not necessarily mean your baby is in distress. The presence of meconium may simply mean that your baby's intestines are mature enough to have a bowel movement. If your baby is postterm, she may be more likely to pass meconium than a term baby, but again, this does not necessarily mean that your baby is having—or will have—a problem. However, sometimes meconium does indicate that your baby has been stressed, and your care provider will want to closely monitor the baby's heartbeat in the hospital. Call your care provider immediately if your amniotic fluid is stained an olive green color.

Meconium may present a problem if your baby has inhaled it, because this waste product, if inhaled, may cause a condition known as *meconium aspiration syndrome*. However, this syndrome is quite rare, since only 0.2 percent of babies will develop it. If the meconium is thick, go to the hospital immediately since your baby is at increased risk of developing problems.

Doctors now believe that meconium aspiration syndrome may be caused by intrauterine fetal distress when the baby is, for some reason, deprived of oxygen in the womb. This distress may be caused if the umbilical cord is compressed—which can occur if the baby is not protected by sufficient amniotic fluid. Doctors theorize that it is the compression of the umbilical cord that causes the lack of oxygen and "fetal gasping" that results in the baby's inhalation of meconium.

To prevent meconium aspiration syndrome from developing, doctors try to identify high-risk babies (such as postterm babies) and then employ an intervention called *amnioinfusion* to put additional amniotic fluid back into the uterus. The added fluid suspends the baby in enough liquid to prevent the compression of its umbilical cord.

If meconium is present in your amniotic fluid, your doctor or midwife will suction the baby's nose and mouth at birth to remove the meconium. If aspiration is suspected, your baby will need to go to the nursery for observation or treatment.

Care providers' responses to meconium-stained amniotic

fluid have changed over the years. In the late 1950s through the 1960s, when meconium was thought to indicate fetal distress, doctors intervened to get the baby born quickly whenever meconium was seen in the amniotic fluid. However, in the mid-1970s, doctors saw the presence of thin meconium as an indication for monitoring the baby by fetal scalp sampling in order to see if the baby was getting enough oxygen. Currently, if the baby has meconium-stained amniotic fluid, some doctors may carefully monitor the baby to make sure the baby is not overly stressed. Other doctors may intervene more aggressively, depending on the medical circumstances of you and your baby and the thickness of the meconium.

Discuss with your caregiver his or her approach to preventing and treating meconium problems so that you will understand what kind of medical treatment is routine—and not a cause for undue concern.

Chapter 24
Augmenting Labor

*The progress of labor is the continued dilation of the cervix . . .
continued descent, and/or rotation of the baby's head. You need
one or more of these things to be happening.*
—Dr. Watson Bowes Jr.

◆ ◆ ◆

Augmentation of labor means assisting a labor that
has already begun. It may mean assisting labor aggressively
with Pitocin to strengthen your contractions. Pitocin is the
drug form of *oxytocin* (the hormone that produces your
uterine contractions), and it is administered intravenously in
a hospital. Since birth center staff do not administer Pitocin,
you will need to go to the hospital for this kind of intervention. Augmenting labor may also include natural, nonaggres-
sive approaches such as walking or changing positions
in order to make your contractions more productive and
to help your labor progress. Getting continuous support
from a labor and delivery nurse or doula could also be considered a form of augmentation, since women supported
continuously through labor have shorter labors and fewer
cesarean sections.

If your labor is not progressing the way that it should, if your cervix is not dilating as well as it should, if your uterus is not contracting as it should, or if the baby's head is not descending as quickly as it should, your care provider may recommend augmenting your labor.

However, the "should" is a subjective criteria. "There are no absolutes about it," says Dr. Watson Bowes Jr., who believes that augmenting labor calls upon "the art of managing a labor. This is where the health care provider needs to use a tremendous amount of judgment regarding how the mother and baby are doing and the therapeutic options."

Augmenting Cervical Dilation

Pitocin should be used carefully to make the uterus behave like it does during normal labor.
—Marion McCartney, CNM and Director of Professional Services, American College of Nurse-Midwifes

* * *

During your first stage of labor, your contractions should make your cervix gradually dilate. If your dilation process is too slow or has stopped altogether, you and your care provider may need to intervene and give nature a boost. Some of the initial interventions are *things you can do* to get your labor started, such as walking around or experimenting with different maternal positions (see Chapter 20). Walking and changing positions may help your baby engage in your pelvis in a position that is advantageous for his birth. As the baby engages, he puts more pressure on your cervix, and this pressure encourages cervical dilation. Other gentle things that you can do to enhance cervical dilation include sitting in a Jacuzzi or standing in the shower.

However, if the noninvasive methods do not work, your care provider may need to rupture your membranes, and if that doesn't start labor or doesn't result in efficient contractions, your care provider may offer you Pitocin to *augment* cervical dilation.

Augmenting Rotation and Descent

During the second stage of labor, as in the first, you can try different birthing positions to assist the descent and rotation of your baby as it moves through your birth canal. You also may help your labor along by the relaxation techniques and supportive methods discussed in Part 7. However, if these methods do not help your labor progress or if your baby needs to be born sooner rather than later, your care provider may offer you Pitocin or other medications to move your labor along by making your contractions stronger, more regular, and more effective.

If administered carefully, Pitocin can strengthen your contractions, make your labor more effective, and help you birth your baby. However, you and your baby must be carefully monitored to make sure your contractions do not become too powerful, and your dose of Pitocin should be adjusted to meet your individual needs.

When Is Pitocin Your Friend?

Pitocin can be your friend if you're having a long, drawn-out labor. Use it if needed. Otherwise, it's like going for nuclear power when all you need is a pop gun.
—Pam Spry, CNM

＊ ＊ ＊

Pitocin may jump-start your labor, decrease the amount of time you spend in labor, and decrease the amount of time your baby spends being born. Because your body needs to be ready for Pitocin-induced labor, care providers recommend that women undergoing Pitocin augmentation should be close to term, with their baby's head engaged, and their cervix effaced and softened. If the cervix isn't soft enough, cervical ripening agents may be used to ripen the cervix and prepare it for the strong contractions brought on by Pitocin.

"Pitocin is a wonder drug sometimes," says nurse-midwife Marion McCartney, since Pitocin augmentation may greatly benefit you in your first or second stage of labor by helping you achieve a vaginal birth. However, Pitocin has its downside; it is a powerful drug that must be carefully administered and monitored to make sure you get just the right dose for you (some women are more sensitive to the drug than other women). Because Pitocin increases the power of your contractions, the drug may also increase your discomfort. To help you adapt to the increased intensity of your Pitocin-stimulated contractions, your care provider may start you on the smallest effective dose of the drug—or in slowly increased doses that mimic the gradually intensifying contractions of spontaneous labor. High doses of Pitocin may make your contractions become abruptly painful, and the change from relatively weak contractions to very strong ones may be difficult for you to adjust to at first. Care providers disagree as to whether Pitocin actually makes labor more painful. Some argue that the drug compresses the work of labor into a short period of time instead of letting it stretch out over several hours and that the labor only seems more painful since you have jumped from mild labor directly into strong labor without having time to adjust. Others argue that the uterus may become overstimulated and that the contractions are indeed more painful and more powerful.

High doses of Pitocin may cause general intense contractions that may be hard on the baby and may lead to fetal distress. However, such fetal problems may be prevented if the drug is carefully administered and monitored. However, for some women, the monitoring is another downside of Pitocin augmentation, since your care provider will put you on a fetal monitor, which means you will be confined to a bed or a chair.

The timing and dose of Pitocin may significantly affect your labor experience, since the drug may assist the natural process of labor and help you achieve a vaginal birth, or it may begin a chain reaction that leads to additional interventions. For instance, some women may need epidural anesthesia to relieve the pain of Pitocin-induced contractions; the epidural, in turn, may slow down second stage labor or interfere with a woman's pushing efforts, and the woman may require further medical interventions such as forceps or vacuum extraction to get her baby born.

A walking epidural may offer a way around potential problems with your pushing efforts, since this lighter form of anesthesia may allow you to voluntarily push during the second stage of labor, and it may give you more freedom of movement to assume positions that may help labor along (unless you have continuous fetal monitoring due to the Pitocin).

Like any other medication, Pitocin has benefits and risks that you should discuss with your care provider.

"Failure to Progress" and Dysfunctional Labor: How Long Is Too Long?

"Failure to progress" begs the point. We aren't getting anywhere, but why?
—Dr. Brooks Ranney, Professor Emeritus of Obstetrics and Gynecology, University of South Dakota

• • •

Normal labor in healthy women lasted longer than many clinicians expect. The criteria for distinguishing normal from

abnormal labor, based on time, need revision.
—Leah Albers, CNM/Ph. D. "The Duration of Labor in Healthy Women." *The Journal of Perinatology* 1999 Mar; 19(2):114–9. Leah Albers is referring to her study of low risk pregnant women receiving care from certified nurse-midwives in nine hospital settings in the United States.

* * *

There is a lot of disagreement about how long labor can be before it is abnormal. How long is too long? Labor must be progressing, but how fast it should go is arguable.
—Dr. Watson Bowes Jr.

* * *

At what point does a long labor become "too long"? There is often no easy answer to the question. Answers to the question also vary depending on whom you ask, their particular philosophy of childbirth, and the individual circumstances of the mother and baby. Some care providers go by strict time limits that define normal progress in active labor and second stage labor. Other care providers are more flexible and will tolerate labors that go beyond such time limits as long as the mother is not exhausted, the baby is not distressed, and the dilation of the cervix and descent of the baby show clear progress. For some care providers, the answer to "how long is too long?" depends on the *reason* for a long labor, since women who have babies in the OP position and women who have epidural anesthesia will typically have longer labors than other women.

The strict time limits that some doctors use to define the length of normal labor are based on "the Friedman curve." The Friedman labor curve was designed by Dr. Emanuel A. Friedman to provide a standard way to evaluate progress in labor on the basis of time, degree of cervical dilation, and rate of the baby's descent down the birth canal.

The Friedman curve is the American standard, and American physicians are taught that a woman's cervix should dilate one centimeter per hour during the active phase of labor and that the second stage of labor should be limited to two hours. According to Friedman, a normal *latent phase* of labor, in women having their first babies, should last approximately eight to ten hours, although he still considered latent labor to be within normal range if it lasted up to twenty hours.

According to the Friedman curve, a normal second stage of labor should last two and a half hours or less for a woman having her first baby, and fifty to sixty minutes for a woman who has previously given birth. Thus, for a care provider who adheres to Friedman's standards, a second stage labor of more than two and a half hours may be seen as a "failure to progress"—and a possible cause for medical interventions such as Pitocin augmentation or an instrumental forceps or vacuum delivery.

Interestingly, Dr. Friedman did not always advocate interventions such as cesarean or forceps delivery for a prolonged second stage of labor and was, under certain circumstances, tolerant of an "abnormally slow" rate of the descent of the baby through the birth canal. In his chapter in the obstetrical text *Cesarean Section: Guidelines for Appropriate Utilization*, published in 1995, Friedman writes that longer-than-average labors may be allowed to continue if mother and baby are doing well: "Thus, allowing patients to proceed into a long second stage is quite acceptable, even if descent [of the baby] is occurring at an abnormally slow rate," although he adds that both mother and baby must be carefully monitored "to insure that continued progress is being made, albeit slowly, and that both mother and fetus remain in good condition." However, if the mother's pelvis is not big enough for the baby to descend, or if the baby's descent is slowed by some "anatomic obstruction," Friedman recommends cesarean section.

Otherwise, Dr. Friedman writes in the abovementioned chapter that physicians allow the labor to continue or that they augment uterine contractions, if necessary: "As long as things continue to go well, and one is reasonably sure that there is no anatomic obstruction that would make fetal descent hazardous, allowing labor to continue is not only acceptable but entirely appropriate."

Some physicians and midwives have more flexible standards than the Friedman curves and think that cervical dilation at half a centimeter per hour during active labor is "normal"— as long as the mother and baby are doing well. Midwifery studies at the University of New Mexico and other medical centers suggest that active labor may take longer than previously thought and that half a centimeter per hour may represent reasonable progress. According to Leah Albers, a nurse-midwife and Professor of Nursing at the University of New Mexico, a "normal" active phase of labor that "lasts longer than many clinicians expect."

The time at which care providers intervene during long labors is based, in part, on their childbirth philosophy. Those with an expectant "wait and see" philosophy think that birth will usually proceed normally—even if some births take a little longer than others—and that the best approach is to let nature take its course. For care providers at the most liberal end of the labor management continuum, a laboring woman is not failing to progress in labor as long as her cervix continues to dilate and her baby continues to descend, and as long as she is not exhausted or dehydrated and her baby is not distressed.

Care providers with an interventionist philosophy are more likely to "do something" to speed up a long labor. Their time limits may be relatively flexible for latent labor, since the beginning of the latent phase is often hard to define. However, for the second stage of labor, these care providers tend to follow the Friedman curves and the interventions that are necessary to keep a woman's labor progressing according to the Friedman curves.

Discuss with your care provider his or her ways of managing long or dysfunctional labor and where he or she falls on the interventionist or expectant continuum of childbirth philosophies.

Some Reasons for Long Labors

Failure of the presenting part to descend may be due to inadequate or incoordinate uterine contractions; to malposition or malpresentation of the baby; or to cephalopelvic disproportion. The cause of this failure to progress must be diagnosed and appropriately treated. Malpresentation, or minor degrees of cephalopelvic disproportion, may sometimes be overcome by encouraging the mother to vary her position. Intravenous oxytocin can be used if contractions are inadequate. Instrumental or manual manipulations, or sometimes cesarean section, may be necessary.
—Dr. Murray Enkin et al., *A Guide to Effective Care in Pregnancy and Childbirth* (third edition)

* * *

Labor can be prolonged or ineffective due to any of the following reasons: a baby that is awkwardly positioned (i.e., OP, breech); a pelvis that is too small to accommodate the baby; a cervix that will not fully dilate; an epidural or spinal anesthetic that interferes with uterine contractions or pushing efforts; and maternal fear or exhaustion. Interventions for these conditions vary, depending on your medical circumstances and your caregiver's style of labor management.

The cause of a long labor is often an important factor in a

care provider's decision regarding when or how to assist labor. In the following examples, Dr. Donna Kirz and Dr. Susan Porto chose expectant management because their patients had awkwardly positioned babies. In each case, patience—combined with experience and good judgment—were key to successful expectant management of childbirth.

Expectant management worked well for Dr. Donna Kirz when she cared for a laboring mother who experienced prolonged back labor with an OP baby. Because the woman's baby was facing the "wrong way," Dr. Kirz understood why the labor was taking longer, and she adopted a wait–and–see approach because it is "normal" for back labors to be long:

"I let her push for four hours. Well, the standard [for the second stage of labor] is two hours, but I thought she was making progress, and she and I were working together on this. She wasn't complaining, and it was fine. It takes longer when the baby is facing up. But I knew that and she knew that. So on an individual basis, I let a woman go longer. By the same token, if a woman has pushed for two hours and I think she has pushed well, and there is no particular explanation for slow progress, then we have a discussion about what is going on and what the choices are."

When Dr. Susan Porto saw that her patient was having a long labor because the baby's head was not sufficiently flexed and was thus in an awkward position for birth, Dr. Porto knew that her patient had a good reason for a long labor, that the position of the baby's head could potentially be corrected, and that a wait-and-see management plan made sense.

"If something happens where there is not enough flexion of the head or there's a little turn here or there that doesn't put the smallest part of the head in the pelvic cavity, you're going to get an obstruction of labor. Now those things can correct," says Porto. Dr. Porto waited, the baby's position was eventually corrected, the labor progressed, and the mother had a vaginal birth.

However, Dr. Porto says that in such cases she intervenes in some way, either by suggesting maternal positions to help the baby descend more easily or by administering Pitocin if the woman's contractions aren't efficient enough to get the baby born. Sometimes Dr. Porto recommends both Pitocin and birthing positions, combining the standard interventions from both obstetrics and midwifery:

"If the woman doesn't have good contractions, this is where you use augmentation [with Pitocin] or if she is already augmented you can use various repositionings. You can put a woman on her hands and knees for a while, depending on what you think the problem is. You can shift her to one side. You can have her stand up."

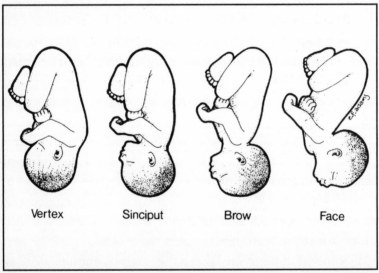

| Vertex | Sinciput | Brow | Face |

Figure 24-1: When the baby's head is vertex—the optimal position for birth—the smallest part of the head passes through the cervix

From Creasy, *Management of Labor and Delivery*. Reprinted by permission of Blackwell Science, Inc.

If your labor slows, assume positions that facilitate dilation or descent, and try to not obsess about the "pause" in your labor. Remember that failure to progress can sometimes be treated with patience.

For many caregivers it's not the fact that the labor is slow but *why* it is slow that determines what action, if any, is taken. Your labor may slow or not progress for any of the following reasons:

- You are having your first baby
- You have abnormalities of the uterus or cervix
- You have had analgesia and anesthesia (pain medications and epidurals)
- You are lying flat on your back and not standing or sitting during labor
- Your labor has been induced
- Your baby is in an awkward position (OP, breech)
- Your baby is too big for your pelvis
- Your uterine contractions are dysfunctional
- You are in your late thirties or your forties and pregnant for the first time
- You have an infection
- You are very frightened

Even if your labor is long for one of the above reasons, you may not need aggressive interventions in order to have a vaginal birth and a healthy baby. Discuss your particular circumstances with your care provider. If birthing positions don't help and your baby needs to be delivered immediately, you can move to your next set of choices: Pitocin, forceps or vacuum delivery, or cesarean section.

Long Labors: What's Age Got to Do with It?

I make individual decisions with clients and don't do things by

a cookbook. The first thing with an older woman is having the patience to allow her body to do things in its own pattern. With a first baby at thirty-eight or forty, there is more dysfunctional labor. The uterus doesn't seem to respond as efficiently and seems to take longer to get into functional labor patterns. Sometimes, it is just a matter of being patient and letting the uterus do its job.
—Laraine Guyette, CNM

• • •

It's my sense that practitioners would find that women close to age thirty-five don't have the problems [with labor] that are purported to exist in the older age group. Any problems related to older women would be rare in a thirty-five-, thirty-six-, or thirty-seven-year-old woman, but you would probably see more problems as you get past age forty. As a woman gets past forty, more and more you'll find doctors unwilling to stress her physically. However, you can't say on the basis of chronological age how a woman will react to labor because the health of the individual woman is what is important. Chronological age can be misleading because of an increase in the health status of women over forty.
—Dr. Allen Killam

• • •

There is . . . no supportive evidence in the literature for the frequently heard argument that older women have less tolerance for (prolonged) labor.
—Drs. Norbert Gleicher, Richard Demir, Jeanne Novas, Stephen Myers, "Methods for Safe Reduction of Cesarean Section Rates." *Cesarean Section: Guidelines for Appropriate Utilization*

• • •

Care providers disagree as to whether or not women over thirty-five have long labors or dysfunctional labors, although some care providers find that women over forty have longer labors than younger women. However, despite conflicting medical opinion, one fact is clear: Women over thirty-five are more likely than younger women to have interventions for "failure to progress in labor" and consequently are more likely to receive Pitocin to strengthen their labor contractions, more likely to have forceps and vacuum deliveries, and more likely to have cesarean sections. But why? Nobody knows for sure.

A possible explanation for the increased incidence of medical interventions in women over thirty-five is increased physician/patient anxiety about a "premium pregnancy." "Because women over forty often have a history of infertility or doctors assume it will be their first and possibly their last baby, I see more aggressive treatments of longer labor in women over forty. It's not that the labor has more problems but that the doctor is less likely to tolerate the problems that do occur," says Dr. Susan Porto.

It is possible that women over forty do have longer labors—but that long labors may be relatively normal as long as the baby and mother are otherwise doing well and the mother is progressing in labor. "Maybe we need a whole other labor curve for older women, " suggests Pam Spry.

One of the reasons cited by medical studies for an increased cesarean rate in older women is a condition called dystocia or "difficult birth." Difficult birth, if it is related to slow or halted progress of cervical dilation or the passage of the baby down the birth canal, may also be called "failure to progress."

Medical studies suggest that abnormalities of the first stage of labor (slow or arrested dilation) occur in approximately 25 percent of women giving birth to their first baby. Prolonged second stage of labor (slow or arrested descent) is also primarily a problem of a first pregnancy that occurs in 5 to 10 percent of these women. A prolonged second stage often involves a persistent failure of the baby's head to rotate to a position advantageous for birth. Some medical studies suggest that maternal age of thirty-five-plus does not significantly affect cervical dilation and the length of the first stage of labor. (The first stage is the part of labor most commonly influenced by dysfunctional uterine contractions.) However, studies point to the second stage of labor—and factors that influence the descent and rotation of the baby—as those affected by increased maternal age.

Some researchers speculate that women over thirty-five may be more likely than younger women to receive medical interventions for prolonged labor due to age-related medical problems and to age-related physiological changes in the uterus or cervix that make labor less efficient.

Although some care providers worry that older women are less able to tolerate longer labor than younger women, other care providers believe that a woman's stamina for long labor is based on her individual health and fitness.

Whether you are forty-five or twenty-five and you experience slow progress during your second stage of labor, what can you and your caregivers do about it? The answer depends, in part, on the reason for your long labor; on the shape and size of your pelvis and your baby; and on how well you, as an individual, tolerate long labor. It also depends on what interventions you and your care provider are comfortable with.

Do not assume that you are automatically destined for a long, difficult labor because of your age! Many women have short, efficient labors in their thirties and forties. However, to be prepared in the event of a long labor, make sure you understand the following interventions:

- Induction of labor by mechanical or medicinal methods
- Augmentation of labor with Pitocin
- Epidural anesthesia
- Forceps delivery
- Vacuum extraction
- Cesarean section

Chapter 25
When Instrumental Assistance Is Necessary: Forceps and Vacuum Deliveries

A major key to minimizing the cesarean section rate is to empha-size the importance of operative delivery [use of forceps and vacuum extraction] as a potential solution to failure to progress in the second stage of labor.
—Dr. Robert L. Barbieri in his foreword to *Current Problems in Obstetrics, Gynecology, and Fertility*, Vol. XVII, No. 3, May/June 1994

• • •

There are times when birthing positions and Pitocin do not offer enough assistance to get your baby born. If your baby is not progressively descending down the birth passage because of its position, if you are unable to continue pushing due to exhaustion or anesthesia, or if your baby is not toler-ating a long labor, your doctor may need to use instruments such as forceps or vacuum extractors to help your baby finish the journey down the birth canal. In such circum-stances, your only way to a vaginal birth may be through a forceps or vacuum delivery, otherwise known as an "instrumental delivery."

The Art of Forceps Delivery

A forceps is kind of like a shoe horn. The shoe horn helps the heel fit into the shoe. That's what a forceps is like. It looks kind of funny, but it helps the baby's head come out by gently cradling the head in the same way that a shoe horn cradles the heel.
—Dr. Donna Kirz

❋ ❋ ❋

"There are problem deliveries in which natural childbirth just doesn't work, and it's not the fault of the mother or anybody—it's just the nature of the delivery," says Kevin, referring to his wife's forceps delivery. Cathy feels pleased with the forceps birth of her daughter, since it helped her have a vaginal birth and avoid cesarean surgery: "I spent three hours pushing this baby, and I couldn't get her out. They tried a vacuum extractor, but they couldn't get a proper grip on the head. They finally tried forceps, and that worked the first time. The forceps didn't hurt at all; they gave me a lot of local anesthetic. The forceps worked. I'd done it! I had the baby. I felt triumphant I was able to have a vaginal delivery. I felt my doctors and I really worked together."

Forceps have been around for a long time and were once a standard obstetrics procedure used as an alternative to cesarean section. By using a forceps, a physician can guide the baby's head through the birth canal or slowly rotate the baby, if necessary. Dr. Joseph DeLee, a major figure in early modern American obstetrics, believed that forceps deliveries were better for the baby. He argued that forceps could shorten the second stage of labor and thus spare the baby the effects of prolonged pressure on its head caused by the forces of labor. Although forceps are no longer as popular (or as overused) as they were in the 1940s and 1950s, they still play a useful and sometimes lifesaving role in delivering babies. Unfortunately, forceps skills have been phased out of some medical training programs, decreasing the number of young American physicians who are learning the art of forceps delivery.

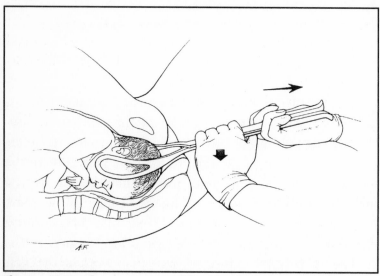

Figure 25-1: The forceps guides the baby's head through the birth canal

From Creasy, *Management of Labor and Delivery*. Reprinted with permission of Blackwell Science, Inc.

Forceps are used nowadays when the baby's head does not completely descend down the birth canal during the second stage of labor or if the baby isn't getting enough oxygen and needs to be delivered quickly. When the baby is relatively low in the birth canal, either an "outlet forceps" or a "low forceps" delivery can guide the baby's head. Either procedure is best performed by a doctor well trained in forceps delivery. Midwives do not usually use forceps (they call in a doctor if forceps become necessary).

In order to make informed decisions about forceps use during childbirth, discuss with your caregiver the possibility of forceps delivery. Have this discussion weeks before your due date. If you wait until you are in labor, you will not be in an

optimal state of mind to learn about forceps, absorb information, and participate in decision-making.

Holly never considered forceps until she needed assistance
during her second stage of labor. Although under normal circumstances Holly is a quick-witted and take-charge kind of
woman, she found herself frightened and confused when faced
with unfamiliar procedures and instruments. However, the outcome was good: Holly's son was successfully delivered by forceps, and Holly avoided cesarean surgery.

Forceps delivery has significant advantages for both mother
and baby. The mother avoids cesarean section and the risks that
accompany even the safest surgery (bleeding, infection, and
anesthesia), and her second stage of labor may be shortened
considerably. With forceps, the incidence of injury to the baby
is very small—especially with the use of *outlet* forceps in the
hands of an experienced physician. In a forceps-assisted birth,
the baby can be delivered quickly if she's in distress; forceps can
also rotate a baby from an awkward position in the birth canal
to a position advantageous for birth and can help your doctor
gently deliver the head of a breech baby.

Disadvantages of forceps delivery for the mother include
some bruising or bleeding of vaginal tissues, the possible need
for an episiotomy, and the use of local or epidural anesthesia.
Other disadvantages depend on how deeply the baby's head
lies within the birth canal. If the baby's head is close to being
born, and the delivery requires an "outlet forceps" or "low
forceps," the chance of serious problems for the baby due to
outlet forceps delivery is quite low. Possible risks to the baby
include bruising and scalp injury. In some cases, however,
more serious problems such as skull fracture, intracranial
bleeding, eye injures, or facial nerve injury may occur. If your
doctor is experienced in forceps delivery, serious problems are
unlikely to occur.

In a "mid-forceps" delivery, when the baby's head lies farther from the perineum, the risk of injury to mother and baby is higher than in a low forceps delivery. Mid-forceps deliveries are complex and require a physician highly skilled in forceps techniques. Although mid-forceps deliveries were popular in the 1940s and 1950s, they are now controversial. Consequently, such deliveries are rare and are largely replaced by Pitocin augmentation or cesarean section, although there may be circumstances when a mid-forceps delivery is advantageous.

Because cesarean section has become a safer surgery than it was twenty years ago, many doctors now choose cesarean surgery as a mode of delivery instead of using mid-forceps if the baby is relatively high in the birth canal. Other doctors base their choice of cesarean over forceps on a medical/legal climate that automatically makes cesarean section a safer legal choice for doctors. Still other doctors choose cesarean over forceps because they did not acquire extensive experience with forceps deliveries during their medical training and, consequently, they are not comfortable doing forceps deliveries.

Cesarean section is not necessarily safer than forceps delivery. Various medical studies have compared the potential risks for mother and baby associated with cesarean and forceps deliveries and found that problems for the mother such as fever, blood clots, and hemorrhage increase with cesarean delivery. Some studies have shown an increased rate of injury to the baby with forceps, but these injuries were rarely serious or life-threatening, and most resolved without permanent problems for the baby. Although cesarean surgery is sometimes seen as the "cure" for difficult birth, such surgery is not a panacea. Although cesarean section can be lifesaving, it will not totally prevent injury to your baby and will not reduce your baby's odds of being born with cerebral palsy or other long-term neurological problems.

Dr. Declan P. Keane, in his chapter on instrumental delivery in the obstetrics textbook *Management of Labor and Delivery*, confirms the advantages of forceps delivery and put the comparative risks of cesarean and forceps deliveries into perspective:

"Thus, even if clinicians resorted to cesarean section for all obstetric complications, maternal and fetal injuries would still occur and not all infants would be born normal. Assistance in the birth process may be desirable, can be life-saving, can prevent the need for cesarean section with its increased maternal morbidity, and should be available . . . We must not lose the art of forceps delivery."

Vacuum Extraction

The vacuum extractor is like a gentle suction cup applied to the baby's head that helps guide the baby out while the mother is pushing.
—Dr. Donna Kirz

❋ ❋ ❋

For a vacuum extraction, your doctor applies a suction cup to your baby's head and leads him through the birth canal by suction or "vacuum" force (see Figure 25-2). The vacuum extractor is sometimes used in a prolonged second stage of labor instead of forceps—a choice that often depends on the training and preferences of your physician. However, vacuum extraction will probably not be used to deliver your baby if your baby is too big for your birth canal, if your cervix is not dilated, if your baby is high up in your pelvis, or if your baby is premature or very distressed.

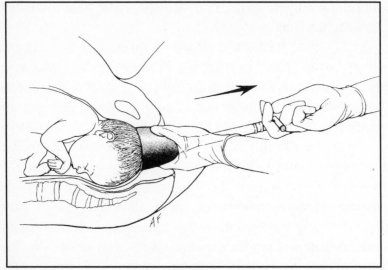

Figure 25-2: The vacuum extractor guides the baby's head through the birth canal

From Creasy, *Management of Labor and Delivery*. Reprinted by permission of Blackwell Science, Inc.

Vacuum extraction is sometimes used in the second stage of labor when the baby is distressed or not progressing down the birth canal. In fact, lack of progress in labor during the second stage of labor accounts for about 50 percent of vacuum deliveries.

When considering vacuum extraction, you and your care provider must balance the potential benefits and risks to mother and baby. According to current medical studies, vacuum extraction may pose less trauma to the mother and more to the infant when compared to forceps delivery. With vacuum extraction, the mother is less likely to have cuts or episiotomy incisions that are as deep or as problematic as those incurred during a forceps delivery. However, vacuum extraction may cause more scalp injuries and retinal bleeding in babies.

Most complications for the baby are not serious and resolve with time. The most frequent complication is called a *cephalhematoma*—a blood bruise underneath the baby's scalp that occurs between 1 percent and 18 percent of the time depending on whether metal or flexible head cups are used to deliver the baby. Intracerebral hemorrhage (bleeding in the brain) also may occur, but the incidence is very, very small—around 0.35 percent. The incidence of bleeding is higher in preterm babies, which is why vacuum extraction is avoided with preemies.

Serious injury to the baby is uncommon with either instrument, although forceps present less risk for the baby, according to Drs. Johanson and Menon in their Cochrane Review of the medical evidence on forceps and vacuum extractors. The reviewers' conclusions were that, "Use of the vacuum extractor rather than forceps for assisted vaginal delivery appears to reduce maternal morbidity [injury]. The reduction of the cephalhematomata and retinal haemorrhages seen with forceps may be a compensatory benefit."

Forceps and vacuum deliveries are, to a large extent, "interchangeable procedures," according to Dr. Murray Enkin et al. in their review of medical studies on the subject in *A Guide to Effective Care in Pregnancy in Childbirth* (second edition). The authors found that the "use of forceps is more likely to result in maternal injury and is more dependent on extensive analgesia or anaesthesia than is vacuum extraction" but found that vacuum extraction "with a forceps backup when required" may more effectively prevent cesarean section than vacuum extraction alone.

Chapter 26
Big Babies, Difficult Births: Cephalopelvic Disproportion and Fetopelvic Disproportion

Fetal-pelvic disproportion may simply be due to a fetus that is too large, a pelvis that is too small, or a fetus in such a position as to interfere with the normal mechanism of labor.
—Dr. Watson A. Bowes Jr., "Dystocia," in *Management of Labor and Delivery*

• • •

Cephalopelvic disproportion (CPD) and *fetopelvic disproportion* (FPD) mean that the baby's head (in the case of CPD) or the baby's body (FPD) is either too big to fit through the mother's birth canal or too big to fit through the canal without injury to the baby. Both conditions complicate childbirth.

FPD is a common cause of difficult labor. In FPD, the baby is too large to fit through the mother's birth canal. Some care providers propose that FPD in the United States is caused by a gradual increase in babies' birth weight. As the population becomes better nourished, people get bigger, but the increase in the size of a mother's pelvis lags behind the increase in the size of her baby by one generation. Consequently, there has been an increase in cesarean section due to FPD resulting from increased fetal weight.

However, other care providers disagree. They argue that FPD is not on the rise and that the high cesarean rate is due to other causes.

CPD is another cause for difficult labor because the baby's head is either too large to pass through the mother's birth canal or that the head is too awkwardly positioned. The most common problems with awkward positioning are the OP position and circumstances in which the baby's head may not be in the optimal chin-tucked or flexed position. Instead of the smallest part of the baby's head coming first through the birth canal as nature intended, a broader part of the baby's head comes first. Brow and face present are less common forms of this malposition but may also create a more difficult birth (see Chapter 24, Figure 24-1). In some cases, CPD causes difficult labor.

Many physicians see FPD and CPD as straightforward problems that can be diagnosed and managed, in many cases, by cesarean delivery.

Midwives tend to see the problem—and the solution—somewhat differently. For instance, some midwives help the laboring mother change positions in order to increase the size of the passage or to find angles that better accommodate the baby and help the baby move down the birth canal. Sometimes midwives suggest that the mother get up and walk during labor in order to help her baby become well aligned in the birth canal and to facilitate the baby's passage.

However, if labor does not progress or if there is a maternal or fetal emergency, the safest solution for FPD or CPD may be cesarean delivery of the baby.

Care providers disagree about whether or not women who have had cesarean birth for CPD or FPD require cesarean births for future pregnancies. Some doctors and midwives choose to evaluate each pregnancy separately and believe that a woman should be allowed a "trial of labor" with the option of having a VBAC (vaginal birth after cesarean), since the size of the baby and its position in the birth canal may be different for each pregnancy (see Chapter 28). However, there are instances when a woman may have an extremely small pelvis or anatomical quirks that predispose her to FPD and may indeed require a cesarean section for each baby. Discuss your individual circumstances with your care provider.

Fetal Macrosomia

I was eleven days overdue. Those last two weeks were really uncomfortable because I was so huge with this big baby. The doctor knew he [the baby] was in the right position, but he wasn't going anywhere. Every few days I had a stress test. The doctor knew I needed to try to have the baby myself, but she scheduled a c-section. I saw her the day before, and she manipulated my membranes to stimulate labor.
—Rhonda

*   *   *

Rhonda labored for hours, but she ended up needing a cesarean section because the baby was too big to enter her birth canal. Her doctor had a conservative attitude toward cesareans, and Rhonda trusted her.

"I could see that things were not happening the way I expected, and I was willing to go with the flow [having a cesarean section]. I was relieved afterward that I had a c-section. I've heard of babies who broke a collarbone on the way out. I was pretty grateful that my doctor realized how big he was and could safely get him out. He was a big baby—the size of a three-month-old. Nurses came in to see him after he was born saying, 'I heard about the big baby.' He was like a sumo wrestler."

Macrosomic babies are *big babies*. A baby is considered macrosomic if it is over 4,000 to 4,200 grams (4,000 grams equals 8.8 pounds), or if its birth weight is greater than the ninetieth percentile for gestational age and sex. About 50 to 60 percent of macrosomic babies are large but not fat: their weight is often appropriate for their length. These babies are at increased risk for birth injury due to difficulty squeezing through the birth canal. Macrosomic babies from diabetic mothers (which account for about 35 to 40 percent of macrosomic babies) are also at increased risk for intrauterine death.

Unfortunately, there is no reliable way to identify macrosomic babies before birth, and ultrasound does not offer a completely reliable way of predicting macrosomia. Fetal weight estimates are frequently inaccurate, and false positives may be as high as 75 percent.

If your caregiver suspects that your baby is macrosomic, he or she may suggest expectant management to see if the labor moves along normally, induction of labor, or cesarean section, depending on your particular circumstances and your care provider's birth philosophy. The benefits of expectant management are (1) you may be able to deliver vaginally, since many macrosomic babies are misdiagnosed, and (2) you may be able to deliver vaginally if your pelvic bones and your baby's head make structural adjustments during the birth process. However, expectant management can pose problems if your baby is truly macrosomic and too big for your birth canal, since the baby may suffer injury in the birth process or become stuck in the birth canal and require forceps or cesarean delivery.

Some caregivers may suggest inducing labor before your baby gets too big. If your baby is term or mature enough to be born, induction may offer a good solution. However, induction may lead to prolonged labor or cesarean section if it is done before your cervix is ripe or before you are forty-one weeks along (see "Inducing Labor" in Chapter 23).

Discuss with your caregiver the advantages and disadvantages to you and your baby of the previous options. You will need to consider your individual circumstances—your medical history, the structure of your pelvis, and the health of the baby—when you make the decision. In some cases, an expectant approach will be safe, and in other cases it may not.

Rhonda and her doctor agreed that she would have a trial of labor with her large baby, because Rhonda and her baby were healthy, Rhonda was not diabetic, her pelvis was roomy, and she wanted a vaginal birth. After many hours of labor, however, it became clear that if labor proceeded, the baby ran a considerable risk of birth injury because he was too big to descend through Rhonda's birth canal. Luckily, Rhonda's doctor had anticipated potential problems and scheduled Rhonda for a cesarean section. The baby was delivered by cesarean, and Rhonda has no regrets.

Shoulder Dystocia

Shoulder dystocia occurs in 0.24% to 2.00% of vaginal deliveries. The incidence depends, to some extent on how the disorder is defined. . . . There is some question on whether the incidence of shoulder dystocia is increasing as a result of the increase in mean birth weight.

—Dr. Watson Bowes Jr., "Dystocia," *Management of Labor and Delivery*

• • •

Shoulder dystocia is a childbirth complication that may occur if the baby's shoulders are too big to fit through your birth canal. Under some circumstances your care provider may offer you a "trial of labor" to see if your pelvis and the baby adjust to one another during the birth process. True shoulder dystocia, however, is a medical emergency where the baby's head is delivered but its shoulders remain stuck. This situation can result in injury to the baby, since the baby's collarbone may be broken in order for the baby to be born vaginally.

If the baby's shoulders are clearly too big to fit through your birth canal, the safest solution may be a cesarean section.

Women who are obese, who are diabetic and carrying a big baby, or who have postterm pregnancies are at increased risk for shoulder dystocia. However, shoulder dystocia is very difficult to predict.

Shoulder dystocia can be prevented by cesarean delivery and may possibly be managed by maternal position during childbirth, advises Dr. Watson Bowes Jr., in his chapter in *Management of Labor and Delivery* on dystocia:

"An opportunity of prevention occurs in the management of labor. If arrest of descent occurs in the setting of other risk factors for shoulder dystocia such as estimated fetal weight above 4,000 grams, operative vaginal delivery should be avoided and cesarean delivery should be recommended. Another alleged but poorly studied and unproven preventive measure for shoulder dystocia is maternal position at delivery. . . . In my personal, but not well-documented experience, patients who deliver in the lateral Sims' position appear to have a lower incidence of shoulder dystocia."

Shoulder dystocia is an obstetric emergency. Once the problem is recognized, a doctor has two options: to perform a cesarean section before the baby's head is born or to follow various hands-on maneuvers to relieve the dystocia. If the baby does not deliver, the physician will need to do an emergency cesarean section.

Chapter 27

"Several Times a Rare Thing Is Still a Rare Thing"

You may have heard that your rate of pregnancy and child-birth complications doubles, or in some cases triples or quadruples, if you are over forty. What you may not have heard is that many of these complications are *rare* for any woman at any age.

For instance, a problem like placenta previa may present a 0.5 percent risk to women under thirty. This means that placenta previa occurs in only 0.5 of every 100 women. If your risk doubles or triples with advancing age, your risk is still small—a 1 or 1.5 percent risk is a very small risk. Even if your risk increases tenfold, it becomes a 5 percent risk.

Looking at your pregnancy from a practical perspective, you have a 95 to 99 percent chance of not having rare conditions such as placenta previa, placental abruption, and cord prolapse. I have included rare conditions in this chapter to inform you about them just in case they arise in your pregnancy. But keep in mind that they probably will not present a problem for you.

Placenta Previa
A number of factors appear to increase the risk of placenta previa, including advancing age, multiparity, African or Asian

ethnic background, smoking, cocaine use, prior placenta previa, one or more previous cesarean births, and prior suction curettage for spontaneous or induced abortion.
—Dr. Steven L. Clark, "Placenta Previa and Abruptio Placentae," *Maternal-Fetal Medicine* (fourth edition)

❋ ❋ ❋

"Placenta previa increases tenfold in older women; but ten times a rare thing is still a rare thing," reassures Dr. Watson Bowes Jr. Placenta previa is a complication of pregnancy that occurs in only about 0.5 percent of the total population. In older women, the rate of placenta previa may increase as much as ten-fold, but with a 5 percent incidence rate, it is still a rare thing.

Placenta previa means that your baby's placenta covers or partly covers the opening of your cervix: the placenta comes first (previa)—before the baby—and can obstruct the birth canal and prevent the baby from descending through your cervix. As your cervix dilates, this misplaced placenta can be separated from the uterine wall. As the placenta separates, you may bleed (usually painlessly), and the baby may be deprived of oxygen.

If the placenta completely covers the cervix, the baby must be delivered by cesarean section. However, if the placenta covers only a small portion of the cervix, the baby sometimes can pass through your birth canal and be born vaginally—it all depends on your specific circumstances.

If your caregiver tells you after an ultrasound early in your pregnancy that you have a "low" or "previa" placenta, this is not necessarily a cause for alarm since a low placenta is relatively common in early pregnancy and may resolve as your uterus lengthens. The area where the placenta has attached may be pulled upward as your uterus expands during the course of pregnancy.

The main symptom of placenta previa is painless bleeding in the second or third trimester of pregnancy. The only treatments for a partial placenta previa are delivery of the baby or bed rest. Your doctor's goal in managing this condition is to minimize risks to you and your baby and to allow for as mature a baby as possible. Depending on your individual circumstances, your caregiver may suggest either a wait-and-see approach if the bleeding stops and the baby is premature or an immediate cesarean or vaginal delivery of the baby if the bleeding poses serious risks.

Placental Abruption

Abruptio placentae has long been known to occur more frequently in older women, but this increase probably reflects the effect of increased parity [having several children]. . . . The incidence is less than 1 percent among primigravidas [women pregnant with their first baby] and rises to about 2.5 percent among grand multiparas [women who have had several children].
—Dr. Steven L. Clark, "Placenta Previa and Abruptio Placentae," *Maternal-Fetal Medicine*

* * *

Placental abruption is a rare complication of pregnancy, occurring in roughly 1 percent of women pregnant with their first baby. Although the rate more than doubles if you are over thirty-five or if you have had several children, your odds of having a placental abruption are still low. However, your odds of placental abruption increase if you have high blood pressure, smoke cigarettes, or use cocaine.

Placental abruption is the separation of the placenta from your uterine wall, resulting in bleeding and pain, although this problem can exist without either bleeding or pain.

The condition can be extremely dangerous to both you and your baby and requires immediate attention by a physician. Treatment usually involves hospitalization. If the abruption is partial and your baby is premature, your doctor may try to forestall labor until your baby is more mature. But if your bleeding is profuse or if your doctor thinks the abruption is significant, your doctor may have to perform an emergency cesarean section as a lifesaving measure for both you and your baby. Under some circumstances, however, if your baby is not in distress and your bleeding is not serious, your physician may think that a vaginal delivery is safe.

Symptoms of an abruption—bleeding or severe abdominal pain—may come on quickly, and the safest response on your part is to immediately call your doctor. If your doctor is not available and you are bleeding profusely, call 911. In any case, seek medical care immediately. Sharlene, pregnant at age fifty-two, went into what seemed like a normal labor that was following the same pattern as her previous labor—until she began to bleed.

"All of a sudden I was not OK," remembers Sharlene. She rushed to the hospital, where her baby girl was delivered by emergency cesarean section. Both mother and baby were fine.

Umbilical Cord Problems

A *prolapsed cord* is a serious but *rare* complication of pregnancy in which the baby's umbilical cord slips through your cervix and down into your vagina. This is a very dangerous place for the umbilical cord to be, since the cord can be squeezed by your labor contractions or pressed against your pelvic bones in such a way that the baby's blood and oxygen supplies are cut off.

If your membranes have ruptured and your baby's head is not yet engaged, or if your baby is in a breech or transverse position, your odds for a prolapsed cord increase—but they are still very small. If you know that your baby is breech or transverse and your bag of waters suddenly ruptures, assume a hands-and-knees position to minimize compression of the umbilical cord. If you suspect a prolapsed cord but cannot see or distinctly feel it, wash your hands with strong soap and hot water (or put on sterile gloves if you have them) before you feel for the cord. Check to see if the baby's cord is in your vagina. Never pull on the cord. If you find a prolapsed cord, call 911 and remain in the hands-and-knees position all the way to the hospital.

Your baby's umbilical cord can also become compressed if you do not have enough amniotic fluid in your uterus to sufficiently surround your baby—and its cord. This complication needs to be dealt with immediately, since the umbilical cord is your baby's lifeline. A compressed cord may be treated with amnioinfusion, a procedure in which your doctor puts amniotic fluid into your uterus to relieve pressure on the baby's umbilical cord.

Uterine and Cervical Problems

Some fibroid tumors may create uterine or cervical problems during childbirth. Fibroid tumors may grow during pregnancy, but most often they do not complicate birth. Even if you have very large fibroids, they may not grow into the birth canal. As one surgeon put it, "sometimes the baby just pushes the fibroids out of the way."

However, occasionally the fibroids are close enough to the cervix to obstruct the birth canal—in which case a cesarean birth may be necessary.

If you have had previous surgery for uterine fibroids, you also may be advised to birth your baby by cesarean section, since the size or placement of your previous uterine incision may weaken your uterus and thus increase your risk of uterine rupture if you go through labor. If your previous uterine incision has "entered the cavity" of your uterus, has weakened the uterine wall in important places, or resembles a classic vertical cesarean incision in your uterus, a cesarean section may be safer for you than a vaginal birth (see Chapter 28).

Discuss your circumstances with your obstetrician and bring your obstetrician *all of your medical records concerning your fibroid surgery* or any other previous reproductive surgeries. You may have a bikini line external scar, but that does not necessarily reveal what kind of incision was made into your uterus.

The drug DES may also create cervical and uterine problems that complicate childbirth in DES daughters. If your mother took DES during the first trimester of her pregnancy with you, you may have certain uterine and cervical abnormalities that increase your risk of preterm labor. Some DES daughters have a small or T-shaped uterus that puts them at increased risk of going into labor before their due date or an incompetent or weakened cervix that begins to dilate before the due date and may lead to premature labor and birth.

In some cases, premature labor can be prevented or postponed until the baby is sufficiently mature. For instance, women with an incompetent cervix may benefit from the use of a cerclage (which involves sewing up or holding the cervix together until the baby nears its due date or bed rest).

If you are a DES daughter, find an obstetrician who has experience with pregnancy in DES-exposed women. You will need a doctor willing to follow you carefully during and after pregnancy. After your baby's birth, discuss with your doctor a plan for your future Pap smears and breast exams. Also discuss pediatric care for your baby (see Chapter 11).

Chapter 28
Cesarean Section and Vaginal Birth after Cesarean

A cesarean birth can be a beautiful birth. I had two cesarean births, so I'm a little bit biased. But if a birth ends up as a cesarean, the world has not come to an end. Most places allow a support person in the room with the mom; whomever she wants is right there with her the whole time. So that's nice. The other thing is that 99 percent of the time, the mom is awake. . . . She hears the first cry. Lots of times we're able to drop the drape and mom can see the baby, and within five minutes she gets to hold the baby.

Maybe it's not her ideal plan, but cesarean birth still can be pretty nice. I just hate to see women crying because they're having a cesarean section.
—Dr. Louise Kirz, an anesthesiologist who specializes in obstetrical anesthesia and has had two babies by cesarean section

• • •

It is becoming more common for the baby to accompany the mother the entire time from birth, through recovery, to her postpartum room. Breastfeeding on the operating table as the mother's incision is sutured or in recovery is also a possible option to promote bonding and help reduce the mother's blood

loss. Ask your care provider about these options.
—Connie Banack, doula and President of ICAN (International Cesarean Awareness Network)

❀ ❀ ❀

A cesarean section, also called an abdominal delivery, is a surgical procedure in which your baby is taken out of your uterus by way of an incision made in your abdomen. As surgery goes, it is a relatively safe and short procedure that takes about an hour: fifteen to twenty minutes to get the baby and thirty to forty minutes to finish the surgery, close the incision, and stitch you up. You are usually in the hospital for two or three days. The total recovery period is usually about four to six weeks.

A cesarean is performed when a vaginal delivery becomes too difficult or too risky for either you or your baby and when the benefits of surgery outweigh the risks. Complications of pregnancy and labor that almost always warrant cesarean delivery include:

- Prolapsed cord
- Complete placental abruption
- Placenta previa that completely covers the birth canal
- True CPD, FPD, or shoulder dystocia
- High-order multiples (quadruplets, quintuplets, and more)
- Serious fetal distress
- Fibroid tumors that obstruct the birth canal

In the above circumstances, cesarean delivery may be a life-saving intervention.

Other conditions may or may not require a cesarean, depending on your individual circumstances, the seriousness of the risk to you or your baby, and the availability of effective alternative ways to facilitate childbirth (e.g., birthing positions, forceps delivery, vacuum extraction). Conditions that sometimes require cesarean delivery are:

- Failure to progress in labor
- CPD
- Macrosomia
- Malpresentation or malposition (breech, transverse lie, brow presentation)
- Fetal distress
- Partial placenta previa or placental abruption
- Serious maternal illness (diabetes, eclampsia)
- Previous cesarean section

Don't wait until your last trimester of pregnancy to discuss with your caregiver his or her reasons for doing a cesarean delivery. Discuss cesarean section early on, preferably as part of your initial visit. If your caregiver is an obstetrician, you will be talking to a person who performs cesarean sections. If your caregiver is a midwife, she cannot perform surgery, but she can refer you to her backup obstetrician if she believes you are having complications that call for a cesarean. If possible, talk to this backup obstetrician early on in your pregnancy to explore the circumstances under which he or she would recommend a cesarean birth.

There are two types of cesarean section—a scheduled cesarean and an emergency cesarean; they are defined by the circumstances under which the surgery is done. If your health or your baby's health requires that the baby be born soon—but not immediately—your doctor may schedule a cesarean for you before you go into labor. However, if you baby needs to be born immediately, your doctor may need to do an emergency cesarean.

One of the risks of a cesarean done before labor begins is that your due dates may not be correct, and your baby may be born when she is somewhat premature. If your cesarean surgery is scheduled before your due date, your doctor may give the baby corticosteroid medication to help her lungs mature before the surgery. Another potential problem in delivering a baby by cesarean before labor begins is that the baby is "deprived" of experiencing labor. Labor is good for the baby: It prepares the baby's lungs for breathing air and stimulates the baby so the baby is alert and responsive after birth. Consequently, your doctor may wait to do a "planned" cesarean until just after you begin labor. A benefit of waiting until labor spontaneously begins is that the chances that your baby will be mature and ready for birth increase.

There are times when your baby must be born immediately by emergency cesarean section because the surgery may save your life or your baby's life. A prolapsed cord, severe bleeding, placental abruption, and a baby in severe distress are all reasons for an emergency cesarean delivery. Under such circumstances, your baby needs to be born within ten, twenty, or sometimes thirty minutes. If you or your baby's medical condition places you at increased risk for emergency cesarean, you may want to deliver your baby in a hospital or at a birth center adjacent to a hospital. Make sure the hospital is capable of performing emergency surgery and that it either has a surgical team and anesthesiologist in the hospital at all times or that a surgical team plus an anesthesiologist is "on call" and can be assembled and ready to go within thirty minutes. Fortunately, most emergency cesareans are not so urgent; a doctor or midwife often has far more than thirty minutes to recognize a problematic labor and to make preparations to get you to surgery.

If You Want Your Partner or Doula with You

If you and your partner wish to share the cesarean birth of your baby, or if you want your doula with you for moral support, discuss your wishes with your caregiver, write down your preferences in your birth plan, and discuss your wishes with the charge nurse on the labor and delivery unit. Even if you are not planning on a cesarean birth, inform the necessary people well in advance of your due date that you want your birth partner or doula with you if you end up needing a cesarean. Get written permission from your doctors, nurses, and hospital administrators. If you need a cesarean when the night shift is on, written permission may make all the difference between having your partner with you or not. Some hospitals will not allow partners or family in the operating room, so check on hospital policy early in your pregnancy. Many hospitals will allow only one person, usually the partner or spouse, in the operating room.

If your partner is interested in being with you but feels queasy about seeing blood, arrange for him or her to look at your face—and not at the surgery. If your partner is not comfortable going into the operating room, and you don't want to be alone, arrange for a midwife, labor coach, family member, or doula to accompany you (if the hospital permits this).

Anesthesia

Your surgery will be done under epidural, spinal, or general anesthesia, depending on your medical condition, your anesthesiologist's and caregiver's preferences, and your wishes. Epidural or spinal anesthesia allows you to remain awake for the birth, to see your baby immediately, and to be more able to respond to and breastfeed your baby shortly after surgery. With general anesthesia, you will "go to sleep" and may remain unconscious or groggy for some time after the birth. Epidurals and spinals are more commonly used for cesarean deliveries than general anesthesia, although there are circumstances where general anesthesia may be used (see "Regional Anesthesia" and "Analgesics" in Chapter 22).

Surgery and Recovery: What to Expect

Doctors and hospitals may differ slightly in their protocol, but you can generally expect the following events:

1. You'll be asked to sign a consent form that sometimes gives the doctor permission to perform a hysterectomy if necessary to save your life. Try not to be alarmed. This is a standard sentence in most consent forms and takes into consideration the remote possibility that a hysterectomy may be necessary in case of uncontrollable bleeding.

2. The nurse will put an IV into a vein in your hand or arm through which fluid or medication will be administered.

3. Sometimes the nurse also will put a catheter into your urethra to keep your bladder empty during surgery. If you are concerned about the procedure and your cesarean isn't a true emergency, you can ask her if she can put in the catheter after the anesthesia has taken effect.

4. If you wish your partner, doula, or friend to be with you—and your doctor has agreed to this—remind the staff of this agreement if your partner is not yet inside the room.

5. Your abdomen will be washed with a disinfectant, and the upper portion of your pubic hair may be shaved.

6. An anesthesiologist will begin the anesthesia. Epidural and spinal anesthesia are commonly used for cesarean

section, although general anesthesia may be used under some circumstances (see Chapter 22).

7. A partition will be put up between your shoulders and the incision, to ensure a sterile field around the area of surgery. If you want to see the baby immediately, ask the surgical team to lower the partition during birth.

8. If you receive epidural or spinal anesthesia, you will be awake and able to greet your new baby.

9. When the baby is born, your partner or the nurse can bring your baby to you after its birth, although you may be too weak or drugged to safely hold your baby.

10. You will be taken to the recovery room until the anesthesia wears off. Try to make arrangements in advance for your baby to be brought to you in the recovery room so you can begin to bond. If you want to breast-feed your baby, ask the nurse or your partner to help you hold the baby (you may be too weak or groggy to safely hold the baby by yourself). Discuss bonding and breastfeeding issues with your care provider before your last trimester of pregnancy.

11. You will be taken back to your room. If your baby doesn't need to be observed in the nursery and you want to nurse or room in with your baby, ask your partner, doula, and/or nurse to make sure the baby is brought to you.

12. Your epidural or spinal will gradually wear off over the next twelve to twenty-four hours, depending on the type and amount of anesthesia used. After the anesthesia wears off, you may still feel considerable pain at the incision—especially when you move and use your abdominal muscles. (You will be surprised at how often you use your abdominal muscles.) You will probably be offered pain medications—anything from mild medications like

Motrin to self-administered IV opiates. Discuss pain medications and their possible side effects with your doctor, since if you are dopey from strong pain medications, you may not be as responsive to your baby (see Chapter 22).

Possible Risks for the Baby

The major hazards of cesarean section for the baby relate to the risks of respiratory distress contingent on either the caesarean birth itself or on preterm birth as a result of miscalculation of dates. Babies born by cesarean section have a higher risk of respiratory distress syndrome than babies born vaginally at the same gestational age.
—Dr. Murray Enkin et al., *A Guide to Effective Care in Pregnancy and Childbirth* (third edition)

* * *

Cesarean birth may pose some risks to the baby, especially if the baby is born before the mother has experienced labor. Many childbirth experts believe that labor is good for the baby and prepares the baby's lungs for breathing air. Cesarean-born infants who do not experience labor tend to have more respiratory problems than vaginally born infants. Cesarean-born infants may have additional breathing problems if they are premature.

Possible Risks for the Mother

Under normal circumstances, a vaginal birth is safer for the mother than a cesarean, because a cesarean involves major surgery for the mother, and any major surgery carries with it risks of bleeding, infection, and anesthesia.

Like any abdominal surgery, cesarean section may sometimes cause long-term problems for the mother such as internal scarring and adhesions that may cause pain or interfere with fertility. Scarring from the surgery (especially from repeat cesareans) may create adhesions around the uterus, fallopian tubes, or ovaries that can compromise future fertility.

Fortunately, cesarean section is a relatively safe and effective surgery, and over the last twenty years it has become even safer due to progress made in surgical techniques, equipment, and anesthesia. Most complications are minor and are easily treated. Rarely—in approximately 4 out of 10,000 births—cesarean section leads to fatality. Although this is a tiny number, it is four times the number associated with vaginal births.

Even the potentially serious complications of cesarean section may be treated if diagnosed quickly. Call your caregiver immediately if you develop any of the following symptoms of possible infection, bleeding, or blood clots.

Infection

You may have a postsurgical infection if you develop a fever or abdominal pain, if your incision becomes hot or red, if it oozes blood or fluid, if you develop red streaks going from your incision across your belly, or if your stomach becomes hard, distended, or painful to the touch. Such infections can be treated with antibiotics, but your caregiver needs to examine you first to see what kind of infection you might have and what antibiotics are best used to cure it. You may not have an infection, but it is better to err on the side of caution and to call your caregiver than to overlook a potential problem. If your midwife or doctor is not available, call someone else in his or her practice. If no one is available, go to an emergency room of a reputable hospital, preferably the one where your caregiver has admitting privileges.

Bleeding

You may have postsurgical bleeding if you have prolonged or heavy bleeding from your vagina or incision or if your abdomen becomes distended, hard, or tender to the touch. Call your midwife—and doctor—immediately. Call 911 in the case of severe bleeding or pain. If the 911 paramedics offer to take you to the hospital, accept the offer. If your care providers are unavailable, go to the emergency room of a good hospital (see Chapter 4).

Pulmonary Embolism (Clot)

Shortness of breath is a rare but dangerous symptom since it may indicate that you have developed a pulmonary embolism (blood clot)—a serious complication. If you develop shortness of breath, call 911 immediately and then call your doctor.

Other Potential Problems

Other symptoms that warrant a call to your doctor are: abdominal pain; trouble urinating; persistent backache; leg pain and swelling of legs or ankles; constipation; and severe headaches. Like all women who have just had babies, you may develop postpartum blues that may be increased by the normal feelings of vulnerability and helplessness that people may experience after surgery. If you feel extremely depressed, anxious, helpless, angry, or afraid, call your care provider. (If you need further emotional support, see the appendix for referrals for postpartum depression.)

Recovery

The duration and difficulty of your recovery from cesarean surgery will depend upon your overall health, the skill of your surgeon, the medical care you receive at the hospital, and the care and help you receive at home. During your first few days of recovery in the hospital, nurses will help you with the baby and with your own tasks of daily living. Aids will deliver meals to your bedside. You will have the time and nursing support to focus on the two biggest priorities in your life: caring for your baby and resting.

However, many women do not realize that when they return home with a new baby (and without the assistance provided in the hospital), they will be thrown back on their own resources at a time when they can barely walk across the room, and these resources may not be adequate to meet the challenge of recovering from surgery—which means resting and eating well—as well as feeding and bathing a newborn, cooking, and washing dishes and clothes. Consequently, many women recovering from cesarean sections find themselves underprepared and overwhelmed once they come home. If you have little help awaiting you at home, or if you are particularly anxious about your recovery, consider staying in the hospital as long as your insurance will allow.

If you want to go home as soon as possible after your cesarean birth because you feel that recovery at home will be more peaceful than in a bustling hospital, plan ahead. Arrange for adequate care at home for you and your newborn to ensure that your recovery will be both peaceful and comfortable.

Hospital Recovery

I left the hospital too soon, because of the way coverage is. You don't have a clue [at the hospital] because you're being helped a lot. The hospital was easy. I had Demerol. I had the nurses. Michael was there, and he could pick up Julia and hand her to me.
—Anna, forty

● ● ◆

After cesarean surgery, expect to remain in the hospital for two to three days. You will need help getting in and out of bed, turning over in bed, sitting up, and holding your baby. Giving your baby a bath or changing your baby may be extremely difficult for the first several days after surgery.

You have just had *major surgery*, and unless you have considerable help at home, you may benefit from the nursing care and help with your baby that are available in the hospital. During your two-day hospital stay, you may face such challenges as difficulty urinating, constipation or fear of having a bowel movement, and gas pain. Some women feel extremely vulnerable during early recovery, and normal bodily functions become challenging and sometimes a bit unnerving. These feelings are normal. Fortunately, most of these new ordeals of daily living can be easily managed. If you are having difficulty urinating, stand in a warm shower with water running over your perineum or sit in a warm bath; urinate in the shower or bath if you need to—it's a "privilege" of the recovering surgery patient.

For constipation, drink plenty of water and eat plenty of high-fiber foods (fresh vegetables, fresh and dried fruits, bran). Avoid foods that give you gas or indigestion. Check with your doctor before you take *any* over-the-counter medicines such as stool softeners. You may or may not have significant gas pain in the day or two following your surgery. If you do, gas pains often subside if you get up and walk around. If you are too weak to walk alone, ask someone to assist you.

By the first day, the nurses will be asking you to cough in order to keep your lungs clear and free from infection. Coughing usually hurts, but it is far more manageable if you hold a pillow to your belly to support your incision and then cough. By the second day, the nurses will want you out of bed. The sooner you are up and about, the quicker your intestines and other bodily systems will return to normal. Getting up, leaning back, or doing anything that uses your abdominal muscles may cause you sharp pain. To minimize pain, support your incision with a pillow when possible. When getting out of bed, roll over onto your side near the side of the bed. Push yourself upright with your arms as you let your feet drop slowly from the bed to the floor.

Home Recovery

You shouldn't be home alone. A woman will need support for two weeks. She needs another person to help out. She should not have sole responsibility for the baby, so she can rest when the baby sleeps. She should not do any housework and only minimal cooking. No lifting, no driving, no shopping. If she doesn't have backup, she'll find herself exhausted and making bad judgments.
—Dr. Allen Killam

• • •

I was afraid to come home. I never cared for a baby before . . . . I was still in a lot of pain, and I was very tired. I was not able to take care of him. Getting up to change his diaper hurt. I needed help breastfeeding. It was like I needed three hands with him.
—Rhonda

• • •

The first one or two weeks after surgery are the most difficult, although every woman experiences pain differently and recovers at her own rate. Do not compare yourself with other women who have had cesarean deliveries, and do not underestimate the length of time your recovery may take or the amount of help you may need during the first two weeks after your surgery. Some women have trouble sitting in a chair, some are constipated, some are tired, and some bounce back with amazing speed and vigor—even if they are over forty-five. Jessica, at age forty-seven, was out of bed after a week and running after a month. However, Anna, at forty, was tired and sore for weeks. For the first two weeks post-surgery, Anna's abdomen was so tender that she hated wearing clothes.

Once you go home, it is natural for you to feel over-whelmed since you are recovering from the surgery and you need care at the same time that you need to care for your baby. If at all possible, recruit someone to care for you—a friend, relative, spouse, postpartum doula, or hired caregiver who will prepare meals, feed your cat, do the wash, and change the sheets so that your only responsibilities can be to recover from surgery and care for your baby. If your baby is big, you may need someone to help you bathe and feed him—at least for the first week. Pushing yourself may slow your recovery, pull on your incision, and leave you feeling exhausted and frustrated. If your doctor advises you to walk, rest, and do no household tasks, follow this advice by taking little walks first around the house, then outside, and eventually halfway down the block. Ask your care provider how long you must wait before you walk up and down stairs, lift, clean, or drive. There are reasons for limiting your activity. You need to allow the incisions in your abdomen and uterus to heal.

Plan for a comfortable recovery. Many women do not prepare their homes for recovering from cesarean birth because they expect a vaginal birth—not surgery—or because they have never had abdominal surgery and do not know what to anticipate. For instance, Sharon and her husband slept on a futon bed on the floor for years, and it never occurred to Sharon that getting up from the floor would be painful after cesarean surgery.

The following adjustments in your daily living make recovering from a cesarean a little bit easier.

Recovery Supplies

1. *Bed.* The closer your bed is to the floor, the more you will use your abdominal muscles to climb into and out of bed. After a cesarean surgery, using your abdominal muscles for this purpose will hurt and may put unnecessary strain on your healing incision. If your bed is on the floor, put it on a platform or bed stand during your recovery from surgery.

2. *Prepared food.* Stock your kitchen with easily prepared or preprepared foods (frozen meals, soups, cottage cheese, cheese, fruit, juices, yogurt). Ask friends and relatives to bring food after your surgery so you do not run out.

3. *Constipation prevention.* The combination of pain medicine and abdominal surgery can lead to constipation—something you want to avoid. Drink plenty of fluids. Take stool softeners if your care provider says it is okay to do so. Avoid laxatives since they cause cramping and may irritate your bowel.

4. *Comfort items for bed and nursing.* Try a foam wedge to help elevate your back and head when you are reclining in bed. Try a nursing pillow to help support and position your baby.

5. *Heating pad (if recommended by your caregiver).* Heat can promote healing and comfort—just make sure to apply heat as directed by your caregiver and not any longer. Do not fall asleep with a heating pad on your abdomen, since some pads can burn your skin if left on too long or at too high a temperature.

6. *A caregiver.* You may think that you can manage by yourself and feel embarrassed asking someone to take care of you. However, these are special circumstances:

You have just had a baby and are recovering from surgery at the same time. Either event by itself merits having someone help you at home for a week or two.

7. *Loose-fitting clothing.* It may hurt to have any pressure around your waist, even though your incision is at the bikini line. Wear drawstring pants or sweat pants, loose dresses, jumpers, overalls, and loosely fitting underwear and pajamas.

What Your Partner, Family, and Friends Can Do

Swan was so great. He took off work. He stayed at the hospital. He slept there.
—Rhonda

* * *

If your spouse can take two weeks off that's fine—if your spouse is useful around the house.
—Dr. Allen Killam

* * *

If you are the partner, friend, or family member of a woman recovering from a cesarean birth, try to fill the niche that is comfortable for you. If you are good at practical things like shopping, cooking, cleaning, and doing laundry, then do practical things to help. If the new mother needs moral support (given her dual challenge of recovering from surgery at the same time she takes on motherhood), and if you feel comfortable in the emotional realm, offer support. Sometimes visits are in themselves supportive—as is food. When in doubt, bring food: fruit, cheese, juice, soup, salad, or whatever else the woman likes and whatever requires *no preparation* on her part. She may be so sore that cooking becomes a major challenge.

If the woman is a single parent, family and friends can take turns providing care. Set up a reliable schedule so that everyone knows who is doing what—and when.

Why Do Cesarean Section Rates Go up in Older Mothers?

The finding of an increased risk of CS [cesarean section] delivery with increasing maternal age appears to be a relatively consistent conclusion of several studies. The reasons proposed for this are not clear, but include an increased risk of malpresentation and a decreasing proportion of occiput anterior positions in older mothers [older mothers have more OP babies—and more back labor]. Others have suggested the increased risk results from increased dysfunctional labor patterns in older women. However, the obstetric/medical factors are unlikely to be the sole explanation. Undoubtedly in some cases, obstetricians may have a lower threshold for performing CS on these older women because their pregnancies are considered to be "precious," that is, the likelihood of having further pregnancies is low.
—Dr. T. J. Broadhead and Dr. D. K. James, "Worldwide Utilization of Cesarean Section," in Flamm and Quilligan, *Cesarean Section: Guidelines for Appropriate Utilization*

* * *

Medical studies show that women over thirty-five years have a higher rate of cesarean section than younger women. Approximately one third of older mothers undergo cesarean birth. In 1999, according to *National Vital Statistics Reports*, overall cesarean rates increased steadily with advancing maternal age and were almost twice as high for mothers aged forty to fifty-four (34.7 percent) than for women aged twenty to twenty-four (17.9 percent).

Interpretations differ as to why the cesarean rates are so high for older women. Some medical experts argue that the higher cesarean rates in women over thirty-five may be justified by the medical conditions and physiological changes that come with age. They say that women over thirty-five have an increased incidence of high blood pressure, diabetes, placental problems, malposition (such as OP babies and back labor), and dysfunctional labor. According to Dr. Watson Bowes Jr., "There is something inherently different in relation to age that predisposes women to cesarean section. A woman who is forty-two and having a baby has a risk of cesarean section—for very legitimate reasons—that is greater than a twenty-two-year-old's."

However, some experts argue that a higher incidence of such problems in older women does not completely explain the high cesarean rates. Medical authorities such as Drs. T. J. Broadhead and D. K. James write in *Cesarean Section: Guidelines for Appropriate Utilization,* that the increased cesarean rates in older women may be due to physicians' concerns about late-in-life "precious" pregnancies. Dr. Donna Kirz, an expert in high-risk pregnancy and advanced maternal age, agrees that the high cesarean rate in older women is related to physician attitudes about "precious" or "high risk" pregnancies and that such attitudes lower a doctor's "threshold" for performing cesarean sections. "The overwhelming majority of studies in the obstetric literature describe a significantly higher rate of cesarean births in older women," writes Kirz in her 1985 article on advanced maternal age ("Advanced Maternal Age: The Mature Gravida," *American Journal of Obstetrics and Gynecology,* May 1, 1985). "It is unclear why this is so. No one specific indication for cesarean birth showed an increase in the pregnancies of women over 34 years. It may be that the increase in cesarean births for older women is a self-fulfilling prophecy. "

Dr. Gertrude Berkowitz, an epidemiologist at Mount Sinai

Medical Center in New York City and coauthor of a March 8, 1990, *New England Journal of Medicine* article on delayed childbearing, writes that the *indications for cesarean section* in the group of women she studied appeared to be *less* than the *rate* of the cesarean sections performed. When Berkowitz examined the reasons for the cesarean sections, she found "no increase in the frequency of any particular indication, with the possible exceptions of elective cesarean sections and those performed for placenta previa or abruptio placenta." She speculates "greater vigilance and more conservative treatment" on the part of physicians may contribute to the high rates in older women. However, Berkowitz says that such vigilance may "be overly cautious." She summed up her view of the studies and what they mean in a 1998 interview:

"C-section is much more common with first and subsequent births—that is the most established complication of older women (almost everyone found this). Women over thirty-five had a 40 percent incidence of c-section compared with 20 percent in younger women. Doctors may be overly cautious when a woman over forty is having her first baby, and this may be her last birth. But 40 percent is really sky high. You probably could safely decrease that c-section rate in the older age group."

Where older women are concerned, physicians may choose cesarean delivery out of a sincere desire to protect the woman's emotional and biological investment in what might be her last—and only—pregnancy. Thus the doctor may opt for cesarean to be on the "safe side" if he or she believes that a cesarean section is the safest mode of delivery for the baby and may protect the baby from injury, stress, or oxygen deprivation.

But when is cesarean section necessary, when is it "overly cautious," and when do its risks outweigh its benefits? These are challenging questions that can be answered neither quickly nor easily. Discuss with your care provider under what circumstances he or she thinks cesarean is the safest form of birth.

The Cesarean Controversy

Some doctors believe that cesarean rates greater than 10% reflect unnecessary surgery and others honestly believe that even a 25% rate is too low. There are actually some physicians who believe that all babies should be delivered by cesarean.
—Dr. Bruce Flamm, "Cesarean Delivery in the United States: A Summary of the Past 20 Years," in *Cesarean Section: Guidelines for Appropriate Utilization*

※ ※ ※

The cesarean section rate varies considerably among countries, from about 5% to over 25% of all deliveries. The optimal rate is not known, but little improvement in outcome appears to occur when rates rise above a minimum level. Despite this, higher rates of cesarean section persist in many parts of the world.
—Dr. Murray Enkin et al., *A Guide to Effective Care in Pregnancy and Childbirth* (third edition)

※ ※ ※

It is important to keep in mind that cesarean sections have saved the lives of many mothers and babies. The surgery can be a quick, relatively safe procedure and a reasonable response to certain complications of pregnancy and birth. However, cesarean surgery is major abdominal surgery that is best performed under specific circumstances when the benefits of surgery outweigh the risks.

Between 1970 and 1999, the cesarean section rate in the United States rose from 5.5 percent to 22.0 percent. Some years in the 1980s and 1990s had a cesarean rate of over 23 percent.

However, in the Netherlands, an affluent and medically advanced country with a very low infant mortality rate, cesarean rates are approximately 10 percent. Although the cesarean rates in the United States have decreased since an all-time high in the mid-1980s, our rates fall short of the goal of both the Department of Health and Human Services and the World Health Organization (WHO) for the year 2000: a 15 percent cesarean section rate.

Why are so many cesarean sections performed in the United States? Over the last twenty years, important factors contributing to the rise in cesarean deliveries in the United States are (1) a medical-legal environment in which patients sue obstetricians if a baby develops medical problems and in which cesarean delivery has been defined, in the courts, as legally safer than vaginal delivery, and (2) a belief on the part of the American public that cesarean sections are "safer" for the baby than are vaginal deliveries.

The notion that cesareans are safer for the baby is based on the outdated theory that cerebral palsy and other disorders are somehow related to birth injuries incurred during vaginal delivery and that cesarean birth somehow prevents these problems. However, several studies have shown otherwise. Doctors now believe that children born by cesarean do not have a reduced risk of cerebral palsy and that cerebral palsy usually occurs before birth—and not as the result of birth injury or vaginal birth.

Consequently, cerebral palsy is no longer believed to be related to the mode of delivery of the baby.

Some health experts believe that educating the public about the causes of cerebral palsy and changing the legal attitude toward cesarean section may help reduce cesarean rates in the United States. Dr. Bruce Flamm, a critic of unnecessary cesarean sections, believes that certain legal reforms may help lower cesarean rates. He writes:

"Unfortunately, in contemporary obstetrics, a discussion of almost any possible indication for cesarean would not be complete without consideration of medical-legal ramifications. Cesarean-related discussions almost always end up focusing on lawyers and lawsuits. Murphy's law states that if anything can go wrong, it will. The obstetrical corollary is that if anything goes wrong, you will be sued. To this corollary it is often added that if you did not do a cesarean you will lose the case. This is commonly rephrased as "the only cesarean I've ever been sued for is the one I didn't do." Many American physicians believe that the single most effective way to reduce unnecessary cesareans would be tort reform that eliminates frivolous lawsuits." ("Cesarean Delivery in the United States: A Summary of the Past 20 Years," in Flamm and Quilligan, *Cesarean Section: Guidelines for Appropriate Utilization*)

⁕ ⁕ ⁕

Adding to the complexity of the cesarean issue are the popularity of cesarean birth among some women and the increasing safety of cesarean surgery due to advancements in anesthesia and in surgical procedures.

Vaginal Birth after Cesarean

"The further you got in your first labor, the better your chances of having a VBAC," says Michelle Brill, a childbirth educator and VBAC mother. Michelle had a cesarean section for the birth of her first child after twenty-four hours of active labor and pushing for four hours with a posterior baby who wasn't descending. She says her VBAC with her next baby was "picture perfect" with only five or six hours of labor.

⁕ ⁕ ⁕

Although 'once a cesarean always a scar' is a truism, it is not true that once a cesarean always a cesarean.
—Dr. Richard H. Paul, editorial. "Toward Fewer Cesarean Sections: The Role of a Trial of Labor." *The New England Journal of Medicine.* (335) 1996

❋ ❋ ❋

Overall, attempted vaginal birth for women with a single previous low transverse cesarean section is associated with a lower risk of complications for both mother and baby than routine repeat cesarean section.
—Dr. Murray Enkin et al., *A Guide to Effective Care in Pregnancy and Childbirth* (third edition)

❋ ❋ ❋

The saying "once a cesarean always a cesarean" is now out of date. Over the last decade, many women who delivered their first baby by cesarean section are delivering their next baby vaginally. Of the women who choose a "trial of labor" (to see if they can labor successfully and have a vaginal birth instead of automatically choosing a "repeat cesarean"), about 70 to 80 percent have vaginal births, according to the American College of Obstetricians and Gynecologists (ACOG) in their July 1999 *ACOG Practice Bulletin.* According to the *Practice Bulletin,* the success rates of VBAC in women whose first cesarean delivery was performed for a condition that does not tend to recur (such as breech presentation) are similar to those of women who have never had a cesarean delivery.

Women's chances of having a successful VBAC are highest if their first cesarean section was done because of the breech presentation of the baby. But even if their first cesarean was due to a problem that may recur—such as failure to progress in labor or dystocia—they still have over a 50 percent chance of having a successful VBAC, according to a review of the medical studies on VBAC by Dr. Enkin and his coauthors presented in *A Guide to Effective Care in Pregnancy and Childbirth* (third edition)—and according to the ACOG bulletin. Some medical studies show VBAC success rates as high as 60 to 70 percent for women whose prior cesarean was due to dystocia (difficult birth). However, according to the 1999 ACOG report, women who choose a trial of labor but who end up having a cesarean are at a higher risk for infection and other postpartum complications than are women who choose a repeat cesarean.

On the other hand, according to Dr. Enkin et al. those women who have VBAC experience fewer complications after childbirth than women who have had repeat cesareans, although with VBAC, women have a slightly increased risk of uterine rupture or *dehiscence* (separation of the uterine scar that may create a "window" in the uterus) before or during labor. However, studies show that rupture and scar separation are rare, occurring in only 1 to 2 percent of women attempting VBAC. In fact, other rare occurrences in childbirth, such as placental abruption, happen in about 1 to 2 percent of *all* pregnancies.

Medical studies show that VBAC is a safe childbirth option for women who, on the basis of their past and current pregnancies, qualify for a "trial of labor." If you have had a previous cesarean section and are interested in attempting a vaginal birth, ask your care provider whether or not you are a good candidate for VBAC. If you had a classic cesarean section—a vertical uterine incision in your uterus—or if you had fibroid surgery that "entered the cavity" and involved vertical incisions or many incisions in your uterus, your uterus may have been weakened by the surgery, and it may be too risky for you to go through labor. In order to determine precisely the kind of incisions that you may already have in your uterus, it is important that you obtain the medical records of prior uterine or reproductive surgery and show them to your obstetrician. The scar on your abdomen does not necessarily indicate the kind of scars you have in your uterus, since it is possible to have a tiny bikini line scar on your belly and have vertical or deep scars in your uterus that are more likely to separate or rupture during labor than are horizontal or transverse scars in the lower portion of the uterus.

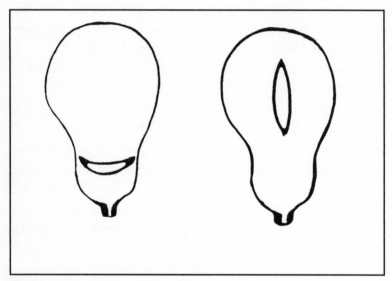

Figure 28-1: Types of Cesarean Incisions
A. Low transverse uterine scar.
B. "Classic" or vertical uterine scar.

Note: To qualify for VBAC, the scar in your uterus should be a low transverse scar.

Illustration by Howard Petote

Criteria for a VBAC

If your caregiver thinks that VBAC is a safe option for you, and you meet the following criteria, then you may proceed with a "trial of labor" that is closely supervised by either a doctor or a nurse-midwife. (If you choose a nurse-midwife, she must work with a backup physician.)

The usual criteria for a VBAC are:

- One or two prior cesarean births with a low transverse incision (see Figure 28-1)
- A singleton (one) baby
- No serious medical complications
- A vertex, or headfirst, baby
- A pelvis large enough to accommodate your baby (no clear-cut macrosomia or cephalopelvic disproportion, although these conditions are often difficult to diagnose in advance)
- No previous rupture
- A physician or nurse-midwife available to monitor you throughout your labor
- A hospital with an anesthesiologist and surgeon in-house who can do an emergency cesarean within ten or fifteen minutes away

Some care providers will insist that, in order to have VBAC, you must give birth in a hospital with an anesthesiologist and surgeon "in-house" (often this will be a Level II or III hospital).

If you meet the standard criteria and your care provider is still not comfortable with VBAC, get a second opinion from a care provider who is experienced in VBAC. You will need someone with experience who believes that VBAC can work well—and that it can work for you.

Exceptions may be made to some of the above criteria, depending on your care provider, your medical condition, and the size and position of your baby. A few doctors will consider VBAC if you are pregnant with twins. Some doctors will consider VBAC if you already have had two cesarean sections; others will not. Currently, it is controversial whether or not VBAC should be encouraged for women with twins, breech presentation, postterm pregnancy, suspected macrosomia, or an unknown uterine scar. If you fall into any of these controversial categories, discuss your individual circumstances with your physician. For further information, contact VBAC organizations (see appendix).

Your VBAC Birth Setting

Many care providers now argue that your safest VBAC option is to birth your baby in a hospital with an "in-house" anesthesiologist and surgical team that can perform an emergency cesarean section within minutes—just in case you are among the group of women who will need a repeat cesarean after a "trial of labor." Although some care providers are comfortable with home or birth center births for VBAC, most are not.

Some hospitals, especially small community hospitals, may not have the capacity to do emergency cesareans, and you may need to go to a Level II or Level III hospital. If your baby is in distress or in need of special care, he may also benefit from a hospital with a Level II or Level III nursery (see Chapter 4).

Although giving birth in a hospital may not be what you had in mind, there are ways you can make the best of it and "humanize" the hospital setting.

Ask for a birthing room if the hospital has one, and ask for a room with a shower or Jacuzzi. Bring familiar objects from home that give you comfort—a shawl, robe and nightgown, pillow, blanket, music, fragrant massage oil. Most importantly, choose a supportive care provider and arrange to have continuous support in labor from a doula or midwife.

Your VBAC Care Provider

Having your VBAC in a hospital instead of a birth center or your home does not mean that you give up a "child-birth-is-normal" approach to childbirth. Choose a care provider who will support your birth philosophy and with whom you feel comfortable. If you and your baby are healthy and the baby is in a good position, your have the same choice of care providers as any other pregnant woman: obstetrician, perinatologist, family practice physician, or midwife. Just make sure that your care provider has considerable experience with VBAC. If you prefer a nurse-midwife, find a nurse-midwife with hospital privileges who will support you during labor. That way, you will have the benefits of midwife labor support and a medical/surgical backup if it is needed. If you choose a physician as your care provider, hire a doula (preferably one with VBAC experience) to offer you continuous labor support (see Chapter 17 and Chapter 4).

Fetal Monitoring, Pain Medications, and Augmentation for VBAC Labor

If you are having a VBAC, many care providers will recommend that you and your baby be carefully monitored during labor. ACOG's 1999 *Practice Bulletin* recommends that "personnel who are familiar with the potential complications of VBAC should be present" to watch for significant changes in the baby's heart rate or in the mother's labor patterns. The ACOG guidelines state that "most authorities recommend continuous electronic monitoring." Since changes in the baby's heart rate are often the first signs of a previous cesarean scar giving way, many care providers prefer continuous fetal monitoring (CFM), so they can pick up the signs of a problem early on—and intervene immediately.

Continuous fetal monitoring is frequently recommended for VBAC women who do not have a care provider at their side throughout labor to monitor both the mother's and the baby's response to labor contractions. However, if your midwife, your physician, or your labor and delivery nurse are willing—and able—to labor-sit and to frequently listen to your baby's heart with a stethoscope or Doppler ultrasound, you may not require continuous fetal monitoring. Some care providers alternate electronic monitoring with listening to the baby's heart rate. Talk to your care provider before labor begins about his or her attitude toward electronic monitoring. Ask if telemetry is available, since this kind of monitoring allows you freedom of movement.

If you are attached to a fetal monitor throughout your labor, change positions from time to time to enhance the progress of your labor. Try sitting up in a chair or rocking chair rather than remaining in bed. Ask if you occasionally can get up to walk around the room.

Many caregivers agree that epidurals are safe for VBAC and that the epidurals do not mask symptoms of scar problems. According to the ACOG findings, "success rates for VBAC are similar in women who do and who do not receive epidural anesthesia, as well as in those women who receive other types of pain relief." However, care providers' opinions differ as to whether or not epidural anesthesia is the best approach to vaginal birth in general (whether VBAC or not). On the one hand, an epidural may slow your labor and may set you up for interventions such as Pitocin (oxytocin) in order to speed up your labor. On the other hand, if your fear of labor pain is the only thing standing between you and a vaginal birth, an epidural may bring you a more relaxing birth experience.

The safety of using drugs such as oxytocin or prostaglandin to induce or augment labor in women having VBAC has been controversial. Some doctors argue that oxytocin puts too much stress on the previous cesarean scar and that the use of oxytocin in VBAC women should "proceed with caution." Some care providers believe that oxytocin is safe—if used in moderation and closely monitored. Other care providers argue that augmenting labor with oxytocin is safe for VBAC, but that inducing labor with the drug is not. Although some studies indicate that the use of prostaglandins (a cervical ripening agent) appears safe, other studies indicate that certain prostaglandin medications may increase the odds of rupture. If you are planning a VBAC, discuss with your care provider his or her philosophy regarding medically inducing or augmenting labor in women having a VBAC.

VBAC and Repeat Cesarean: Weighing Benefits and Risks

Neither repeat cesarean delivery nor trial of labor is risk free. When VBAC is successful, it is associated with less morbidity than repeat cesarean delivery. The advantages include fewer blood transfusions, fewer postpartum infections, and shorter hospital stays, usually with no increased perinatal mortality.
—*ACOG Practice Bulletin*, No. 5, 1999

❋ ❋ ❋

When you are deciding whether or not to have VBAC, ask your care provider for information about the risks and benefits of *both* VBAC and repeat cesarean section. Then carefully weigh the benefits and the possible risks of morbidity (i.e., infection, injury) and mortality associated with each option, keeping in mind the words of the above ACOG statement that neither option is risk free.

The Benefits
The benefits of a VBAC, as compared to a cesarean section:

- Greater odds of uninterrupted bonding time with your baby following birth
- Increased alertness and lung maturity for the baby (labor

is good for the baby, and spontaneous labor often means your baby is ready to be born)
- Decreased risk of bleeding
- Decreased risk of blood transfusion
- Decreased anesthesia risks
- Decreased risk of infection
- Decreased risk of surgical scarring that could impair future fertility
- Decreased incidence of postpartum fever
- Decreased length of hospital stay and shorter recovery time
- Increased sense of accomplishment (achieving a vaginal birth)

The benefits of a repeat cesarean are:

- Convenience and planning (being able to plan the date of birth)
- Decreasing the fear of uterine rupture
- Alleviating fear of long or difficult labor
- Decreasing the small risk of uterine rupture
- Avoiding the possibility of going through labor only to have another cesarean
- Maintaining a sense of control over how and when medical interventions occur

Remember that some apparent benefits may not seem as attractive when you weigh them against risks. For instance, the benefit of convenience does not usually outweigh the risks of anesthesia and major abdominal surgery.

The Risks of VBAC

. . . [I]t is worth remembering that labor following cesarean delivery does carry a greater risk to the patient, that is, greater

than if the previous labor had resulted in vaginal delivery. The main risk to mother and fetus is the risk of scar rupture or dehiscence.

—Declan Keane, "Operative Procedure," in *Management of Labor and Delivery*

* * *

The main risk of a VBAC is rupture or separation (dehiscence) of your previous cesarean scar. Although uterine rupture is a serious problem, most babies can be safely delivered by immediate cesarean section, and ruptured scars often can be repaired. The odds of your uterus rupturing are less than 1 percent according to some medical studies, and less than 2 percent according to others, which means that you have approximately a 98 to 99 percent chance of *not* having your previous scar rupture or separate. However, women with a low transverse uterine incision have only about a 0.2 to 1.5 percent chance of rupture. Interestingly, according to medical studies reviewed by Dr. Enkin et al. in *A Guide to Effective Care in Pregnancy and Childbirth* (third edition), evidence of uterine scar dehiscence was found in 0.5 to 2.0 percent of women undergoing planned cesarean section—before labor even started.

In some studies, rupture and scar separation have been lumped together, which confuses the true risk involved, since *mild forms of dehiscence* are often without symptoms and without serious consequences for mother and baby. In any case, scar rupture and separation are rare complications of VBAC. To put the fear of rupture and dehiscence into perspective, Dr. Enkin and his coauthors write that the possibility of requiring an emergency cesarean section for other emergencies such as fetal distress, cord prolapse, or maternal hemorrhage in *any woman* giving birth "is approximately 2.7 percent, or up to thirty times as high as the risk of uterine rupture with a planned vaginal birth after cesarean."

However, the low level of risk does not minimize the potential danger of uterine rupture if it should occur. "It's not something that happens a lot. But if a rupture does happen and you don't take action, it is potentially catastrophic for the baby," says Dr. Edward Quilligan, an expert in high-risk pregnancy. However, if cesarean section is done within ten to fifteen minutes, the baby is often safely delivered.

Discuss the risks and benefits of VBAC with a care provider who has considerable experience with VBAC, and then make the decision that is best for you. Since research continues into VBAC, check with your caregiver and with nearby university medical centers to find out what the current research shows about the benefits and risks of vaginal birth after cesarean.

If you decide to have a VBAC, attend a childbirth class designed for VBAC mothers. These classes will help you address your concerns about a vaginal birth, dispel myths about VBAC, and bolster your confidence that your body still knows how to give birth and that you can have a healthy vaginal delivery of your baby.

The Risks of a Repeat Cesarean

No medical procedure is without risks. With a second cesarean, you have all the usual risks of surgery and anesthesia. These risks may be small, but once again, it is a matter of what kind of risks are acceptable to you, and what risks seem small or loom large. With major abdominal surgery, no matter how safe that surgery is, you face risks of bleeding, infection, and blood clots. "Putting a scar in your uterus has consequences," says Dr. Edward Quilligan, who thinks that VBAC "makes more sense" than cesarean section for women who are planning a large family (that is, of course, if they meet the criteria for

VBAC). With cesarean surgery, you have the risk of additional scar tissue and adhesions forming in your pelvis, which could interfere with your future fertility or complicate future births. Scarring may cause adhesions that entrap your fallopian tubes and ovaries and prevent them from working as they should. Uterine scarring from multiple cesarean surgeries may also create placental problems such as placental abruption and placenta previa in future pregnancies, especially if you have a new scar for each cesarean.

Surgical anesthesia brings its own unique risks. With epidural and spinal anesthesia there are risks of low blood pressure, headaches, and some small risks of persistent nerve pain. With general anesthesia there are also risks.

Chapter 29
Breech and Malpresentation

Although babies move around within the uterus throughout pregnancy, they usually find their way to a head-first, chin-tucked position before birth. This position is called *cephalic presentation,* and it is an advantageous position for the baby's passage down through the birth canal. Babies that are *breech* (bottom or feet first), *transverse* (lying horizontally cradled in the uterus), shoulder first, or head extended and tipped back all come under the heading of *malpresentation* and are awkwardly positioned for birth. In the case of malpresentation, the "passenger"—the baby—may block its own passage by awkward positioning, no matter how much power is exerted by your uterine contractions.

Factors contributing to breech presentation, such as previous uterine surgeries, fibroid tumors that crowd the uterine cavity or birth canal, placenta previa (where the placenta is between the baby and the birth canal), abnormalities causing reduced fetal movement and tone, and pregnancy with twins or triplets, may increase slightly with maternal age.

Pregnancy with multiple babies, which is on the rise in women aged thirty-five to fifty-four, may result in breech presentation or other forms of malpresentation, since one of the babies may be lying sideways (transverse lie) or in a breech position to accommodate the other babies in a crowded womb. If you are pregnant with twins or more, you may want to talk with your care provider about the possibility of breech presentation and his or her approaches to breech delivery.

If you are told in your last trimester of pregnancy that your baby is breech, it means that your baby is positioned in one of three ways: as a frank breech, a complete breech, or an incomplete breech.

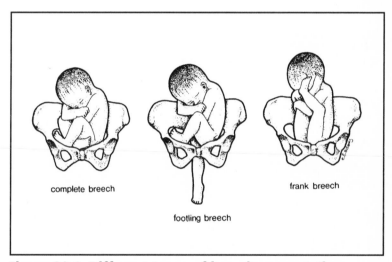

complete breech

footling breech

frank breech

Figure 29-1: Different types of breech presentation

From Creasy, *Management of Labor and Delivery*. Reprinted by permission of Blackwell Science, Inc.

The *frank breech* is a bottom-first presentation in which the baby's legs are flexed at the hip and extend up toward the head. In a *complete breech* the baby's knees are flexed, and she sits cross-legged in the uterus. In an *incomplete breech* one of the baby's feet or knees extends down toward the birth canal; this can easily become a *footling breech* if a leg actually drops through the birth canal and becomes the first presenting part of the baby at birth.

Even if your baby is breech in your last month of pregnancy, the odds are in your favor that your baby will eventually turn to the cephalic position. During your last twenty-eight to thirty-eight weeks of pregnancy, your baby may move from cephalic to breech and then back to cephalic position several times before birth. This is normal. Roughly one third (24 percent to 33 percent) of all babies are in the breech position during the late second and early third trimester. By thirty-three weeks gestational age, only 10 to 14 percent of babies are still breech and about one half of these will spontaneously turn to the normal, cephalic position before birth.

Doctors disagree about whether or not breech presentation increases slightly in women over thirty-five. Some doctors think that older women may have more breech babies because of uterine fibroids that obstruct the uterine cavity or an increased incidence of placental problems. However, others think there is no increase in breech babies in older mothers. Dr. Edward Quilligan, Emeritus Professor of Obstetrics and Gynecology at the University of California, Irvine Medical School, says that to the best of his knowledge, there is no increase in breech presentation, although "older women might have more prematurity." In fact, many doctors believe it is the baby's prematurity that causes an increased incidence of breech presentation, since babies frequently assume a breech position, at least temporarily, during the last trimester of pregnancy. "Premature labors carry a high incidence of breech presentations, and the earlier the labor, the higher the incidence of breech presentations," says Dr. Luis Cibils, Professor Emeritus of Obstetrics and Gynecology at the University of Chicago.

Birthing a Breech Baby: Options

The reasons for the rise in rates of CS [Cesarean Section] for breech presentation are complex. Part of the explanation may be a reflection of reduced training opportunities. New obstetricians are less often exposed to vaginal delivery and are unlikely to feel competent to attempt such a delivery, thus a spiral of falling vaginal delivery rates ensues.

—T. J. Broadhead and D. K. James, "Worldwide Utilization of Cesarean Section," in *Cesarean Section: Guidelines for Appropriate Utilization*

* * *

Breech presentation and transverse lie are associated with a much higher than average incidence of premature rupture of the membranes, premature labor, prolapsed cord, traumatic deliveries, cesarean section . . . and various birth injuries. Judicious use of gentle external cephalic version [turning breech babies to a head-down position before labor begins] permits the careful obstetrician to prevent the occurrence of some of this trauma. . . .

—Dr. Brooks Ranney, "The Gentle Art of Cephalic Version," *American Journal of Obstetrics and Gynecology*, 1973

* * *

How to manage breech babies before and during delivery has been the subject of heated medical debate for the last twenty years. Care providers disagree about the mode of delivery—whether breech babies should be delivered vaginally or by cesarean section—and about when and if the baby should be turned to cephalic position within the womb in order to prevent a breech delivery. However, in the year 2000, a large, international study of over 2,088 breech deliveries quieted this debate, since the study showed that cesarean section is safer than vaginal delivery for breech babies. However, these findings do not rule out vaginal delivery as a reasonable mode of delivery in certain cases, especially if the delivery is done artfully by an experienced care provider.

Care providers' solutions to breech presentation vary, depending on when and how they were trained, their attitude toward breech birth, their experience, and the physical condition of the mother and baby. Doctors who have been well trained in the vaginal delivery of breech infants can confidently maneuver the baby bottom first, and sometimes feet first, through the birth canal. Before cesarean sections were as safe as they are today, vaginal delivery of breech babies was often the first choice. In the 1960s, only about 10 percent of breech deliveries were done by cesarean surgery. Medical schools trained generations of doctors in the subtle manipulations of a baby's limbs and head that are required to slip the baby safely through the birth canal.

But times have changed. Since the late 1970s, this kind of classical obstetrical training has been phased out in some medical schools. As a result, increasingly fewer young obstetricians feel comfortable doing vaginal breech deliveries. Consequently, cesarean section has become the most common mode of delivery for breech babies in the United States. "Early in my career 80 percent of the breech births were delivered vaginally; now, over 90 percent are delivered by cesarean section," reflects Dr. Allen Killam, who thinks it's a pity that the skills to do vaginal breech births are being lost.

When Dr. Killam started delivering babies in the early 1960s, the cesarean rate for breech babies was 10 percent. By 1980, the cesarean rate for breech presentation was 67.2 percent. By 1999, the rate was up to 90 percent. Some doctors choose cesarean delivery for breech presentation 100 percent of the time, especially if they went through their training relatively recently and if they believe that vaginal breech deliveries increase the risk of injury to the child.

At times, the risks of a vaginal delivery lie not so much in the procedure itself but in the inexperience of the person who delivers the baby. An obstetrician experienced in breech delivery will be technically superior to one who has done only a few such deliveries during training.

When training in breech birth fades from obstetrics training programs, both obstetricians and pregnant women end up with fewer options. Canadian physician Murray Enkin and his coauthors reflect on this medical catch-22 in *A Guide to Effective Care in Pregnancy and Childbirth* (second edition): "A key factor is the experience of the attendant. The use of caesarean section for breech delivery in the belief that it is safer may be a self-fulfilling prophecy as attendants become less skilled at breech delivery."

Some prominent American obstetricians argue that vaginal breech deliveries are safe, although these are often older doctors who were trained to deliver breech babies when they were in medical school. Dr. Edward Quilligan is such a doctor, and he once passionately argued for vaginal breech delivery. But Quilligan has changed his views, and he now thinks that elective cesarean section is a reasonable and safe mode of delivery for breech babies given the current realities of medical training, the medical-legal environment, and the increasing safety of cesarean surgery.

"Having a high c-section rate for breeches—80 to 90 percent—is probably the right way to go now," says Quilligan.

However, Quilligan believes that vaginal delivery of breech babies is an art that still has its place. "There are some breeches that will come in that are 'in delivery,' and you will have to deliver them. That kind of delivery can be easy—or it can be goofed up if you get panicky," says Quilligan, who advises that obstetrics training programs continue to provide young doctors with experience in vaginal breech deliveries.

Your doctor's training and philosophy will determine what tack he or she will take toward delivering a breech baby. It is best not to ask your doctor to do something that he or she is uncomfortable doing. "I'd seek out someone who I thought would be honest about their comfort zone and would give me the facts," advises Dr. Quilligan.

Discuss with your caregiver his or her attitude toward and experience in breech delivery. Ask your caregiver to explain the benefits and risks to you and your baby of both vaginal and cesarean modes of delivery. Also ask about ways of turning your baby from the breech to the cephalic position before birth.

Turning a Breech Baby: What You and Your Health Care Provider Can Do

It is much easier for the baby, the mother, and the caregiver when a baby is in the cephalic or head-down position as labor begins. By turning your baby to a headfirst or cephalic position before birth, your care provider may avoid a breech delivery altogether.

There are three approaches to turning a breech baby: (1) the care provider performs external cephalic version to gently turn the baby, (2) the mother assumes positions that encourage the baby to turn, and (3) an acupuncturist or physician uses a Chinese technique called moxibustion to get the baby to turn. External cephalic version is the most popular of the three techniques in the United States and the technique most thoroughly studied. The effectiveness of positional change and moxibustion for turning breech babies has not been determined by large controlled medical studies.

The Gentle Art of Cephalic Version

ECV [external cephalic version] is becoming acceptable again. It should be the recommended standard of practice. All women with breech babies should be offered ECV.
—Eileen Hutton, Assistant Professor of Midwifery Education, McMaster University, and Research Fellow, the Institute of Medical Science, University of Toronto

❖ ❖ ❖

One should approach the gentle art of external cephalic version with a flexible attitude. The brain, nerves, muscles, and fingers of the obstetrician should be sensitively elastic. This is no place for a hasty or domineering approach, which is futile and possibly dangerous.
—Dr. Brooks Ranney, Emeritus Professor of Obstetrics and Gynecology at the University of South Dakota, in "The Gentle Art of External Cephalic Version," *American Journal of Obstetrics and Gynecology,* March 15, 1973

❖ ❖ ❖

Some caregivers attempt to turn breech babies by external cephalic version (ECV)—a hands-on technique by which the baby is turned from breech to the cephalic, head-down position by gentle external manipulation. By placing his or her hands on your pregnant belly, your caregiver locates your baby's head and buttocks and then gently presses against them to help the baby flip over to a head-down (cephalic) position in your uterus. If the version is successful, the baby can be delivered in the normal manner, and cesarean surgery or a vaginal breech delivery can be avoided.

Three essential ingredients are required for a successful version: sufficient amniotic fluid to enable the baby to turn; a skilled, gentle caregiver experienced in cephalic version; and sufficient relaxation on your part to allow the process to occur. Currently, doctors prefer women to have this procedure done in a hospital or in a doctor's office near a hospital, in the event of any cord or placental problems. However, if you are in the hands of a skilled and experienced practitioner, such problems are uncommon.

ECV has been in and out of favor over the last fifty years, but the technique is once again becoming popular. In the 1960s, some European studies found cephalic version risky, but many obstetricians now believe that some of these risks were created by the techniques used in Europe at that time: versions were performed too forcefully, while the woman was under anesthesia. In the early 1970s, a gentler form of the technique was brought back into American medical practice, and it is once again being taught in American medical schools.

One of the doctors who reintroduced cephalic version to American medicine was Dr. Brooks Ranney. His often-cited medical journal article, with its poetic title, "The Gentle Art of Cephalic Version," influenced a generation of young obstetricians to learn the "art" and then pass it on to the next generation. Ranney practiced cephalic versions with great success and found the procedure safe if practiced patiently and gently, without forcing the baby.

"Cephalic version is safe if it's done gently and carefully, with constant reference to the fetus inside, and with a willingness to discontinue the procedure and try again next week," says Dr. Ranney. If he met with resistance while turning the baby, if the mother experienced pain, or if the baby's heartbeat indicated distress, Ranney would stop the version, allow the baby to turn back to breech, and try again at the next office visit. "With experience, one learns to be gently persistent within reasonable physiologic limits, almost coaxing the fetus around and never exceeding safe limits of pressure or tension," Ranney advised in his 1973 article.

To what extent versions are successful is the subject of debate. Some experts say that success rates vary widely from doctor to doctor but average about 63 percent. However, skill and experience may bring success rates up to 80 percent or 90 percent. Some doctors say that tocolytic drugs that relax the uterine muscle make the procedure easier, especially if it is done late in the pregnancy when there is less room for the baby to move. However, other doctors contend that tocolytics are not always necessary to ensure success.

Risks of Cephalic Version

The risk of attempted external version to the mother is extremely small. It consists of the possibility of adverse effects from any of the drugs used to facilitate versions and the hazards of placental abruption, a rare but recognized complication.
—Dr. Murray Enkin et al., *A Guide to Effective Care in Pregnancy and Childbirth* (second edition)

* * *

Reported risks for the baby are small, but they include umbilical cord injuries, placental abruption, fetal distress, Rh factor problems in Rh-negative mothers if bleeding occurs during version, and premature delivery of the baby.

Although ECV is not without risks, a skillful physician can minimize them. Some physicians believe that the potential risks have been exaggerated or that they result from undue force and lack of careful monitoring of the responses of baby and mother. According to Dr. Luis Cibils, "It is hard to escape the conclusion that in these cases overzealous determination of the operator must have played a major role in the complication."

Gentleness and skill are key to the safety of ECV, says Dr.

Brooks Ranney, who found no evidence that gentle external version causes any fetal or maternal damage in his 1973 study of 860 pregnant women who underwent one or more cephalic versions. Some of these women required several attempts at version before their babies finally settled into a head-down position. Out of the 1,240 total versions he performed during the course of his study, Dr. Ranney found no increase in problems with the placenta, the umbilical cord, or Rh factor that adversely affected the baby or the mother.

When to Turn the Baby

If you look at the research data, it is pretty clear that there are benefits to starting ECV [external cephalic version] at thirty-seven weeks. . . . Right now we don't have good evidence to support doing ECV early [at thirty-four to thirty-six weeks], although it is a promising option that is being explored. If your baby is breech, don't wait until thirty-nine weeks: get ECV at thirty-seven weeks.
—Eileen Hutton, Assistant Professor, Midwifery Education Programme, McMaster University

• • •

Although doctors agree that the timing of cephalic version is important, they disagree as to the optimal time during pregnancy to most effectively and safely perform a version. Many American physicians prefer to turn your baby at or after your thirty-seventh week of pregnancy. Others may start versions as late as thirty-eight to thirty-nine weeks. Some physicians use cephalic version at the time of labor (if your membranes have not broken). A few, like Dr. Brooks Ranney, believe it is safe to begin the procedure by the thirty-fifth week of pregnancy, since at this point the baby can be turned with the most ease, the baby has the least chance of injury, and the mother has the least chance of discomfort. However, most American and Canadian physicians do not support turning babies before the thirty-seventh week.

Central to this debate about timing is the fear that version may necessitate prompt delivery of the baby and the fact that babies often spontaneously turn by themselves before the thirty-sixth week of pregnancy. Consequently, most American doctors prefer to do versions in the thirty-seventh or thirty-eighth week, arguing that the baby is less likely to flip back into the breech position, that the version procedure is less likely to cause premature delivery of the baby, and that if an emergency does arise, the baby will be mature enough to thrive.

The benefit of doing versions later, after thirty-seven weeks, is if there is a problem, your doctor can intervene with a cesarean section and you will still have a baby that is full term. However, a drawback of turning the baby late in pregnancy, at thirty-nine or forty weeks and close to its due date, is that the window of opportunity for easily turning the baby gets smaller and smaller.

In the thirty-sixth or thirty-seventh week, your baby floats in enough amniotic fluid to facilitate flipping relatively easily from breech to cephalic position. By the thirty-eighth week, however, the baby has grown, and it has less room to turn around in your uterus. At this point, versions may become more difficult and more apt to meet with physical resistance. Although tocolysis (drug-induced relaxation of uterine muscle) can help reduce resistance, it cannot solve all the problems encountered in turning a baby late in pregnancy.

Dr. Brooks Ranney argues that versions are safe when started at the thirty-fifth week of gestation when there is sufficient room and amniotic fluid in the womb to easily turn the baby. By turning the baby early, says Ranney, complications such as prematurity, cord or placental problems, and maternal discomfort can be avoided. If the baby reverts to breech, Dr. Ranney suggests that the doctor turn it again—as many times as necessary—between the thirty-fifth and thirty-eighth week. During his years of performing ECV, if a woman felt pain or if he encountered resistance to the version, Ranney tried again another day—most often successfully.

An ongoing Canadian study is comparing ECV done early, at thirty-four to thirty-six weeks, with ECV done during the currently recommended period, thirty-seven to thirty-eight weeks, to investigate whether there is an advantage to doing cephalic version early. When the study results are in, we should have additional answers to the questions about timing.

Home Remedies: What You Can Do

I asked if there was anything I could do to make her turn. "You can lie upside down on an ironing board at 45 degrees." They didn't have any hopes of it working. I went home and got the ironing board. It's very uncomfortable to stand on your head.
—Sharlene's baby had turned to the normal head-down position by the time she went into labor, three days late.

* * *

Midwives, more often than physicians, use techniques that you can use at home to encourage your baby to turn. The theory behind these techniques is that if you work with gravity and assume certain positions, you may dislodge the baby from a breech position and give him an opportunity to move into the cephalic position. The following are the most common methods that you can do at home.

The Ironing Board Method: Take an ironing board and place it at a 45 degree angle by leaning it against a couch or other solid, stable object. Then lie down on your back with your head at the lower end of the board. A variation of this involves placing a cushion against a chair, and propping up your hips and feet can have the same effect. Some care providers believe that the positions use gravity to encourage your baby to disengage from breech and turn. Maintain this position for twenty minutes once or twice a day until the baby moves. Do not persist in this position if you get headaches or have extremely elevated blood pressure or a tendency to have seizures. Consult your care provider before you attempt this method or any other home remedy for turning a breech baby.

The Knees-to-Chest Method: Get on your knees on the floor. Bring your chest and head toward your knees (as close as you can get). Some midwives suggest that if you do this for fifteen minutes at a time every two hours during the day for five days, your baby may turn to the cephalic position. This position is also recommended by some acupuncturists as part of the Oriental moxibustion treatment for breech presentation.

Although some care providers and women believe in the effectiveness of the above positions for turning breech babies, there is currently not enough medical evidence to prove that they work, say medical reviewers for *The Cochrane Library.* More studies need to be done to prove that "postural management" of breech presentation is effective.

Acupuncture and Moxibustion

The method is introduced from ancient records. To help turn a breech baby around, we use moxibustion on the baby toe on the urinary bladder (UB) meridian #67; we also use the knee-chest position afterwards . . . the two practices work together to turn the baby.

—Dr. Z. J. Chen, Carolina Center for Acupuncture. Dr. Chen is a medical doctor and acupuncturist who has practiced in China and the United States.

※ ※ ※

. . . moxibustion for 1 to 2 weeks increased fetal activity during the treatment period and cephalic presentation after the treatment period and at delivery.

—F. Cardini and H. Weixin, "Moxibustion for Correction of Breech Presentation: A Randomized Controlled Trial," *Journal of the American Medical Association,* October 13, 1999, 282(214): 1329

• • •

Moxibustion (burning herbs to stimulate acupuncture points), a traditional Chinese method to promote version of fetuses in a breech presentation, has recently been evaluated in a randomized control trial. Despite the fact that more subjects in the control group received subsequent external cephalic version, significantly more fetuses in the intervention group had a cephalic presentation at birth.

—Dr. Enkin et al., *A Guide to Effective Care in Pregnancy and Childbirth* (third edition)

• • •

According to an October 1999 medical study published in the *Journal of the American Medical Association* (*JAMA*), *moxibustion* has been shown to be a useful method for turning a baby from breech to a head-down position.

Moxibustion is an ancient Chinese medical technique that involves the use of a stick of burning herbs near—but not on—the acupuncture point. The warmth stimulates the acupuncture point and, according to Chinese medicine, the process stimulates uterine contractions or fetal activity that helps the baby turn to cephalic position. (The specific mechanism by which moxibustion works is not fully understood.)

Dr. Z. J. Chen, an acupuncturist and Chinese physician practicing in North Carolina, begins moxibustion for breech presentation weeks before the baby's due date. He also uses the technique several times over a period of weeks if the baby does not turn. "This is not a onetime thing," says Dr. Chen. Dr. Chen applies moxibustion to the acupuncture point BL 67 (beside the outer corner of the fifth toenail) over a period of time—from seven to fourteen days—to increase fetal activity and encourage the baby to turn.

Moxibustion is widely used in China and in some European countries, but not in the United States. However, since the article on moxibustion was published in *JAMA*, some American physicians have learned the technique. Ask your doctor if he or she practices moxibustion. If your doctor does not use the technique but does not object to you trying it, seek an experienced and certified acupuncturist. Do not attempt this technique without a trained professional.

Vaginal Breech: A Vanishing Skill

The younger obstetricians are no longer trained to do vaginal breech deliveries. In order to learn to do it right, they need experience.
—Dr. Watson Bowes Jr.

❉ ❉ ❉

The amount of training that an average resident has in delivering a breech baby is considerably less than it was in the 1970s. My current feeling is that if someone doesn't feel adequately trained, they should attempt a version [turning the baby to a headfirst position] in the thirty-seventh and thirty-eighth weeks. If the version is unsuccessful, they should schedule the woman for a cesarean section.
—Dr. Edward Quilligan

❉ ❉ ❉

A breech baby can make a vaginal delivery challenging for your caregiver, since your baby needs to be carefully maneuvered through the birth canal in such a way that its widest anatomical parts—its head or shoulders—do not get stuck. If your birth canal isn't large enough to deliver the baby's head and if this doesn't become clear until the last stages of labor, an emergency cesarean section may need to be performed.

Only those physicians who are experienced in vaginal breech delivery will allow vaginal delivery only if your pelvis is roomy enough to accommodate the size of your baby, your baby isn't too big, and your baby shows no signs of fetal distress. Some will not attempt a vaginal delivery for a first baby, since in this case your pelvis would be "unproven" in its capacity to accommodate the size of a baby.

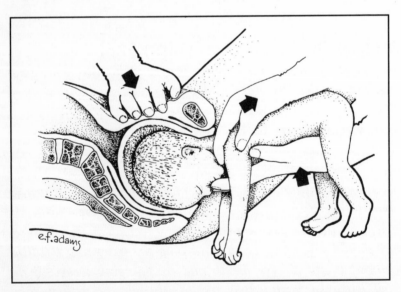

Figure 29-2: The vaginal delivery of a baby in the breech position

From Creasy, *Management of Labor and Delivery*. Reprinted by permission of Blackwell Science, Inc.

Up until recently, vaginal breech delivery was a standard part of obstetrical training at many medical schools. But no longer. Some medical schools are phasing out vaginal breech delivery or doing too few to give young doctors sufficient experience and comfort with the procedure. Consequently, if your baby is breech when you go into labor, only a few young doctors will offer you the option of delivering that baby vaginally.

"Young doctors may choose cesarean delivery because they do not have the skills or experience for vaginal breech," says Dr. Murph Goodwin, Professor of Obstetrics and Gynecology at the University of Southern California Medical School. "Six years ago all our residents were comfortable doing vaginal breech and forceps deliveries. But in 1998, we will have no senior residents who will go out and offer breech or forceps deliveries when in private practice. There isn't going to be experience with breech delivery—it's going to be vanishing," says Goodwin, who teaches at one of the largest obstetrics training programs in the United States.

Other reasons that a growing number of doctors will not attempt a vaginal delivery and will opt for cesarean section instead are that (1) the doctor believes that a cesarean section is safer for the baby than a vaginal delivery and (2) the medical-legal climate makes a vaginal breech birth legally riskier for the doctor than a cesarean section.

Since opinions and training vary widely, discuss breech birth with your care provider early in your pregnancy in order to evaluate the options available to you given the background of your particular doctor. If you are under the care of a midwife, she may refer you to a physician for a breech delivery. Most midwives will not perform vaginal breech deliveries alone, so they will either refer you to a physician or work in concert with a physician if the decision is reached to attempt a vaginal delivery.

In the case of a breech baby, home birth is not your safest option—*especially* for a first baby—since quick surgical intervention may be necessary in case the baby's umbilical cord becomes compressed or in case the baby's head is too large to pass through the birth canal (in which case you would need immediate cesarean to deliver the baby).

Playing It Safe: Balancing Risks and Benefits for Mother and Baby

When cesareans had a major risk in the past we were willing to take a little risk to the baby [in the case of breech] to make sure the mother was okay. Now that there is so little risk in doing a cesarean, most mothers say, "I don't want even a little bitty risk to the baby. I'll go ahead and have a cesarean, and I'll be okay."
—Dr. Allen Killam

◆ ◆ ◆

A long-standing global debate in the obstetric community concerns the safety of vaginal delivery of the term or near-term breech fetus. Many experts embrace fervent opinions on both sides of this controversial and complex issue. It is unlikely that this controversy will ever be resolved definitively.
—James A. Thorp, "Malpresentations and Special Situations," *Management of Labor and Delivery*

◆ ◆ ◆

Experts agree that vaginal breech delivery carries fewer risks for the mother than does cesarean section. But is vaginal breech delivery as safe for the baby as cesarean section? The answer may be found in a large international study by Dr. Mary Hannah et al., and published in the British medical journal, *The Lancet*, in October 2000. The study showed that planned cesarean delivery is better for the baby than planned vaginal delivery. Breech babies delivered by cesarean section had a 1.6 percent risk of injury or other bad outcomes whereas babies delivered vaginally had a 5 percent risk. However, some researchers say that the debate remains unresolved and that questions about the safety of vaginal breech delivery for premature babies and twins remain unanswered. Furthermore, some doctors firmly believe that vaginal delivery of breech babies is extremely safe—and, in experienced hands, this may be the case. Dr. Brooks Ranney, for instance, believes that the debate about the safest mode of delivery for breech babies "is not a debate which can be resolved by a statistical analysis method. Each individual mother and each individual fetus is different. What a mother should hope for is that she has a trained and experienced obstetrician caring for her who is capable of recognizing these variable differences and who is then capable of choosing a proper, balanced method of caring for her and her fetus." Ranney thinks a skilled doctor can see if a certain mode of breech delivery is not working and then modify it "on the spot" for better results.

For the time being, the prevailing thinking among many doctors is that cesarean delivery of breech babies is a little safer for the baby than vaginal delivery and that cesarean birth reduces the risks of fetal injury and death.

Discuss the pros and cons of cesarean and vaginal breech delivery with your doctor. Although most physicians will recommend cesarean section because they believe it is the safest option for your baby, some physicians are sufficiently skilled at vaginal breech delivery to offer you a reasonably safe alternative to cesarean birth.

Part Nine

Motherhood

When you're older, you know your limits. You're more adept, more flexible, and don't get as upset. I think that being older is much better mentally. And I have a lot of energy. I'm in better shape now than I was in my twenties.

—Jessica, fifty-two, is pregnant with her second child. She has a five-year-old daughter.

• • •

You're at this stage of life where you're ready to be less selfish and more flexible.

—Miriam, forty-nine, has a twelve-year-old daughter

• • •

Many midlife mothers discover that instead of being too rigid, too tired, or too old to keep up with a baby, they are energized by the birth and the daily presence of a child in their lives. Much to their surprise and the surprise of their friends and colleagues, these mothers find themselves becoming more flexible, more able to go with the flow, and less bound by habit and rigid daily schedules than they were in their twenties and early thirties.

"It's more of a change to have a child than it is to get married," says Joanne, who married at age forty-five and had her first and only child when she was forty-nine. But Joanne feels energized by the changes that came with the birth of her son. "I walk in the door, and I'm so excited to see that little face. It's just so joyful. I think it's because I've had that single life so long."

Many midlife mothers feel that older is better, since they find themselves free from the anxiety, ambition, and self-absorption of their twenties and early thirties. Says Eileen, pregnant at thirty-eight, "The advantage that older women have is that we may not be as rigid and fixed as when we were younger. We can change and shape our lives. We're more resourceful when we get older."

Of course, the adjustment to parenthood will not happen overnight. You may find yourself unnerved, at least initially, by the changes you must make in your familiar routines. And such changes are inescapable. If you try to manage parenthood the way you managed your career and weekly schedule, you are bound for frustration and disappointment. "Mothering can teach you to ride life instead of direct it, to be open to unexpected opportunities and ready for sudden turns in the road, " writes Gale Pryor, in *Nursing Mother, Working Mother.* This advice is especially useful as you are making the transition to motherhood.

Although the process of mothering *teaches* you flexibility, you may benefit from "practicing" in advance by anticipating the changes that come with parenthood. Your new baby will change your routines, your partner's routines, and your relationship with your partner. You will need to recreate and reorchestrate many aspects of your life: when you sleep, wake up, go to work, socialize, and relax. Since you cannot predict the personality of your baby, her sleeping and feeding patterns, or her reactions to new people and places, you will need to develop coping strategies as you go along.

This section on motherhood offers you strategies created by other midlife parents to adjust to life with their baby or babies, addressing such topics as sleep, bonding, the "baby blues," social isolation and social support, your relationship with your partner, time for yourself, returning to work, and staying at home.

Chapter 30
The Transition Period: Uncharted Territory

Those first months were like landing on Jupiter. It wasn't bad. It wasn't good. The gravity was just totally different. There is this complete strangeness about having a new baby: an alien being, two feet tall, doesn't speak English, completely dependent, comes to live with you.
—Leslie

. . .

You start from ground zero. Having a baby alters everything: conversational patterns, sleeping patterns. There's nothing it doesn't touch in some way. It's daunting. We love having kids, but it does alter everything.
—Kevin

. . .

As you adjust to your new role and the personality of your infant, you may experience a wide range of "normal" emotions such as joy, awe, sadness, and fear. You may find yourself happy and sad at the same time, as are the 80 percent of women who develop the "baby blues," or the numerous women who find themselves surprisingly ambivalent toward their new baby. On the other hand, you may feel like a "natural" at motherhood.

For some women, early motherhood is exhilarating. Joanne, a first-time mother at age forty-nine, was so thrilled at finally having a child that she savored every moment and felt reenergized. For Auben, at forty-six, early motherhood was a time of "continuous amazement." For her, the transition from the scheduled life of a clinical psychologist to the more unpredictable life of a new mother was a relatively easy one. She adjusted her expectations and adapted to her new life:

"I used to make lots of lists. Now I have very short lists. I get happy if I do the laundry and make three phone calls. I'm learning to adapt and be flexible—that's the challenge. Part of it is being more reasonable about my expectations and being more able to change midstream."

However, Auben decided to maintain some important routines that she and her husband, Rick, had developed over the course of their twenty-one-year marriage—but to include their young son Joe. Now the whole family goes out for coffee, and takes in a weekly movie together. Auben and Rick still go on their yearly fly-fishing trip. Joe accompanies them, although he spends several hours a day with a baby-sitter while his parents spend time together casting for trout.

"We need to feel that our life is still normal. We go for coffee at Peet's (an Oakland coffee shop). We need to go to Peet's. We need to realize that our lives are both different and still the same. We went fly fishing in Canada. We were able to hire somebody to baby-sit for two hours here and three hours there—just enough so I could go fishing for a little bit."

Jessica used similar strategies to make her transition to motherhood a relatively graceful one. For Jessica, life as a first-time mother at age forty-seven didn't look much different from her previous life. She simply fit the baby in. She didn't want her life to change too much—and it didn't. Jessica literally was off and running after the birth of her daughter, despite the fact that she was recovering from a cesarean section. She spent a week in bed after her cesarean section and was jogging three weeks later. During the first two months of her baby's life, Jessica brought the infant along on a sea-faring research boat and took her camping. "I thought, 'I want a child who's going to fit into our life.' I nursed her in a boat when she was one month old. My husband and I went camping in the Pacific Northwest with her when she was seven weeks. Sometimes I'd take her in a basket to my office and let her sleep." Later, she brought the baby, in a daypack, to the university where Jessica was a professor. The baby grabbed at erasers and chalk from her perch on Jessica's back. Now, at age four, the child still accompanies her mother to work and "works" at colorful crayon drawings while her mother writes reports at her desk. Jessica believes she plunged back into her life more quickly than she might have if she'd had her baby twenty years earlier because she developed more confidence in herself: "It may be easier when you're older and you know you can do it," says Jessica.

Recovery from childbirth and adjustment to life as a new mother appears more related to confidence, good health, good timing, financial security, a strong support system, and a baby with a mellow disposition, than it is to age. At forty-seven, Jessica had a solid career, a good marriage, financial stability, and a nanny to help her care for the baby.

Cathy, also a college professor, had a much different experience. She made the transition to motherhood without the help of a nanny or daily child care. For Cathy, the greatest challenge of early motherhood was meeting the needs of a demanding baby who required considerable attention. Consequently, Cathy had less time for sleep and for her relationship with her husband, Kevin.

Cathy had grown accustomed to a flexible academic

schedule that gave her a lot of time to herself, but with the birth of her first baby, Amy, time alone became a luxury. Even simple tasks such as taking a shower became a major challenge, since Amy would begin to howl when Cathy stepped into the shower and continue screaming until Cathy could once again pick her up. Fortunately, Cathy's supportive marriage and relaxed, resourceful personality allowed her to adjust to this major change in her lifestyle.

However, such continuous demands for mom's attention by needy babies may leave some new mothers overwhelmed and frustrated, creating mixed emotions about motherhood. Although these mixed feelings usually include joy, they may also include bewilderment, fear, and self-doubt. Unfortunately, these normal mixed feelings are considered taboo. Because motherhood is supposed to be a happy time— not an ambivalent time—many women and their care providers avoid discussing the many conflicting emotions. The unfortunate consequence of keeping ambivalent feelings under wraps is that new mothers remain isolated and unable to discuss coping strategies with their friends during the stressful transition period.

"Sometimes people don't want to admit how hard it is, because it is supposed to be something you wanted. Women tend to gloss over some things," says Leslie. After years of working a five-day week, Leslie found herself at home alone with an inconsolable infant. Leslie began to feel that her whole sense of self-worth was tied up in making her baby happy—which was not an easy task in the early months. "Her deep helplessness scared me. . . . Seeing her inconsolable was a blow; sometimes I would just weep with her," says Leslie. Fortunately, for Leslie—as for most new mothers—these normal but distressing feelings usually pass as the baby develops.

Your baby will not remain inconsolable. You will all move to something better. . . . Even if it goes on for a few months, it seems very long. The first year or two seems very long, but the next years seem to fly by.
—Leslie

• • •

Of course, the joys of motherhood make the changes well worth the effort. Mary, who at age thirty-eight was the mother of a demanding and inconsolable baby, says: "The best part is putting him to sleep at night. There's something so sweet about this little hand fondling you. The smiling really gets to you, too. And a child is so curious and alive. You just wonder what he'll become. That's the draw for me. What this little person is and what he will become. It's very magical."

Mary found motherhood so magical that she had two more babies—the second when she was forty and the third when she was forty-two. "The first year is so hard. The second year is stressful. The third is a piece of cake," says Mary.

Coping with Isolation

One thing that's been really helpful is my mothers' group. It was advertised at the Women's Center.
—Mary

• • •

Many new mothers stress the importance of having someone with them during the first week or two after the birth, says anthropologist Robbie Davis-Floyd. "Those who were left alone reported that feelings of bewilderment, confusion, isolation, and exhaustion often came to define this period far more strongly than the special magic felt by those women who did have the supportive and reassuring presence of a companion—mother, significant other, or friend," writes Davis-Floyd in her book, *Birth as an American Rite of Passage.*

Although some societies offer support to the new mother from family or from postpartum nurses, American society does not routinely offer women the kind of support that would ease their transition from "pregnant woman" to "mother." Consequently, the first weeks of motherhood are often isolating for many women. The isolation is especially intense for women recovering from cesarean sections and struggling with postsurgical fatigue and pain, although women who have had vaginal births may also feel isolated from their coworkers and friends and cut off from the world as they had known it before they had a baby.

When Leslie was recovering from her cesarean section, she felt extremely cut off from the world. She had taken leave from the printing job she had had for fifteen years, and she missed the daily contact with her coworkers and friends. Furthermore, she had no contact with women who had had children and who could share their mothering experiences with her. Since her daughter was a fussy baby, Leslie says she could have used some support from friends and advice from experienced mothers:

"My daughter was very hard to please. No matter what I did, she seemed inconsolable. I also was alone a lot. In other societies maybe more people come, and you have the benefit of someone's experience. Sometimes I'd call Paul and ask him to come home, or I'd call just to weep on the phone."

It took Leslie several months to adjust to motherhood. By maintaining important aspects of her identity and her prebaby life, such as swimming and reading books, she stayed connected to an adult world and did not become totally immersed in "babyland." Since reading books was an important part of Leslie's life before she became a mother, she read and nursed at the same time, bringing together her "old self" and her new one.

Anna also found herself isolated and without social support after she gave birth. Like Leslie, Anna was recovering from cesarean surgery and caring for a demanding baby at the same time. Aside from a visit from her mother, Anna was alone in the house while her husband was at work. Her mother stayed two weeks, which, from Anna's point of view, was not nearly long enough. Her isolation and lack of help with the baby during the day when her husband was at work left Anna exhausted for months following the birth.

Anna's friends worked, and none of them had children, which added to Anna's sense of isolation. During the months when she was housebound with her baby, Anna's friends kept calling and asking her to go out with them, but she felt that going out with a potentially fussy baby was too difficult for her. She kept turning them down. Eventually, Anna decided she could spend time with friends if they came to visit her at her home. Consequently, Anna overcame her social isolation by explaining the problem and asking her friends to visit her at home.

However, she still felt isolated when grocery shopping or running errands, since people who had opened doors for her when she was pregnant no longer opened them or offered to help her in any way—even when she was laden with heavy grocery bags and a newborn baby: "Everything is done in preparation for the big event—the pregnancy and birth. During this time there is enormous support. People hold doors for you when you're pregnant. But two weeks later you're walking around with this bucket with a child in it—and you're on your own. You are abandoned afterward."

One way to manage potential isolation is to anticipate it. Your friends may be afraid to "bother" the parents of a newborn. If you want company, make your wishes clear to friends and family: ask them to visit you or to keep in touch by phone.

If you need help shopping or doing errands, arrange joint shopping trips with friends or neighbors. If neither friends nor family are available, consider hiring a postpartum doula to help you with daily tasks and to offer breastfeeding support.

Some women find that joining a mothers' group gives them social and emotional support as well as offering them the wisdom and coping strategies of other mothers. Mothers' groups may be available through your local women's center, churches or synagogues, childbirth education classes, neighborhood play groups or baby-sitting co-ops, or birth centers.

Enlisting Support: Friends, Family, Doula, Postpartum Nurse

Some people brought some soup and chicken to us. We were tired. We had nothing to eat. I still remember that—it's the nicest thing you can do for someone. Just to be there and help and save them some work and show them your support.
—Lucy

* * *

You're gonna be exhausted. When you're feeding the baby, you need someone to bring you food. It's a huge change in your life. I was very unhappy for at least five weeks. I felt I was a mess. I couldn't accomplish anything.
—Anna

* * *

Along with social support, you will need support at home since it is exhausting to care for your baby and your household at the same time.

For some couples, the transition to parenthood is made easier by the arrival of other mothers, mothers-in-law, or other supportive family members and friends who can cook and clean while you care for your new baby and recover from childbirth or cesarean surgery. However, sometimes the arrival of relatives makes life more complex, especially if the relatives expect you to take care of them.

Kevin and Cathy preferred to be alone as a couple the first weeks after the birth of their first child in order to get to know their new baby and establish their new life and routine as parents. Fortunately, Kevin's job allowed him to take a few weeks off to cook for his wife and help with the baby and household tasks. However, when Cathy and Kevin had their second baby, Cathy asked her family to arrive before the baby was born in order to baby-sit during labor and birth and to care for the toddler during those first weeks when she and Kevin would be busy with their new daughter, Susan.

Pete and Lucy cherished their time alone before the family arrived when they had their first baby. They, too, could focus on getting to know their child and adapting to the rhythms of life as parents. When their family did arrive, their stress and fatigue level increased exponentially, since family members expected Lucy to cook for them and act as hostess. Lucy found the experience exhausting.

If your family is supportive and willing to help around the house so that you can care for your baby, they may be a welcome addition to your household as you adjust to motherhood. However, if your family is more demanding than helpful, you may make your life easier by inviting them to come a month or two *after* the baby is born.

Unfortunately, the American tendency to "go it alone" frequently extends into the realm of motherhood, leaving many new moms spending weeks or months unnecessarily tired and alone with their baby because they assume they should be able to make the transition by themselves. However, leaving mothers to fend for themselves is unheard of in some cultures. For instance, some Chinese families take for granted that a new mother must concentrate on her baby for the first several weeks after birth and provide for the new mother in a variety of ways. In some cases, women relatives experienced in birth and parenting help the mother for two or more weeks. In the Netherlands, an affluent, industrialized country with a sophisticated health care system, new mothers are routinely offered the help of a baby-nurse for one to two weeks after birth. This societal support continues in the form of educational sessions on child development and parenting provided for mothers at their baby's doctor visits over a period of years.

Postpartum nurses and doulas are also available in the United States, although they are underutilized. To arrange for a postpartum doula, call doula and childbirth education resources (see appendix). For postpartum nurses, call your pediatrician or your HMO for referrals. Some American insurance companies and HMOs will cover the costs for a nurse or for other forms of home help for the first few days after birth, although not for two weeks.

If hiring a nurse or doula is not an option, piece together your own network of helpers by enlisting your friends, family, and/or partner to take turns with household chores and cooking. If your partner can take off two or three weeks from work, and if he or she is a supportive person and able to help around the house, the physical and emotional backup may make early motherhood much easier for you.

It is important for you to practically assess your resources for help and plan accordingly. If your friends and family are not able to help after the baby is born, stock your refrigerator in advance with prepared or easy to prepare foods. Collect take-out and home delivery menus from your favorite restaurants. Prepare the house in advance and, if at all possible, avoid moving or renovating your house around the time your baby is due.

Sleep Deprivation

I was so tired. Getting awakened in the middle of the night was like Chinese water torture.
—Holly

* * *

Our baby was very alert and kept us awake every night. She woke up every ninety minutes. We finally brought her into bed with us.
—Lucy's husband, Pete, built a little platform for the baby beside the bed—that way, Lucy could nurse the baby without having to get up at night. This practice is referred to as "the family bed."

* * *

Sleep deprivation is often one of the greatest challenges for new mothers. Most mothers (and many fathers) will face nights of little or no sleep as they adjust to nighttime feedings and as their baby adjusts to the adult sleeping schedule. Because such disruptions in your sleep patterns over an extended period of time can cause depression as well as exhaustion, it is important to develop some coping strategies to help you get enough rest.

Adjusting your sleeping arrangements to your needs and the needs of your new baby can help you minimize stress and maximize your hours of sleep. It is common in American culture (but definitely not in the majority of cultures in the world) for parents to keep the baby in a crib in his own room. But if your baby cries every two or three hours, keeping you awake, exhausted, and stumbling down the hall to his room to nurse him or give him a bottle, you might consider bringing his crib into your room and setting it up next to your bed—with the railing down on your side. (Make sure the crib is stabilized or attached to your bed frame so the baby doesn't slip through the crack.) That way, when your baby gets hungry, you can simply reach over and draw him to you to be fed. Some parents bring the baby into bed with them, an approach known as the family bed, in order to keep the baby close at hand to feed or comfort.

If you take the baby into your bed, take certain safety precautions: make sure his head is far away from your pillows (since pillows could smother a baby) and that he can't slip off the bed. Do not bring the baby onto a waterbed. Although you may fear that you will roll over on the baby, it is very unlikely that you will.

The family bed has been credited with soothing the baby and helping the parents get more rest at night. The family bed may decrease the incidence of SIDS (Sudden Infant Death Syndrome), since some researchers theorize that the rhythmic respiration of the mother stimulates the baby to breathe.

If you find that having the baby in your bed or in a crib in your room is too disruptive to your sleep, you might want to keep him in a crib during most of the night but bring him into bed for a morning feeding. That way you may soothe the baby and sneak in a few more hours of sleep for yourself and your partner.

Caring for Your Older Children

The first baby is not as hard because you don't have another child to take care of. With the second baby, you cannot postpone taking care of your older child. In that case, you really need some help. . . . It would have been helpful to have someone our older child knew to be there to help out for about two or three weeks. That would have been ideal. So find someone the child knows— and not at the last minute.
—Lucy

For a first baby, it was really nice to have it be just Kevin and me for the first few weeks. I liked that, and I would do it that way again. But when we had a second child, I wanted someone to be there when we got back from the hospital, because I needed someone to take care of Amy [the toddler].
—Cathy

● ● ●

When Cathy and Kevin were expecting their second baby, they invited Cathy's parents to come before the birth in order to help care for their older child, two-year-old Amy. Although Amy may have felt jealousy after the birth of her sister, Susan, she did not feel totally displaced or resentful since she had her doting grandparents to rely on for comfort and attention.

You will probably need someone to help you care for your older child when you bring home a new baby, and if grandparents are not an option for childcare, arrange for someone the child knows—one of your friends or a familiar baby-sitter—to look after her and provide her with continuity and comfort. In the event that you have no regular baby-sitter, you may want to introduce the child to a potential caregiver weeks or even months in advance of the birth and allow the child time to become comfortable with him or her.

Of course, your older child will still need reassurance and love from you and your partner, since the introduction of a new family member will be a dramatic change, if not a traumatic one. From this point onward, the child must share your love with the baby. Many children regress to earlier behaviors after the birth of a baby. Your child may "forget" potty training and once again start wetting her pants or the bed. The child may resort to thumb sucking, tantrums, or even aggression toward the baby.

The best thing you can do for your older child is to understand that such behaviors represent normal reactions and to try to address your child's feelings by including him or her as much as possible. By acting in ways that make the older child feel like a special and valued member of an expanding family, you can help the older child adjust. Even if you have a family member present to care for your older child during your first week at home with the new baby, spend some time alone with her doing the things she likes to do. Listen to her needs, acknowledge her feelings about the baby's crying and constant need for attention, and let the child know that she still is very important to you.

Avoid dismissing your child's concerns with statements such as, "You are so lucky to have such a sweet little brother" or "Isn't it nice to have a new playmate?" since your child may not feel at all lucky and may have trouble seeing a tiny, helpless baby as a welcome playmate. When people bring gifts for the baby, arrange to have some gifts for the older child, so she does not feel left out. Consider buying gifts before the birth (since you will not have the time or energy afterward), and put them in a closet until the appropriate moment. Such gifts may take on a special meaning for your child since they provide comfort during a time of stress.

The Baby Blues

You go for almost a year without sleep that's uninterrupted by crying—that alone can cause you to be depressed. . . . But you can be depressed and happy at the same time.
—Anna

⊛ ⊛ ⊛

During the transition to motherhood, about 80 percent of new mothers develop the baby blues—a mild version of postpartum depression—for a few weeks or months after the birth of their child. This condition is caused by the hormonal changes that normally occur after childbirth, although the sleep deprivation and isolation of early motherhood may also contribute to the blues. Luckily, the blues tend to go away within a month or two. Kathleen R. experienced the baby blues after the birth of her son. She felt "miserable and helpless and incompetent" for about a month, but at five or six weeks after the birth she began to feel human. "It was directly correlated with the amount of sleep I was getting," says Kathleen, who felt better after she could sleep for at least three hours at a time instead of in thirty-minute naps. Soon thereafter, Kathleen's baby blues disappeared and her delight in motherhood took over. "By twelve weeks, things were fine. I realized how much love and affection there was coming from me toward this beautiful little person who was responding to me."

If your baby blues last longer than a few months or involve serious depression, you may have postpartum depression.

Recognizing, Preventing, and Treating Postpartum Depression (PPD)

Oh, I had that [postpartum depression]! I think it is probably a natural phenomenon. When Jennifer was born, there were a lot of people around—a steady stream of neighbors, friends, and relatives coming over to see the baby. It was a happy occasion. I felt great. My only responsibility for two months was to love my baby. When Brent was born, my mother came and stayed for one week. Then she left, and I was overwhelmed. I had a new baby, a house, a three-year-old, and a husband who was a disinterested father. He was in law school and was studying all the time. I started off positive. Then the weight of it all wore down on me: the responsibility of the diapers, the laundry, and a three-year-old who went into a regression about potty training. I felt heavy, unenthusiastic, and a lack of joy. It all lasted three months. The baby had seemed very fragile, and I had to be on alert twenty-four hours a day. After three months I knew he was going to be okay.

I had never heard of the baby blues, and I didn't know how to name the feelings.

—Katie had her first baby in her hometown in South Carolina. She had her second baby in Colombia—away from her family and close friends.

* * *

The last time I saw Linda, we were standing over a crib, admiring her five-week-old daughter, Soshana. Linda, at age thirty, was smiling and energetic. She whipped up a meal of corned beef and cabbage, joked throughout dinner, and handled her attention-seeking five-year-old son with her usual calm.

But Linda remembers nothing of this. She doesn't recall seeing me because her memory of events following the birth of her daughter is blurry. Although I saw no outward signs of it, Linda was depressed. Two of her women neighbors must have noticed some of the signs, since Linda says they came over to help her and make sure she was never alone. But no one discussed the obvious. No one gave the depression a name, partly because Linda had a "smiling depression" that concealed her feelings and partly because the subject is taboo. Finally, after about eight months, her depression gradually subsided. At the time, Linda did not know about postpartum depression, but now she wishes she could have given her feelings a name: "It would have made me feel less crazy," she says.

Like 10 percent of new mothers in America, Linda had developed postpartum depression—a potentially serious form of the baby blues. Luckily, this kind of depression is easily treated and cured (usually within six to eight weeks by antidepressant therapy and/or counseling). But the depression needs to be diagnosed before it can be treated. The longer you wait to get help, the longer it may take to treat the depression.

Because feelings of sadness or panic after childbirth run counter to most women's expectations—especially women who are giving birth late in life to long-awaited babies—they may feel embarrassed and confused by their feelings.

You may have postpartum depression if you feel unusually:

- Exhausted
- Hopeless
- Muddled
- Numb
- Irritable
- Obsessive

- Paranoid
- Anxious
- Angry
- Phobic
- Incompetent
- Out of control

If you have any of these symptoms, do not postpone getting help. The trick is to recognize the symptoms and treat the depression before it intensifies. If you are depressed, tell your doctor. If you are not satisfied with your doctor's response, contact a therapist, preferably one who has had some experience with postpartum depression.

Jennifer developed the classic signs of postpartum depression after the birth of each of her two boys:

"I got postpartum depression with my first baby. I got these feelings. I was afraid I was going to hurt him. Something was wrong in my world, and I didn't know what it was. I got depressed when the baby was a month old, and it lasted six weeks. I felt afraid—something that I don't feel on a day-to-day basis. I went and talked to a therapist.

"Women should be warned about postpartum depression. Not enough is said about it. It could be serious.

"I had it again after my second child, but it still took me two or three weeks to figure out that I had it again. The depression was like magnified PMS. I felt panicky, paranoid, depressed, hopeless—like things wouldn't get better again.

"Doctors should follow up on it two weeks after a birth to see if a woman feels okay."

Jennifer sought out a therapist as soon as she realized that she was depressed, and she found the counseling helpful. The good news for her, and for most women, is that postpartum depression is temporary and treatable. Sometimes counseling is adequate; other times, the depression may require medications or short-term hospitalization. Unfortunately, many women go undiagnosed early on, when the depression can be most quickly treated, because (1) they do not know that postpartum depression is a common—and treatable—problem, (2) they are too embarrassed to discuss the depression because everyone expects them to be happy, or (3) their doctor is not sensitive to the symptoms of true depression and dismisses them as the passing baby blues.

The cause of postpartum depression is the subject of debate. Some experts believe it results from a combination of biological, hormonal, societal, and psychological factors. The mother's changing hormones and her biochemical predisposition to depression have been identified as possible biological causes.

Psychosocial causes may include a woman's degree of social isolation, unrealistic expectations of birth and motherhood, and level of stress. "The stresses, strain, and exhaustion might be the final straw for a woman already vulnerable to depression," writes Susan Roan, author of *Postpartum Depression, Every Woman's Guide to Diagnosis, Treatment, and Prevention.* "The task of becoming a mother can lead to serious introspection, and sometimes, a cascade of negative emotions," writes Roan.

Some experts believe that postpartum depression is caused by lack of social support for new mothers, especially in some western societies where women are left to their own devices and not offered sufficient help in making the transition to the demanding role of mother. These experts suggest that rituals like a baby-naming ceremony, a *bris* (circumcision ceremony), or a Christening may provide a means of defining and valuing motherhood, integrating the mother and baby into society, and making the transition to motherhood less stressful—and thus less likely to generate depression.

You may minimize your risks for developing postpartum depression by creating a support system for yourself during and after pregnancy. Avoid becoming isolated. Arrange for friends and relatives to share the burden of household chores in the week or two after the birth in order to free you to spend time caring for your new baby. Invite people to celebrate your new baby by having some kind of ceremony or baby-naming party—but do not overwhelm yourself with cooking and preparation. You may want to have a potluck, in which case you will be relieved of spending energy on food. This is also a way of structuring social support in the form of food and human contact. Gradually rejoin the world of friends, grocery stores, and work with your baby in a front pack, sling, or buggy. Form a play group or child care group with mothers from your childbirth class or neighborhood.

Stealing Time for Yourself

Finding time for yourself away from the kids is the hardest thing. I haven't solved the problem completely. You have to get some time for yourself, and you have to figure out some way of doing it. When I couldn't stand it anymore, I would just plop the kids in a stroller and go for a long walk. Amy would calm down and look out at the world. She liked being strolled.
—Cathy

Parents of all ages say that finding time for themselves is one of the biggest challenges of parenthood. You may not experience your prebaby kind of solitude for a long time, but you can steal moments of solitude or create time for yourself even when your baby is with you. For instance, to steal some moments "alone," Cathy put her verbally demanding toddler and her infant into the stroller and took a long walk. The toddler was happily distracted by the world around her, the infant slept, and Cathy enjoyed some quiet moments during which she was left to her own thoughts. Riding in the car may have the same effect as Cathy's stroller, since it may lull your baby to sleep and give you time to think or unwind.

Time for yourself will be fleeting, and you will need to be resourceful in order to make the most of it.

Midlife Fatherhood

A midlife father may parent differently at age fifty than he did at twenty-five, but that does not necessarily mean that he will become a less active participant in his child's life. My father still took me on daylong muskie fishing expeditions when he was sixty-five—and I was fifteen.

However, a man's *style* of fathering may change in midlife. Reyn, age fifty-three and a father for the third time, found that his *style* of parenting changed, but not his capacity. Whereas Reyn had been an active, athletic father when he was in his twenties, he became a relaxed and accepting father in his fifties. Reyn says he played more baseball as a young father, but he feels he was less patient and more controlling. As a midlife father, Reyn skis with his four-year-old son, but he also engages in non-sports-oriented forms of male bonding, such as playing board games and building things.

Becoming a father in midlife may, in some respects, be less

stressful than if a man were younger, especially if he is settled and secure in his career. Young men must often put in longer hours at work to ensure job security, achieve tenure or seniority, or become a partner. Once job security is attained, some midlife fathers feel like they can relax and enjoy their children.

Your Relationship with Your Partner

We go on family dates. Soren has seen more plays, more concerts, and more dance than any seven-year-old. He does enjoy things you wouldn't think a small child would like. Soren and I go on a Monday night date. We've jogged together in the dark with flashlights. But I'm missing time by myself and time together with Dick as a couple.
—Holly and Dick became parents ten months after their marriage

* * *

We found that we had to find time to talk to each other. When we didn't have child care, we thought we might have to lose a little sleep in order to touch base.

When we have child care, there's a lot to be said for a romantic date in the middle of the week. We go to lunch and talk to each other or rendezvous here at home. And home has the advantage that you can have sex—and that's very nice.

If you've had years together and a routine, it's hard to work a child into that routine. It's good to remind yourself that you're both in this together. You have to work it out together.
—Cathy

* * *

Some new parents believe that parenthood limits their relationship with their partner, especially when it comes to their previous activities as a couple. They think that parenthood means being confined to quarters: no movies, no dinners out, no late-night visits to friends, and no vacations. But limits on such activities are arbitrary. The true limits should be set by the comfort levels of you and your baby—and the advice of your pediatrician as to what is or is not healthy for your baby given its age and medical history. As your baby becomes a toddler, the same principles hold true.

Creating the Life You Want

It takes imagination, resourcefulness, and energy to maintain the relationship with your partner after your baby is born. But you can create the life you want to the extent that the temperament of your baby allows for flexibility. Some children are by nature fussy, in need of constant stimulation, or in need of a very structured and predictable environment. Others are able to go with the flow and travel to Mexico, go to the movies, or make the scene at a party as long as they are strapped snugly to their mother's back or ensconced in a familiar blanket in a comfortable stroller. Sharlene and her husband have been lucky, since their daughter Ryan travels well and adjusts easily to new environments:

"We've done a lot of things we wanted to do [before the baby was born]. Now we say, 'Oh let's do that again, and let's do it with Ryan.' We want to go back to Europe, and we want to do it with Ryan. She's been to Mexico six times, and she's been on two cruises. She is a wonderful child. She has always been this easygoing baby we can take anywhere. We went out to a five-star restaurant when she was two."

Even if your baby is not easygoing, continue activities that allow you to stay connected as a couple. Continue some of your own familiar routines, favorite pastimes, or romantic rituals: order favorite take-out meals, rent videos or listen to music together, have your daily coffee at the corner cafe. Make an effort to integrate the baby into your relationship by taking the baby with you to a restaurant or on your evening walk. You will learn what is tolerable to your baby and what is comfortable for you as a couple. Susan Porto and her husband took their daughter to restaurants even though she had an apnea monitor (to detect breathing problems), because the baby tolerated the excursions and Susan and her husband could feel like a normal couple.

Take time out from the tasks of childrearing to spend some time alone when the baby is sleeping or get a baby-sitter—even if it is just for a few hours. Stay up after the baby goes to sleep at night, even if it means getting a little less sleep, in order to touch base, have an adult conversation, make decisions about the household, or make love. If you are not a late-night person, try lunchtime dates with your partner.

About Making Love

Some women temporarily lose interest in sex after the birth of their baby due to a combination of factors: painful episiotomy incisions, vaginal tears, fatigue, mood changes, and the all-encompassing demands of a new baby. In addition, many women feel overwhelmed by being touched all day by a dependent baby and want some physical privacy by the time their partner comes home at the end of the day.

Cathy didn't want to be touched at night and needed to be by herself for a while when her husband came home from work. Mary's fatigue, as well as feeling her body was no longer her own, depleted her sexual energy for several months. She recalls, "The minute the baby would fall asleep, I would lie down and fall asleep. The sex life really went down the drain. It's very hard on the marriage. When I'd have this kid on me all day and clinging to me, I wouldn't want to be touched."

If you have lost interest in sex, explain your feelings to your partner and explain your need for some physical independence. Rest assured that your interest in sex will return as your baby becomes less dependent and as you adjust to your baby's needs. You may feel less burdened if your partner or another family member holds the baby for long stretches at the end of the day to give you a break. However, you may simply need time and patience, and your sexuality will gradually return. Consult a counselor if you experience long-lasting disinterest in sex, and your obstetrician if you continue to have pain during intercourse.

Even if sex is not on your immediate agenda, there are other ways to feel close to your partner. Focus on other things you enjoy doing together to maintain your sense of being a couple during this period. Foot rubs and back rubs to relieve tension are good ways of maintaining an intimate physical connection—as long as you aren't overwhelmed by all forms of touch.

Sometimes feelings of sexuality decrease due to stress. Consequently, the better your strategies for dealing with the changes in your life and your relationship, the sooner your sex life will return to normal.

Your Relationship with Your Friends

Parenthood definitely shifted our circle of friends. One thing I did notice when I got back to the university was that I'd been accepted into this secret fraternity of dads. People started coming out of the woodwork. Older faculty who hadn't said very much to me (though they were always cordial) now were congratulating me and telling me about their kids. I sort of felt this: "now you are one of us." This curtain was drawn back, and the family lives of these older men were revealed to me in a way they had not been before.

I think that when you have kids, you tend to gravitate to

other people with kids. Some of your friends who chose not to have kids don't particularly like kids, and don't particularly like to hear about your kids. You spend more time with couples who have young children and considerably less time with friends who do not.
—Kevin

• • •

I made new friends—professional women who had children later in life. Anytime I saw a woman with a little gray in her hair who had a baby with her, I'd strike up a conversation.
—Holly

• • •

Your single or child-free friends may drift away from you after you have a baby, although sometimes this is due more to miscommunication than to disinterest in the friendship. If your friends invite you to go out with them to the movies or dinner before you are ready to go out with the baby or to get a sitter, tell them that you aren't ready to go out yet. If you'd like them to come visit you at home, invite them. They may not want to intrude on your new family, assuming that you are too tired or too absorbed in your new life, and they may need an invitation to feel welcome.

Make an effort to contact your friends. Do not expect friends to automatically understand the needs of a new parent. For instance, if you are too tired to cook for them but would like their company for dinner, suggest take-out food. Some people—especially those who have had children themselves—automatically understand the needs of new parents. Pete and Lucy know from experience that new parents are usually too tired to cook and shop. "For friends with a new baby, bring a meal. It's the best thing to do for people—to do something that saves them work," advises Pete.

Do not assume that your friends will be put off by the interruptions of a new baby. They may—and they may not. Friends who do not have children may be fascinated with yours (though not as fascinated as you are) and those whose children are grown may want to vicariously experience a new baby, even though they might not want to have another baby themselves.

Some of your friends may not be able to relate to parenthood and babies and may drift away unless you maintain the basis of your friendship with them. For instance, you may solidify your friendships with people from tennis, bowling, or work once you begin those activities again. Visit the tennis court or workplace with (or without) your baby in tow to reassure your friends that you have not totally disappeared from their world and that you wish to stay in touch. If you are housebound, stay in touch by phone or e-mail.

Sometimes friends will drift away after you have a baby— in which case you will need to make new ones. You may already have the basis for new friendships with women from your childbirth class, mothers' group, neighborhood play group, or your La Leche meeting or Mothers of Twins group. If you feel isolated and are not part of such a group, check out the local women's center for mothers' groups. If you are not a joiner of organizations, start conversations with parents at playgrounds, the pool, or the YMCA.

Holly looked for women her own age and struck up conversations with women who had some gray hair and a young child in tow. (However, sometimes she ended up meeting grandmothers.) Other midlife mothers find that their group of friends suddenly includes younger mothers, since older mothers are not always easy to find. Men also find their old friends dropping away, and men may find themselves even more isolated than women, since they do not have the option of as many support groups and play groups.

Sometimes parents find a whole new social world opening up for them as they become parents. Kathleen R. found herself a contented member of what she calls the "club" of mothers. Kevin was pleasantly surprised to be brought into the world of older male colleagues, what he refers to as a "secret society of dads."

The First Month Survival Checklist

• Social support
(friends, family, mothers' group)

• Household support
(family, friends, doula)

• Breastfeeding Support
(mothers' group, La Leche League,
doula)

• Sleep strategy

• Relationship strategies

• Friendship strategies

Chapter 31

Coping with Motherhood and Career

You can fit kids into your life—you just can. We almost have an obligation to society and to other women to show that this can and should be done. Like breastfeeding in public. You have to say: "This is what I'm doing." The more we can bring kids into the workplace, the better it is for everybody—even the men.

—Jessica, fifty-two, a college professor, brings her daughter to her office and classroom

• • •

The longer you can stay with your baby, the easier the transition is. I took six weeks off. Then I went back to work for two to three days a week, and I took him with me. Then, when I went to work full-time, I took the baby with me to work until he was too big to be carried in a sling—at about six months or so. I got a cleaning woman to do child care and transitioned slowly. . . . I would have liked not to work; but it wasn't going to work out. If I would have had to leave him at six weeks, I would have had regrets. But I had six months of being with him at all times.
—Joanne

• • •

The above statements from midlife mothers represent common responses to juggling motherhood and career from women who have demanding careers and well-established relationships with their partner, friends, and coworkers long before their baby's birth.

Some women have more to juggle than others, depending on the degree of support they get from their coworkers and their partners, on how well they personally adapt to change, and on how well their baby adjusts to the work schedule and child care. Some mothers are anxious to return to work quickly, while others negotiate flexible schedules or a gradual return to work. As a working mother, you must be resourceful in order to juggle the demands of your job and the needs of your child. To handle your new dual role as mother and working woman, you will need to devise strategies for nursing schedules, child care, and breast pumps.

You may also need to adjust your work schedule to the unique personality of your baby. Your baby may be demanding or mellow—factors that will influence your concentration, your job performance, and your working hours. Your baby's needs may also require you to redefine "success" as you go along and change your expectations of just how much you can accomplish in a given day.

Part-time or Flex Time

Depending on your individual circumstances and the temperament of your baby, you may need to job share, work part-time, utilize flex time (such as four 10-hour days or different hours), or work at home.

If you can negotiate for more flexibility in your job when your child is very young, do so, since flexibility can become an important asset as you are learning to integrate work and motherhood. After becoming a mother your priorities may shift, at least temporarily, and you may find it difficult to leave your baby for extended periods of time. A flexible work environment can make the difference between an easy and a difficult juggling act, allowing you to adjust your work schedule to your baby's needs. Unfortunately, such an accommodating workplace is the exception rather than the rule. Support jobs, service jobs, and factory jobs often allow for less flexibility than professional jobs; consequently, women with modest incomes may find themselves caught in a catch-22 of needing day care because they are working full-time, but needing to work long hours to afford day care. However, even in a rigid workplace, there is sometimes room for negotiation regarding hours, schedules, or bringing your baby to work.

Rhonda, who had worked nine to five as a recycling specialist, negotiated for an extended maternity leave and a transitional period of part-time work in order to spend as much time as she could with her son. She believes that she had more confidence to negotiate at thirty-eight than she would have had as a younger mother. She says:

"I arranged to stay home for five and a half months. I didn't think the baby should be apart from me before that. It was really hard to convince my boss of that. But I was adamant. I had saved up as much sick leave and vacation leave as possible. . . . I promised that I would work part-time [at home] during some of my leave. At age twenty-five, I would have felt more vulnerable and I wouldn't have had the power to ask for so much time off.

"For me, as a professional woman, I was ready to get back to work. I needed the challenge and stimulation of work and the company of grown-ups."

Cathy's part-time job teaching at a university allowed her to participate in the working world. At the same time, she was available to her child on an almost full-time basis because she brought her child to work. She describes her experience:

"I was very much involved in the lab when Amy was a baby. I brought her in a backpack or a front carrier. I did computer work and went to lab meetings with her on my lap. She started walking at nine months, but I could still bring her in. I was involved in work, and I found ways of staying involved. But as she got older, I no longer brought her in with me. Then I got child care."

When the baby was young, Cathy brought her to her office and the laboratory, but not to class. Cathy hired a student to tend the baby during class hours and office hours—which amounted to about six to ten hours a week.

Cathy remained part-time because she decided to make her child a priority, continue to teach part-time, and turn down a demanding, tenure-track job. "I didn't want an all-consuming career. I wanted the luxury of being a mom," said Cathy. However, she also wanted to maintain ties with her profession, her colleagues, and adult companionship. Working part-time allowed Cathy the luxury of motherhood, intellectual stimulation, and adult conversation. Working part-time also gave Cathy the advantage of keeping current in her work and leaving the door open for returning to university work once her children were grown.

Working part-time is a good strategy if you are interested in keeping up your skills so you can return to work full-time at some point in the future. Lucy looks back on her years as a mother and wishes she had remained working part-time instead of closing the door completely on her career. Like Cathy, Lucy worked part-time as a college instructor when her first child was a baby. But later on she stopped working and stayed home with her two children because she wanted to, and she could afford to. Now, as her children enter adolescence, Lucy considers re-entering the workforce and, in so doing, she must face the downside of staying at home for more than a decade: falling out of step with her profession by not keeping up her skills and her confidence. "The obstacle is the confidence—you don't believe in yourself anymore," says Lucy.

For maintaining both confidence and competence while raising children, Lucy thinks it is wise for a woman to work a little, even if it is only one day a week, in order to not lose too many options if she wishes to return to work after her children are grown:

"Working part-time is ideal. You have to go back to work as soon as possible; otherwise, you'll lose your skills and your confidence. Even working one day a week will help. Get a baby-sitter for a full day."

Lucy suggests that mothers maintain contacts with their acquaintances from the job world to maintain friendships, avoid isolation, and stay in touch with new job-related developments.

Full-time Work

Having a baby in midlife may prove to be an advantage, since women in their thirties and forties often have gained confidence in their ability to integrate motherhood and career and have achieved enough seniority or experience on the job to negotiate for flexibility during the first months of motherhood. Joanne, Miriam, and Jessica had worked their way up their respective career ladders and "arrived" in their respective jobs before becoming mothers.

Joanne, the director of a small private school, confidently integrated motherhood with her professional life. She took her baby to work with her and wore him in a sling until he was six months old. She even took him to board meetings and acknowledged his presence by making jokes about the little arms and legs protruding from the sling strapped over her shoulder. The child was quiet, content—and his presence was well received by both men and women board members. Joanne, by her example, demonstrates that babies and board meetings can mix—given the right work environments, job security, and a can-do attitude.

Joanne's work environment was flexible enough to allow her to transition slowly from being a full-time mother at work to leaving her son with her housekeeper for progressively longer and longer periods of time. This gradual separation method made transition easier for both mother and baby. Luckily, Joanne's flexible schedule minimized the potential conflicts between work routines and motherhood.

Miriam worked full-time, but at home. She created firm boundaries between work and motherhood that allowed her the best of both worlds. While a baby-sitter watched the baby, Miriam worked from eight to four in her home office. She says, "I felt great. I didn't know what to expect; I guess ignorance is bliss. I worked at home. I was always there. I had a baby-sitter from eight to four.

"Motherhood was very intuitive for me. I never found it overwhelming. I never got crazed about it. I had my own business, and it was doing well. Consequently, I don't think I had pressures at work. I tried to draw a firm line between work and motherhood. I have a whole office that's on the other side of the apartment. My daughter stayed up until 11:00 P.M., so I had a whole day with her after the sitter left at 4:00."

Because Miriam's baby was a night owl and liked to stay up until 11:00 P.M., and because Miriam had considerable energy, she was able to have a complete workday plus a seven-hour day with her child.

Jessica found that being older and settled in her work helped her integrate motherhood and career. As a woman in her late forties she was confident enough to bring her baby with her while she wrote reports in her office and to wear her baby in a sling or front pack when she taught classes.

"I brought her in a front pack or day pack to class and just wore her. Later on, I sat her on the desk with crayons. I couldn't have done that when I was younger."

However, Jessica was also freed to pursue her academic career by the presence of a nanny, who could take over child care whenever necessary.

Holly, at age thirty-six, was still building her career as a lawyer when her son, Soren, was born. She integrated mother-hood and career—but not without considerable conflict and "gut-wrenching guilt" every time she dropped Soren off at day care. After she took her three-month maternity leave, Holly's law firm offered no flex time, no job sharing, and no flexibility for the needs of mothers and their babies. She compensated for her separation from Soren by making frequent calls to his day care and looking at his picture on her desk—none of which eased the pain of leaving him. She managed to continue nursing him by using a breast pump and leaving breastmilk in bottles for him to drink during the day. However, despite the conflicts, Holly loved her work and needed it to feel fulfilled:

"Even the most wonderful small child cannot meet the complex needs of a grown-up. In that respect, I was happy to go to work. In some respects, work became my solace. It was the only place where I could be alone. I used to love driving in the car. It was the only time all week when I was by myself."

Dr. Susan Porto returned to her full-time job as an obstetrician after each of her babies was a few months old, but she would have preferred to follow Lucy's prescription: to work one to two days a week to keep her medical skills current and spend the rest of her time at home with her kids until they were grown. Although she had already built a solid career as a physician,

Susan didn't have the luxury of staying home because her family needed the income and the health insurance.

However, despite the demands of her medical practice, Susan manages to spend time with her children, Lorelei and Emilio. She and her husband work around the needs of their children and resourcefully snatch time within a busy day to spend with their family. For instance, when Susan is at the hospital, sometimes she meets her daughter, Lorelei, and husband in the doctors' lounge or takes Lorelei for a walk on the maternity ward. She says that integrating motherhood and her professional life is not easy, especially with a toddler and an infant.

"It's hard to integrate motherhood and career. Basically, it's work and kids—and that's it. There are many days when my husband brings my daughter to the hospital. He'll bring her toys, and he'll pack her a lunch. There's an attending physician's room with reclining chairs and a television. He'll put her toys on the floor, and she'll play with them. He'll sit in the room with her. Sometimes he'll read a book.

"While one of my patients is still in labor, I will come and play with my daughter. Once in a while I take her out on the unit and walk around. On Halloween I brought her in to the hospital all dressed up and showed my patients. They all got a kick out of it."

Integrating work, your professional identity, and your identity as a mother is a challenge that requires courage and imagination. It also requires the flexibility to deal with unforeseen circumstances as they arise. Fortunately, there are as many "right ways" to do this as there are mothers and babies. Whether you decide to return to full-time or part-time work or to integrate motherhood and career by focusing first on motherhood and then easing yourself back into the workforce, there is no "right way"—just the way that is right for you and your baby.

Maternity Leave and "Phase-back" Policies

When planning your return to work, note that in certain jobs you have the right, granted by the Pregnancy Disability Act and the Family Medical Leave Act, to maternity leave. According to Gale Pryor, in *Nursing Mother, Working Mother,* women have the right to "six weeks of maternity leave with disability pay plus six more weeks without pay—if your employer has 50 or more employees, and if you have worked for that employer at least 25 hours per week for the preceding leave year." If you want more time or a gradual increasing of your hours, you may have some negotiating to do.

Some employers recognize that the first weeks of working full-time may be difficult for mothers. Rather than lose long-standing employees, some employers have developed "phase-back" plans to help women gradually return to the workplace. Employers with "phase back" plans include Aetna Life and Casualty Company, AT&T, Chase Manhattan Bank, IBM, and Patagonia.

If you are interested in "phasing back" to work, talk to your employer during your pregnancy to arrange for your maternity leave and your return to work. You may want to negotiate for returning part-time or for working a three- or four-day week for the first month or two. If your employer wants you to work more than part-time, try to negotiate for working at home as well as at the office. That way, you can go to the office three or four days a week and work at home for a day or two, thus avoiding the drive and the separation from your baby for at least part of the workweek. However, if you have a fussy baby, you may need to hire a baby-sitter or enlist the help of a family member in order to concentrate on work when you are at home.

Staying Home

The conditions of my employment were no longer worth the sacrifice. I didn't want to look back on my life and say I woulda, shoulda, coulda, stayed home with my kids.
—Stacy worked twelve-hour days when her twins were small but, after the birth of a third baby, she decided to stay home to raise her children.

* * *

I don't regret staying at home, but sometimes I wish I got more credit for it one way or another. In Finland, women are subsidized for up to three years when they stay home with their kids. They don't lose their jobs. We're in the dark ages when it comes to family policy.
—Eileen stayed home with her son, Neal, for seven years.

* * *

For some women, staying home with a child is part of their philosophy of childbearing. However, many midlife women who never considered becoming stay-at-home moms are surprising themselves and those who are close to them by deciding to leave work and stay home with their new baby. Leslie had always worked and had intended to go back to her job at a printing press after three months. So far, she's been home with her daughter for nine years, but it was a decision made gradually. She says:

"I was working up to the last day of my pregnancy. I had some arrangement to go back after three months. Then three months went by. I had been at the press more than fifteen years. After three months, I called and said maybe it would be six months. At six months it was clear; I wasn't going back. I could never bring myself to write a formal letter of resignation."

Becoming a mother involved a surprising revelation for

Kathleen R.: she no longer wanted to be a scientist. Kathleen had worked hard for her Ph.D. and never dreamed she would give up a promising career as a scientist to stay home with her baby, but she did:

"Have a baby. Get a degree. Put the baby in day care. Everything will be fine. I never even once considered not working. After we found day care, I felt like I was giving him away. I wouldn't do the drop-off. I was very surprised. I was in a culture where you work hard, get a post-doc, and get a job. There were women around me who came back to work in four weeks. Plus David and I felt we couldn't afford for me not to work. But I didn't want to go back to work. My professional self was gone. I didn't care anymore. I had no interest."

Fortunately, Kathleen's husband, colleagues, and boss were surprised, but understanding. Her boss gave her time to think through her decision, and he supported her choice to become a full-time mother:

"I told my boss before Christmas that I wanted to be a full-time mom. I went through torture with myself to get to that point. He said, 'Are you sure?' I said, 'No, I'm not sure.' He told me to think about it over the holidays. I felt like I was falling off a cliff over the holidays. Later, I told him I knew this was what I wanted to do. He said, 'My wife stayed home with our children.'"

Kathleen had never imagined that she would feel this way, but she has no regrets. She has been home for four years. When her child is grown, Kathleen says she will look for a new career rather than returning to science.

Auben also unexpectedly considered staying at home with her baby. Despite her fulfilling career as a psychologist, Auben so loved caring for her son, Joe, that when he was ten months old, she began cutting back on her work and talked about becoming a stay-at-home mom—much to her surprise and the astonishment of her friends and colleagues: "I'm working two afternoons a week, and I'm turning down a lot of work. I decided that I'm not going back to work full-time—probably ever. I think that being with Joe is very important. I want to be home when he comes back from school. . . . All of this stuff is surprising me. The depth of my feeling surprises me."

Because Auben's coworkers can't understand her decision, Auben is "teaching" them what the decision means to her and confronting their misconceptions about women who stay home with their children: "I've been telling my colleagues that I want to leave work. They say, 'But don't you want to have a life?' I say, 'I'm not thinking of sitting around eating bonbons. I'm just not thinking of being a psychologist.'"

Although staying home may seem like an ideal situation where you can give your baby your undivided attention and care, it comes with potential problems such as decreased social contact with friends and coworkers, decreased income, and decreased mental and social stimulation.

Fortunately, you can anticipate and minimize some of these problems with some strategic planning. If you decide to stay home with your baby, continue your favorite activities such as reading or watching videos—even if you have to do them while nursing or feeding the baby. Maintain contact with your friends, your colleagues, and your previous "world." Have lunch with your friends and coworkers or invite them for a walk with you and the baby. Continue familiar routines like your morning swim at the YMCA or your daily coffee at a local cafe. Do not isolate yourself at home with your baby. Meet other new mothers and socialize with them and their babies through exercise classes and play groups through the local women's center. Join La Leche League or other breastfeeding support organizations, since they can be the source of a social life as well as breastfeeding advice. Start a group with other women from your childbirth class. Seek out women in your neighborhood who are home with children and form a child care network or play group. If you have twins or triplets, join a Mothers with Twins group for companionship and support.

Kathleen R. stayed in touch with her coworkers, maintained friendships, gained ongoing support from her mothers' group, and joined informal play groups with neighbors who had small children. She also maintained some of her earning power by doing medical transcribing while her baby slept, which still left her many hours with her baby.

Not all stay-at-home mothers are as fortunate as Kathleen in receiving social support from friends and colleagues for staying home. In the 1950s and 1960s in the United States, staying home was expected and valued. Nowadays, people's reactions to women who stay home vary widely. Some women find that their decision to stay home may generate admiration, disapproval, or envy. At the YMCA where Leslie swims, she sees tension between the working and the stay-at-home mothers. "I actually find it heartbreaking that we aren't nicer to each other." Leslie finds two conflicting and equally unempathic points of view: (1) working women who think that it is boring to stay home, and (2) stay-at-home moms who think working women don't pay enough attention to their children:

"The working women think: 'Oh, how boring staying home must be.' There's this contempt that may be born partly of jealousy and insecurity. On the other side, the stay-home mothers think: 'Oh, how can she leave her child all day and then get to see him for only two hours?' These are karate-chop statements—why make them? I see women giving each other a hard time whichever end of the spectrum they are. Either way, we should cut each other some slack."

Your own attitude about staying home can make a big difference in how others respond to you. When family and friends ask Leslie if she is working, she says "No" and leaves it at that. She feels she doesn't need to defend herself. Other women, like Auben, try to "teach" their friends to bypass the stereotypes and to understand what staying home means for them.

Re-entering the Workforce

Unfortunately, in the United States, some women who stay home feel that the value of their years at home is not sufficiently appreciated—especially when they try to reenter the work-force—and that their previous skills and work experiences are overlooked. Eileen chose to stay home, has no regrets about doing so, and believes that her son benefited from her presence, but she says she "took a hit" when, after seven years at home, she tried to get a job:

"When you go around looking for normal type jobs, you get the impression that they think you're from an alien planet. Anything you've done, any potential you had, because you've taken time off, is reduced to zero. You have to get recredentialed. You don't have any contacts or any referrals. You end up starting with entry-level jobs, but you're older and you're more educated than some of the people who interview you. It's a very awkward situation."

However, despite the job problems, Eileen felt that she personally benefited from staying home and that the experience gave her an opportunity to make important changes in her life. She became part of a neighborhood through a network of her child's friends, and she came upon a new career:

"You have a ready-made way of changing your life. I had a breather. Things that seemed to count, like status, were replaced by midlife concerns like what feels good. . . . I was going to go into survey research. But I got into teaching through my child. I would never ever have gotten involved in

Montessori if I hadn't had a child. How would I have known about it?"

When Eileen went back to school to become a Montessori teacher, she found she was more energetic, more focused, and more efficient than she had been in her twenties and early thirties:

"When you stay home, you don't have any adult company for the major portion of your day. That's why if you go back to school, you are great at it. You are great at all sorts of things because you really appreciate the outside world. You have more zest! The other thing is you are more efficient than you have ever been."

Breastfeeding and Returning to Work

I had a breast pump at work. I would close myself off. I had to pump twice a day for twenty to thirty minutes. I found it very easy. I nursed him before I left in the morning and when I got home at night. I left a bottle of breastmilk for him during the day.
—Joanne, forty-nine

❀ ❀ ❀

Going back to work was hard. I was breastfeeding. Lorelei was premature and in a NICU . . . and I was [breast] pumping every three to four hours. When I finally got her to breastfeed, I was starting to go back to work again. I was pumping and giving her breastmilk in a bottle. With the second baby [Emilio], it was better because he was a good feeder off the bat. I didn't introduce the bottle until a few days before I went back to work. I've been back to work a month now and I've had to give him formula only once.

The most challenging thing is if you're breastfeeding and trying to find a time and place to pump. You have to make the time.

I have a small hand-held breast pump for when I'm at the hospital. I carry it in a shoulder bag. I have an electric pump at my office.
—Dr. Susan Porto

* * *

If you've been breastfeeding your baby during maternity leave and you wish to continue breastfeeding once you return to work, you can continue nursing your baby—with a few possible modifications. You will need to either breastfeed your baby during the workday or use a breast pump to provide milk and store it for him while you are at work.

Joanne and Jessica nursed their babies during the workday in their private offices at work. Other women traveled from their offices to a nearby day care center to nurse their babies at lunch and at various times during the day. Still others used breast pumps at work and at home to store milk for their babies so the babies could drink bottled breastmilk while their mothers were working. Even though most of these women returned to work full-time, they successfully continued their babies on a diet of breastmilk.

Breastfeeding your baby after you return to work is most effective if you have already established a successful breastfeeding routine at home. Although some mothers and babies make a smooth and immediate adjustment to breastfeeding, many women and their babies experience problems—most of which can be overcome with good coaching from a lactation consultant or a La Leche League leader.

Some nursing mothers find invaluable information, support, and a potential network of friends and play groups at La Leche meetings, and many women continue going to meetings for months after their baby's birth in order to better meet breastfeeding challenges that may appear as the baby develops and the mother returns to work.

With a little expert help, breastfeeding can be successful for women regardless of their age or their return to full-time work. To make the transition from home to work easier on you and your nursing baby, gradually increase your hours at work if possible. You will need some time to become accustomed to your new routine of working, nursing, and pumping and storing breast milk. Do not expect to achieve a harmonious routine right away. This transition is not always a graceful one, so give yourself several weeks for your body to adjust. You might also try finding day care for your baby near your workplace so you can nurse your baby at lunch and, if your job is flexible enough, during a morning or afternoon break.

To pump milk, find a private place in an office or restroom and then refrigerate the milk until you are ready to go home. If you have a long commute from work, bring a cooler to preserve the milk. Once at home, you can pump your milk and then place it in bottles in the refrigerator to store for your baby for the next day. You may also freeze milk for future use. When you are anticipating going back to work after a maternity leave, it is a good idea to start freezing and storing milk one or two weeks in advance. Ask a lactation consultant or a La Leche League leader about how best to store your breastmilk. Breastfeeding expert Gale Pryor recommends that you carefully store your breastmilk in the back of the freezer, where the temperature is constant, and not in the door of the freezer, where temperatures may vary as the door is opened and closed. Never thaw and refreeze breastmilk.

If you are unable to nurse during the day, make arrangements at work for a private place to pump milk and take enough time—fifteen to thirty minutes—to effectively utilize it. For privacy, use your office, a friend's office, a storage closet (that you can lock from the inside), a conference room, or a restroom. For an electric pump you will need an electrical outlet, a flat surface, and a place to sit and relax. When no other options are available, some women pump in a parked car with a sunshade or towels across the windows.

You will need an array of bottles, either plastic or glass, in which to store the milk; a refrigerator at work in which to keep the milk cool; and, if you have a long drive home, a cooler in which to transport the milk.

For more information, call La Leche League at (800) 525-3243, International Lactation Consultants at (312) 541-1710, or see the appendix for more referrals.

Chapter 32
Child Care

It was hard to put Soren in day care. It was horrible. How would you feel if you went to work one day and you left your arm at home? Soren was so much a part of me. Driving to work I would feel him pulling on me. I would worry about him, and I would call. After the first hour I would get so busy I would forget. I'm a lawyer, and I had to keep my job.
—Holly

* * *

Day care is a real tricky issue. At first, because my job is flexible, I had no day care. . . . Kevin filled in, or I had a college student take care of Amy for two hours at the office while I lectured and saw students. I picked somebody whom I knew already. That wasn't stressful. Then I got part-time home day care. Part-time is hard to find. Also, a home day care person can quit any time he or she feels like it. My woman quit in August when all the child care centers were filled up.
—Cathy

* * *

Child care is a challenge for most parents, since many of the options are not ideal and they are something over which you have limited control. You have three main options for child care:

1. In your own home
2. In someone else's home
3. In a day care center

Within these options, you may find variations in setting and caretaker that may greatly enhance or detract from the care your child receives. Whatever day care you choose, make sure the provider is receptive to your calling or stopping by to check on your baby.

In-home Care

My husband doesn't work. He goes to school part-time, so he and my sister-in-law take care of the kids. My sister-in-law comes to the house. . . . I wouldn't have it any other way. Kids get sick a lot at day care. My sister-in-law's kids were in day care, and they were always getting sick.
—Dr. Susan Porto

• • •

You may prefer that someone come into your home to care for your child. The advantages of "in-home" child care are that the child is in a familiar environment and that you can provide your child with the food he requires and his favorite toys. You also have considerable control over the health, cleanliness, and safety of his environment. Your child will not be exposed daily to sick children, head lice, or dirty floors, and both you and your child will be spared the stress of one cold after another and the tedious washing and disinfecting that comes with bouts of head lice.

With in-home care, you can also handpick his caretaker and choose a trusted family member, neighbor, or baby-sitter. The drawback is that such care may be expensive, your caregiver and child may be relatively isolated and lonely, and your caregiver can quit without much, if any, notice.

An au pair may be a good choice, especially if you contract with an agency for a year, and if you get an experienced au pair who is good with your child. Some au pairs are intelligent, enthusiastic young women who enhance your child's environment and help free you from shopping and cooking so you can spend more time with your child. However, other au pairs are inexperienced or immature and may take up your time by requiring considerable supervision. Some children become confused when they get a new au pair every year and lose the au pair to whom they have bonded.

A nanny may be a better choice if you can find a mature person who can stay with your family for more than a year and provide continuity for your child.

Family members are sometimes a good source of in-home child care, provided they have the energy and desire to take care of the child and aren't doing it reluctantly out of obligation to you. If your relative is a good caregiver, this form of day care can work exceptionally well, since the child can have an ongoing relationship with a relative that lasts for many years.

Baby-sitters or baby-sitting co-ops may provide adequate child care if you are not away from the home on a daily basis. However, since baby-sitters are in high demand, you will need to develop some strategies to find a dependable and available sitter. Eileen developed two useful strategies: (1) she joined a neighborhood baby-sitting co-op with other parents who took turns baby-sitting for each other's children, and (2) she found responsible high school baby-sitters and secured their services by paying them well:

"Getting a baby-sitter is a major hassle. These teenage kids have busy social lives. It's expensive, too. I paid well because I always wanted to make sure I had a baby-sitter. I used to pay them more than anybody else paid.

"We do a baby-sitting co-op. Families band together. Each person starts out with so many hours of baby-sitting time—and then you trade it. I would call and ask someone to baby-sit for me. Then I would baby-sit in return. We had fifteen people in the co-op. It's good for married couples because one person stays home with your kid and the other would go off and baby-sit."

Family or Home Day Care

In a family day care, your child becomes the addition to another family. The ideal situation is that. But there are all sorts of tensions that arise when your child bonds with the caregiver and enters into the routine and procedures of another household.
—Eileen

• • •

Home day care is the kind of thing that's hit or miss. My friend Sally takes her child to a woman who lives down the street, and her son is really part of the family. But if you don't like the home situation, there is nothing you can do about it; there is no board to complain to. It's "Take it or leave it. This is how we live. This is how we run our home."
—Amanda

• • •

In a family or home day care, your child goes to someone else's home. Here you will often find children of different ages—

which can be an asset, especially if you have an infant. Make sure that the home doesn't have too many small infants at the same time, since it will be difficult for the caregiver to adequately meet the needs of several young babies. However, if the caregiver is taking care of older children who can play together and do not require as much attention and cuddling as a small baby, the caregiver will be freer to attend to the needs of your baby.

Interview the family day care provider carefully, asking questions that will reveal her knowledge and interest (or lack thereof) in child development and education. Observe her behavior with infants to see if she is warm and nurturing. Ask the provider about the details of a child's typical day, which means inquiring about activities, meals, snacks, amount of television, cleanliness, bathroom and diaper-changing arrangements, safety, pets, and general supervision. Ask how often she will feed your baby and whether she would consider carrying him around in a sling if he is used to constant contact. If pertinent, ask if she feels comfortable with you nursing the baby at her home in the middle of the day. Since your child will be in contact with other children throughout the day, inquire about the care provider's policy on children with infectious diseases: Are they allowed to stay at the home and in contact with other children? Are they sent home? Does the care provider wash her hands after touching a sick child?

Make sure you get several references from the care provider, and check each one. Check on the home yourself by asking other parents about it and by popping in a few times at different times of day to get a better feel for the way the home is run. Observe carefully to see if the children are well cared for, playing happily, and receiving adequate attention and supervision from the care provider. Tour the grounds to check for potential outdoor hazards. Once your child is there, make surprise visits to get a sense of how the children are cared for throughout the day.

Day Care Centers

Institutional day care seems to differ dramatically from center to center. You have everything from employee-sponsored to big franchise day care. Employee-sponsored ones are often on-site, and all of the people coming in and out are keeping an eye on things. Maia went when she was one and a half to a center in Research Triangle Park [near Raleigh, North Carolina] about five minutes from my work. Cleanliness was a big thing there. The workers put on rubber gloves to change diapers in order to prevent the spread of infection. However, the kids were constantly getting ear infections and other viruses. The center had a rule that children should not come if they had a fever within twenty-four hours, but kids are often contagious before they are symptomatic. . . .

I was pretty pleased with the place at work. The two teachers that Maia had both had degrees in early childhood education. The center paid for them to go to conferences and update their skills.

—Amanda

• • •

Day care centers have more children than a group home and more caregivers. They can be homey or institutional; the staff can be well trained or incompetent; and the environment can be stimulating or dull. Start researching day care centers early on in your pregnancy since many have long waiting lists. Ask lots of questions about the training and philosophy of the staff and observe carefully to see if the children are engaged in play, given adequate attention, and well fed. Notice how the infants are treated: Do they spend long hours alone in their cribs (a bad sign) or are they affectionately held and talked to?

An advantage of day care centers is that they are usually subject to stricter regulation than home day care. Day care centers are more likely to have more professional staff.

A good day care center that provides your child with a safe, stimulating, nurturing environment can help socialize your child as he grows older and give him a sense of continuity and community. However, even a good day care center will expose your child to more infectious diseases than he would be exposed to at home, resulting in more illness for your baby, more doctor visits, possibly more illness for you and the rest of your family, and missed work for you (unless you have a backup day care plan).

A poor day care center can have lasting negative effects, which means that you will need to put considerable time and energy into researching your options.

Choosing Day Care for Your Child

When you are looking for childcare, utilize all the resources available in your community: ask your friends, neighbors, co-workers, and health care providers for their recommendations for day care and contact local child care referral organizations (CCROs) for guidance. You also may contact Child Care Aware on the Internet *(www.childcareaware.org)* or call the Child Care Connector at (800) 424-2246.

When you begin to visit child care homes or child care centers, the Child Care Aware organization recommends that you note your first impression of the place and look carefully to see if the place seems safe and clean, if the care providers enjoy talking and playing with children, and if there are toys and learning materials within a child's reach. Visit the home or center more than once and stay as long as possible to get a feel for what the interactions are like between the care provider(s) and the children.

Note how the place "sounds." Do the children sound happy and engaged in play or other activities? Are the children overly quiet or agitated?

Since you may feel very anxious about leaving your child in someone else's care, look for a child care provider who lessens your anxiety by being responsive and responsible and who provides a safe, nurturing, and appropriately stimulating environment for your child.

Evaluating a Child Care Provider

The following list from Child Care Aware is a useful tool for measuring the quality of a child care center.

Caregivers/Teachers

- ❏ Do the caregivers/teachers seem to really like children?
- ❏ Do the caregivers/teachers get down on each child's level to speak to the child?
- ❏ Are children greeted when they arrive?
- ❏ Are the children's needs quickly met even when things get busy?
- ❏ Are the caregivers/teachers trained in CPR, first aid, and early childhood education?
- ❏ Are the caregivers/teachers involved in continuing education programs?
- ❏ Does the program keep up with the children's changing interests?
- ❏ Will the caregivers/teachers always be ready to answer your questions?
- ❏ Will the caregivers/teachers tell you what your child is doing every day?
- ❏ Are parents' ideas welcomed? Are there ways for you to get involved?
- ❏ Do the caregivers/teachers and children enjoy being together?
- ❏ Is there enough staff to serve the children? (Ask local

experts about the best staff/child ratios for different age groups.)

❏ Are caregivers/teachers experienced?

Setting

❏ Is the environment pleasant, safe, and clean?

❏ Is there a fenced-in outdoor play area with a variety of safe equipment? Can the care providers see the entire playground at all times?

❏ Are there different areas for resting, quiet play, and active play? Is there enough space for the children in all of these areas?

Activities

❏ Is there a daily balance of playtime, story time, activity time, and rest time?

❏ Are the activities appropriate for each age group?

❏ Are there enough toys and learning materials for the number of children?

❏ Are toys safe, clean, and within reach of the children?

In General

❏ Do you agree with the discipline practices?

❏ Do you hear the sounds of happy children?

❏ Are children comforted when needed?

❏ Is the program licensed or regulated?

❏ Are surprise visits by parents encouraged?

❏ Will your child be happy there?

Reprinted (and adapted) from the Child Care Aware Web site, *www.childcare.org*, a program of the National Association of Child Care Resource and Referral Agencies, funded through a cooperative agreement with the Child Care Bureau, Administration for Children and Families, and the U.S. Department of Health and Human Services.

Postscript

There is clearly good news for healthy women who become pregnant after thirty. According to medical evidence gathered over the past twenty years, women in their thirties and forties are capable of having normal pregnancies, normal births, and healthy babies.

The key ingredient for having a healthy baby is a woman who is in good health before she becomes pregnant. For women who eat balanced diets, maintain healthy lifestyles, receive appropriate prenatal care, find skilled care providers and have no serious pre-existing medical problems, midlife pregnancy and birth are safe for both mother and baby. However, even women with pre-existing or pregnancy-related health problems such as diabetes and hypertension may have healthy babies as long as the problems are carefully managed by a doctor before and during pregnancy.

The major obstacle to pregnancy in midlife, especially in your late thirties or forties, is waning fertility. Although modern medical technology continues to progress, creating increasingly successful treatments for infertility that have fewer and fewer side effects, we can't entirely change Mother Nature. At least, not yet. Consequently, getting pregnant may become more difficult in your late thirties or forties—but pregnancy is still possible! Conception may take a little longer or require help from medical technology, but as the women in this book show, you need not give up on getting pregnant and giving birth. National health statistics confirm that increasing numbers of women in the United States become pregnant after age thirty-five. The rate of women becoming pregnant in their late thirties has more than doubled since 1978. From 1981 to 1999, the birth rate for women in their forties increased by 95 percent.

Thus, midlife pregnancy is possible, it's safe, and it's becoming increasingly common. But is it a good idea? Most importantly, is it a good idea for you, given your personality, your health, and your priorities in life?

After finishing this book, I called the women and men I had interviewed over the past three years to see how they were faring as later-in-life parents, hoping that their stories would give you a glimpse into their evolution as parents—and a glimpse of what your future may look like. I called them on a Saturday—when most of them were immersed in child-related activities. Frequently, I had to call back. I asked the women how they dealt with the demands of young children, the generation gap, waning energy levels, work, retirement, aging parents, and looking ahead.

Some of them are "drunk" with motherhood. Some are going full steam ahead with motherhood and career and enjoying a busy—but happy—combination of their child's activities and their own blossoming professional lives. Some almost "have it all." Here are their stories:

In Love with Motherhood

Auben

Auben, now age forty-nine, is now the mother of three-year-old Joe. When I called Auben Saturday morning, she was "knee-deep in chocolate" and other preparations for Joe's third birthday party, and she was unable to come to the phone. I talked with her husband, Eli, who told me that their perspective on financial matters such as retirement and savings accounts had changed since Joe's birth. "I'm going to die on the job and continue working until I'm fired," quipped Eli, who at age fifty-one is trying to save money "so Joe can get a good start." As we spoke, Eli had to quickly get off the phone before Joe could destroy his parent's potted Norfolk pine tree with a toy saw.

When Auben and I spoke, she told me that she changed her mind and decided to work part-time as a psychologist instead of becoming a stay-at-home mom. She loves being a mother and is so "drunk on motherhood" that she's perfectly happy "playing puppy"—a game in which Auben, on all fours, becomes Joe's puppy, and he takes her for short walks around the house.

Like many women of her generation, Auben found herself torn between caring for a small child and an aging parent at the same time. When her mother became seriously ill and was hospitalized in a critical care unit, Auben made plane reservations for herself and her son to fly across country to be at her mother's bedside. Unfortunately, Joe developed an ear infection the day before the flight. Since the changing pressure in an airplane cabin can be both painful and dangerous to someone with an ear infection, Auben put her child's health before her mother's and postponed the flight for a week. It was an excruciating choice. "I felt really bad that I was not there with her, but I wasn't going to travel with a sick child. If it was just me [without a child], I would have gotten on the plane."

Sharlene

When I asked Sharlene, age fifty-four, if she had time to talk to me about life as the parent of a two-year old and a six-year old, she said, "Time?" in an ironic tone that answered my question. No, she had no time that Saturday. She and her husband were out in their backyard building a green and yellow paper mache dragon for their six-year-old's school book fair. Her husband, an engineer, had designed the wire structure for it. Ryan, their six-year-old girl, was making paper mache pumpkins. It was the family's first paper maché adventure.

Sharlene's involvement with book fair preparations had kept her up past midnight all week. She suggested I call her back after 10 or 11 P.M., when she could talk. When we spoke late that night, Sharlene was energetic and clearly going strong, despite her struggle with rheumatoid arthritis. She was nursing Arin, the two-year-old.

Sharlene is pleased with the way her life has worked out and pleased that her only job is mothering her daughters. She's traveled, she's worked hard at various jobs, and now she's enjoying being a stay-at-home mom. "Before I was a workaholic," says Sharlene. "Now I'm so completely happy I don't have a job." For Sharlene, there is no downside to parenthood, only "another side" when children become willful and begin to have a mind of their own. On the whole, she thinks that motherhood gets easier as the children grow out of the toddler stage. Mostly, motherhood makes her happy: "I can be sitting there and one of the children will do something that is so funny or endearing that it fills me with joy just to watch her."

Fortunately, Sharlene is not isolated as a stay-at-home mom, since she socializes with the moms from her daughter's elementary school and work with the PTA. Some of the mothers are young, and some are not, but for Sharlene age is not a problem. But sometimes people stop and ask her: "Oh, you have the grandkids?" Sharlene corrects the mistake: "No, they're mine."

Having It All—Almost

Cathy and Kevin

The last time I saw Kevin and Cathy, they were playing "catch the butterflies" with their two young daughters, Amy and Susan, and chasing the girls around their neighborhood cul de sac. Susan (age three) and Amy (age six) were wearing their Halloween butterfly outfits complete with homemade gauzy wings, and Kevin, age forty-one, and Cathy, age thirty-nine, were waving whimsical butterfly catchers.

When I first interviewed the couple two years before, Cathy was distracted by the demands of two children and yearning for adult conversation. Cathy had decided to put mothering before her career, and she was working part-time. Kevin was worried that fatherhood would put a serious crimp in his academic career. He was delighted to be the father of two daughters, yet he feared that his productivity would inevitably decrease. We talked about the trials of trying to write in the presence of a baby who is intent upon getting her parents' attention. Kevin declared that the notion of plunking away at your computer while your baby quietly sleeps beside you was a nice idea, but not part of the reality of parenting.

But Kevin's fears did not materialize. When I spoke to Cathy last Saturday, she told me that she and Kevin had written a scientific paper, they were about to publish it in a top journal, their daughters were thriving, and life was going very well indeed.

A Mixed Bag

Rhonda

Rhonda, forty-four, the energetic mother of a five-year-old boy, Ian, and an adopted three-year-old girl, Fiona, finds satisfaction in work, motherhood, and many other activities.

"Motherhood is more important and more fulfilling than anything I've done in my life. It's made my life complete—and I already had a full life and lots of adventures," says Rhonda. For her, the ups and downs of parenting in midlife are the same as those at any time of life, although she thinks she has less energy at forty-four than she had at thirty-four.

Although Rhonda says she puts motherhood first and structures her work schedule, her workout schedule, and her volunteer work around her kids' schedules, she still needs to keep up her outside activities. She works out, swing dances, and makes jewelry. "If I were with kids twenty-four/seven, I'd go bonkers."

To spend time with her children, Rhonda has arranged flex-time at work that allows her to pick up her children at school or daycare at 3:00 P.M., take them home, and finish the remaining part of her day's work at home. As our conversation neared its end, Rhonda told me two stories that neatly sum up the ups and downs of parenthood at any stage of life. First she described her children's excitement about Halloween: "Last night they were dancing. Ian was wearing his vampire cape and Fiona was wearing the princess dress I got for her. And both of them are wearing the new slippers I bought for them. They were singing and twirling around." Then she described those other moments—usually brief but not always—when children are less than charming: "Sometimes it's horrible to be trapped on a long car ride in a car with them. They both want to talk at once. They scream, 'It's my turn to talk!' They want me to serve them drinks while I'm driving. It jangles the nerves."

Dion

Dion, age fifty-four, is "busy all the time" with work and her twin boys, Alex and Matthew. When I called Dion on Saturday afternoon, she was on the phone with the pediatrician to find out if eight-year-old Matthew had a strep infection. She told me later that he'd been "vomiting buckets all morning." In her philosophical yet straight-from-the-shoulder New York City style, Dion told me that motherhood was "going good," but that it was "such a mixed bag. You get part of what you want. The good things . . . and you get a down-side that you didn't expect."

As we talked, I could hear Dion's son, Alex, clammer for her attention. "Give me two minutes. And I'll be all yours," said Dion, trying to bargain with him. A minute later I hear her say to him: "I'll get the train set down in a minute . . . One . . . Two . . . I'm talking to my friend." Dion tells me she fears Alex will bring the closet shelf down on top of himself if he gets the train set on his own.

Although Dion finds herself "slowing down a little" at age fifty-four, she still runs, lifts weights, does wind sprints, and stays fit. But she can't change the fact that she is older than many other parents who have children her sons' age. A few weeks earlier, when she kissed one of the boys good night, he told her that he was embarrassed by her and by his father because his father was "old" and because his mother had hair color that was different from his. Matthew's hair is blonde—and Dion's is gray-white. "I could dye my hair like some of the other mothers," she told him. "But I have white hair and that's just how it is." After she left his room, she cried. She thought about that day sometime in the future when she would tell her sons they were conceived using donor eggs and sperm.

Adding It All Up

How much age becomes an issue for you and your children will depend upon your individual personalities, your health, and your stage in life. When I was ten, my mother was forty-nine and my father was sixty. As my mother entered menopause, I entered adolescence—which, as you might imagine, caused some emotional turbulence. Although both my parents seemed old to me at that point in my life, by the time I was twenty they seemed to have grown younger. My mother, now ninety-two, is youthful and flexible in mind and spirit, but she is ill and requires considerable care. However, many of my friends have lost parents who were many years younger than my mother even though the odds were in their favor.

Some experts say that midlife mothers frequently have a more mature perspective, more flexibility, and fewer anxieties than younger mothers. Furthermore, midlife moms are confident, financially stable, and resourceful.

Dr. Margaret Bates, a Los Angeles obstetrician who sees many patients in thirties as well as their mid to late forties, is optimistic about pregnancy later in life. "Older parents have more flexibility. Older women should be encouraged: You have a lot to offer a child that you couldn't offer when you were a teenager or in your twenties. A lot of women I see in the older age group—between forty-eight and fifty—have a much easier time being parents that women in their thirties. When you get to your forties, you are able to organize your priorities," says Bates.

If motherhood is one of your top priorities, you will find a way to bring a child into your life whether you become pregnant or you adopt, and, in so doing, you will add a challenging and fulfilling new dimension to your life.

Bibliography

Author's Foreword and Introduction

• • •

Personal interviews (taped) with: Anna, Auben, Dr. Margaret Bates, Dion, Holly, Jessica, Joanne, Dr. Allen Killam, Dr. Donna Kirz, Leda, Miriam, Rhonda, Sarah, Susan, Dr. Mark Sauer, the late Dr. Manuel Spiegel, and Edith Spiegel Winkelman

American Society for Reproductive Medicine. *Media Fact Sheet on Infertility*. Washington, DC: May, 1999.

American Society for Reproductive Medicine (ASRM). Multiple Pregnancy Associated with Infertility Therapy. *A Practice Committee Report: An Educational Bulletin*. November, 2000.

Berkowitz GS, Skovron ML, Lapinski RH, Berkowitz RL. Delayed Childbearing and the Outcome of Pregnancy. *N Engl J Med* 1990; 322:659–64.

Bianco A, Stone J, Lynch L, Lapinski R, Berkowitz G, Berkowitz R. Pregnancy Outcome at Age 40 and Older. *Am J Obstet Gynecol* 1996; 87:917–22.

Bobrowski RA, Bottoms SF. Underappreciated Risks of the Elderly Multipara. *Am J Obstet Gynecol* 1995; 172:1764–70.

Buehler JW, Kaunitz AM, Hogue CJ, Hughes JM, Smith JC, Rochat RW. Maternal Mortality Aged 35 Years or Older: United States. *JAMA* 1986; 255:53–57.

Cnattingius S, Brendes HW, Forman MR. Do Delayed Childbearers Face Increased Risks of Adverse Pregnancy Outcomes After the First Birth? *Obstet Gynecol* 1993; 81:512–6.

Curtin SC, Martin JA. Births: Preliminary Data for 1999. *National Vital Statistics Reports* August 8, 2000; 48(14).

Czeizel A. Maternal Mortality, Fetal Death, Congenital Anomalies and Infant Mortality at an Advanced Maternal Age. *Maturitas,* Suppl.1 (1988):73–81.

Dildy GA, Jackson GM, Fowers GK, Oshiro BT, Varner MW, Clark SL. Very Advanced Maternal Age: Pregnancy after Age 45. *Am J Obstet Gynecol* 1996; 175:668–74.

Enkin M, Keirse MJ, Neilson J, Crowther C, Duley L, Hodnett E, Hofmeyr J. *A Guide to Effective Care in Pregnancy and Childbirth* (3rd ed.). New York: Oxford Press, 2000.

Enkin M, Keirse MJ, Renfrew M. Neilson J. *A Guide to Effective Care in Pregnancy and Childbirth* (2nd ed.). New York: Oxford University Press, 1995.

Forman RF, Meirik O, Berendes HW. Delayed Childbearing in Sweden. *JAMA* 1984; 252:3135–9.

Gordon D, Milberg J, Daling J, Hicock D. Advanced Maternal Age as a Risk Factor for Cesarean Delivery. *Obstet Gynecol* 1991; 77:493–7.

Haines CJ, Rogers MS, Leung DHY. Neonatal Outcome and Its Relationship with Maternal Age. *Aust NZ J Obstet Gynaecol* 1991; 31(3):209–12.

Hollander D, Breen JL. Pregnancy in the Older Gravida: How Old Is Old? Review. *Obstetrical and Gynecological Survey* 1990; 45(2):106–11.

Keefe DL. Reproductive Aging Is an Evolutionarily

Programmed Strategy That No Longer Provides Adaptive Value. *Fertil Steril* 1998; 70(2):204–5.

Kirz DS, Dorchester W, Freeman RK. Advanced Maternal Age: The Mature Gravida. *Am J Obstet Gynecol* 1985; 152:7–12.

Kitzinger S. *Birth Over Thirty-Five*. New York: Penguin Books, 1994.

Lavin ER, Wood SH. *The Essential Over 35 Pregnancy Guide*. New York: Avon Books, 1998.

Lehmann DK, Chism J. Pregnancy Outcome in Medically Complicated and Uncomplicated Patients Aged 49 Years or Older. *Am J Obstet Gynecol* 1987; 157:738–42.

Maroulis GB. Fertility, Pregnancy, and the Older Woman. *Contemporary OB/GYN* May 1993:101–23.

Martel MM, Wacholder S, Lippman A, Brohan J, Hamilton E. Maternal Age and Primary Cesarean Section Rates: A Multivariate Analysis. *Am J Obstet Gynecol* 1987; 156:305–8.

Martin JA, Hamilton BE, Ventura MA. Births: Preliminary Data for 2000. *Month Vital Stat* Rep 2001; 49.

Narayan H, Buckett W, McDougall W, Cullimore J. Pregnancy after Fifty: Profile and Pregnancy Outcome in a Series of Elderly Multigravidae. *European Journal of Obstetrics & Gynecology and Reproductive Biology* 1992; 47:47–51.

Prysak M, Lorenz RP, Kisley A. Pregnancy Outcome in Nulliparous Women 35 Years and Older. *Obstet Gynecol* 1995; 85:65–70.

Resnick R. Editorial. The "Elderly Primigravida" in 1990. *N Eng J Med* 1990; 322:693–694.

Robinson EG, Garner DM, Gare DJ, Crawford B. Psychological Adaptation to Pregnancy in Childless Women More than 35 Years of Age. *Am J Obstet Gynecol* 1987; 156:328.

Rodriguez N. Reproduction in the Older Gravida. *The Journal of Reprod Medicine* Dec 12, 1999.

Sauer MV. Extending Reproductive Potential in the Older Woman. In *Treatment of the Postmenopausal Woman: Basic and Clinical Aspects*, Lobo RA, ed. New York: Raven Press, Ltd., 1994.

Sauer MV, Paulson RJ. Human Oocyte and Preembryo Donation: An Evolving Method for the Treatment of Infertility. *Am J Obstet Gynecol* 1990; 163(5):1421–4.

Sauer MV, Paulson RJ, Ary BA, Lobo RA. Three Hundred Cycles of Oocyte Donation at the University of Southern California: Assessing the Effect of Age and Infertility Diagnosis on Pregnancy and Implantation Rates. *Journal of Assisted Reproduction and Genetics* 1990; 11(2):92–95.

Sauer MV, Paulson RJ, Lobo RA. A Preliminary Report on Oocyte Donation Extending Reproductive Potential to Women Over 40. *N Engl J Med* 1990; 323:1157–60.

Sauer MV, Paulson RJ, Lobo RA. Reversing the Natural Decline in Human Fertility. *JAMA* 1992; 268:1275–79.

Schroetenboer-Cox K, Weiss JS. *Pregnancy Over 35*. New York: Ballentine Books, 1985.

Shapiro H, Lyons E. Late Maternal Age and Postdate Pregnancy. *Am J Obstet Gynecol* 1989; 160:909–12.

Stein ZA. A Woman's Age: Childbearing and Child Rearing. Reviews and Commentary. *Am J Epidemiol* 1985; 121:327–40.

Stoval DW, Toman SK, Hammond MG, Talbert LM. The Effect of Age on Female Fecundity. *Obstet Gynecol* 1991; 77:33–6.

Ventura SJ, Martin JA, Curtin SC, Mathews TJ. Report of Final Natality Statistics, 1996. *Monthly Vital Statistics Report* (Suppl.) June 1998; 46(11).

Ventura SJ, Martin JA, Curtin SC, Mathews TJ, Park MM.

Births: Final Data for 1998. *National Vital Statistics Report* March 2000; 48(3).

Winkelman, CF. "The Fertility Gods." *Southern Exposure,* Summer 1996.

Winkelman, CF. "The Fertility Gods: Making Babies." *The Chapel Hill News,* 24 June 1995.

Winkelman, CF. "Science Outstrips Meaning of the Name 'Mom.'" *The Chapel Hill News,* 30 June 1995.

Part One: Changing Times, Changing Options
Chapter 1: Changing Perspectives: Midlife Mothers and Fathers

• • •

Personal interviews (taped) with: Anna, Dr. Margaret Bates, Dr. Gertrude Berkowitz, Dr. Watson Bowes Jr., Dr. Mark Dwight, Holly, Joanne, Dr. Allen Killam, Dr. Donna Kirz, Leda, Dr. David Meldrum, Miriam, Dr. Brooks Ranney, Dr. Mark Sauer, Dr. David Walmer

1995 interviews for *The Chapel Hill News,* "The Fertility Gods": Dr. Maria Bustillo

Berkowitz GS, Skovron ML, Lapinski RH, Berkowitz RL. Delayed Childbearing and the Outcome of Pregnancy. *N Engl J Med* 1990; 322:659–64.

Bianco A, Stone J, Lynch L, Lapinski R, Berkowitz G, Berkowitz R. Pregnancy Outcome at Age 40 and Older. *Obstet Gynecol* 1996; 87:917–22.

Bobrowski RA, Bottoms SF. Underappreciated Risks of the Elderly Multipara. *Am J Obstet Gynecol* 1995; 172:1764–70.

Buehler JW, Kaunitz AM, Hogue CJ, Hughes JM, Smith JC, Rochat RW. Maternal Mortality Aged 35 Years or Older: United States. *JAMA* 1986; 255:53–7.

Cnattingius S, Brendes HW, Forman MR. Do Delayed Childbearers Face Increased Risks of Adverse Pregnancy Outcomes After the First Birth? *Obstet Gynecol* 1993; 81:512–6.

Curtin SC, Martin JA. Births: Preliminary Data for 1999. *National Vital Statistics Reports* August 8, 2000) 48(14).

Czeizel A. Maternal Mortality, Fetal Death, Congenital Anomalies and Infant Mortality at an Advanced Maternal Age. *Maturitas* (Suppl.) 1988; 1:73–81.

Dildy GA. Very Advanced Maternal Age: Pregnancy after Age 45. *Am J Obstet Gynecol* 1996; 175:668–74.

Forman RF, Meirik O, Berendes HW. Delayed Childbearing in Sweden. *JAMA* 1984; 252:3135–9.

Kirz DS, Dorchester W, Freeman RK. Advanced Maternal Age: The Mature Gravida. *Am J Obstet Gynecol* 1985; 152:7–12.

Sauer MV. Extending Reproductive Potential in the Older Woman. In *Treatment of the Postmenopausal Woman: Basic and Clinical Aspects*, Lobo RA, ed. New York: Raven Press, Ltd., 1994.

Sauer MV, Paulson RJ, Lobo RA. A Preliminary Report on Oocyte Donation Extending Reproductive Potential to Women Over 40. *N Engl J Med* 1990; 323:1157–60.

Ventura SJ, Martin JA, Curtin SC, Mathews TJ. Report of Final Natality Statistics, 1996. *Monthly Vital Statistics Report* (Suppl.) June 30, 1998; 46(11).

Ventura SJ, Martin JA, Curtin SC, Mathews TJ, Park MM. Births: Final Data for 1998. *National Vital Statistics Report* March 28, 2000; 48(3).

Winkelman, CF. "Science Outstrips Meaning of the Name 'Mom.'" *The Chapel Hill News,* 30 June 1995.

Part Two: Preparing for Midlife Pregnancy
Chapter 2: Prepregnancy Health Plan

* * *

Personal interviews (taped) with: Dr. Watson Bowes Jr., Dr. Alice Domar, Dr. Allen Killam, Dr. Donna Kirz, Dr. Gideon Koren (Motherisk), Dr. Sandra Kweder (FDA), Naravi Payne, Dr. Susan Porto, Dr. Brooks Ranney, Dr. Katherine Shaw

Barbieri RL, Domar AD, Loughlin KR. *6 Steps to Increased Fertility.* New York: Simon and Schuster, 2000.

Curtis GB, Schuler J. *Your Pregnancy Over 30.* Tuscon, AZ: Fisher Books, 1996.

Domar AD, Clapp D, Slawsby EA, Dusek J, Kessel B, Freizinger M. Impact of Group Psychological Interventions on Pregnancy Rates in Infertile Women. *Fertil Steril* 2000; 73:805–12.

Domar AD, Dreher H. *Healing Mind, Healthy Woman.* New York: Dell Publishing, 1996.

Gibbs RS, Sweet RL. Maternal and Fetal Infectious Disorders. In *Obstetrics: Normal and Problem Pregnancies* (3rd ed.), Gabbe SG, Niebyl JR, Simpson JL, eds. Philadelphia: Churchill Livingstone, 1996.

Graedon J, Graedon T. *The People's Pharmacy.* New York: Graedon Enterprises, 1996.

Jewell D, Young G. Interventions for Nausea and Vomiting in Early Pregnancy (Cochrane Review). In *The Cochrane Library*, 1, 2001. Oxford: Update Software.

Johnson TR, Walker MA, Niebyl JR. Preconception and Prenatal Care. In *Obstetrics: Normal and Problem Pregnancies* (3rd ed.), Gabbe SG, Niebyl JR, Simpson JL, eds. New York: Churchill Livingstone, 1996.

Jones KL. Effects of Therapeutic, Diagnostic, and

Environmental Agents. In *Obstetrics: Normal and Problem Pregnancies* (3rd ed.). Gabbe SG, Niebyl JR, Simpson JL, eds. Philadelphia: Churchill Livingstone, 1996.

Kitzinger S. *The Complete Book of Pregnancy and Childbirth*. New York: Alfred A. Knopf, 1997.

Lee RV. *Medical Care of the Pregnant Patient*. Philadelphia: American College of Physicians, 2000.

Leiter, G, Kranz R. *Everything You Need to Know to Have a Healthy Twin Pregnancy*. New York: Dell Publishing, 2000.

Merck & Co. *Drugs in Pregnancy. The Merck Manual*. Whitehouse Station, NJ: Merck & Co. Inc., 1995–2000.

Motherisk. (*www.motherisk.com*)

Niebyl JR. Drugs in Pregnancy and Lactation. In *Obstetrics: Normal and Problem Pregnancies* (3rd ed.). Gabbe SG, Niebyl JR, Simpson JL, eds. Philadelphia: Churchill Livingstone, 1996.

Payne NB. *The Language of Fertility*. New York: Harmony Books, 1997.

Payne NB. *The Whole Person Fertility Program*. New York: Three Rivers Press, 1997.

Physicians' Desk Reference (Edition 54). Montvale, NJ: Medical Economics Company, Inc., 2000.

Reece AE, Hobbins JC, Mahoney MJ, Petrie RH. *Handbook of Medicine of the Fetus & Mother*. Philadelphia: J.B. Lippincott Company, 1995.

Reprotox. (*www.Reprotox.org*)

Simkin P, Whalley J, Keppler A. *Pregnancy, Childbirth, and the Newborn*. New York: Meadowbrook Press, 1991.

TERIS (Teratology Information Services). (888) 285-3410.

Young G, Jewell D. Interventions for Preventing and Treating Backache in Pregnancy (Cochrane Review). In *The Cochrane Library*, 1, 2001. Oxford: Update Software.

Chapter 3: Lifestyle

* * *

Personal interviews (taped) with: Louise Aucott CNM, Dr. Watson Bowes Jr., Michelle Brill MPH, Dr. Alice Domar, Laraine Guyette CNM/Ph.D., Kathleen R., Dr. Allen Killam, Dr. Donna Kirz, Miriam, Dr. Susan Porto, Dr. Katherine Shaw

Abrams B, Pickett KE. Maternal Nutrition. In *Maternal-Fetal Medicine* (4th ed.). Creasy RK, Resnik R, eds. Philadelphia: W.B. Saunders Company, 1997.

Andres RL. Social and Illicit Drug Use in Pregnancy. In *Maternal-Fetal Medicine* (4th ed.). Creasy RK, Resnik R, eds. Philadelphia: W.B. Saunders Company, 1997.

Artal-Mittelmark R, Wiswell RA, Drinkwater BL, eds. *Exercise in Pregnancy*. Baltimore: Williams & Wilkins, 1991.

Barbieri RL, Domar AD, Loughlin KR. *6 Steps to Increased Fertility*. New York: Simon and Schuster, 2000.

Brown, JE. *Nutrition and Pregnancy: A Complete Guide from Preconception to Postdelivery*. Los Angeles: Lowell House, 1998.

De Swiet M. Pulmonary Disorders. In *Maternal-Fetal Medicine* (4th ed.). Creasy RK, Resnik R, eds. Philadelphia: W.B. Saunders Company.

Domar AD, Clapp D, Slawsby EA, Dusek J, Kessel B, Freizinger M. Impact of Group Psychological Interventions on Pregnancy Rates in Infertile Women. *Fertil Steril* 2000; 73:805–12.

Domar AD, Dreher H. *Healing Mind, Healthy Woman*. New York: Dell Publishing, 1996.

Institute of Medicine. *Nutrition During Pregnancy*. Washington, DC: National Academy Press, 1990.

Lee RV. *Medical Care of the Pregnant Patient*. Philadelphia: American College of Physicians, 2000.

Payne NB. *The Language of Fertility*. New York: Harmony Books, 1997.

Payne NB. *The Whole Person Fertility Program*. New York: Three Rivers Press, 1997.

Reece AE, Hobbins JC, Mahoney MJ, Petrie RH. *Handbook of Medicine of the Fetus & Mother*. Philadelphia: J.B. Lippincott Company, 1995.

Simkin P, Whalley J, Keppler A. *Pregnancy, Childbirth, and the Newborn*. New York: Meadowbrook Press, 1991.

Chapter 4: Choosing Your Medical Care Provider: The Best Person and Place

* * *

Personal interviews (taped) with: Leah Albers CNM/Dr.PH, Amanda, Auben, Louise Aucott CNM, Dr. Watson Bowes Jr., Michelle Brill MPH, Dr. Michael Fisher, Laraine Guyette CNM/Ph.D., Jean, Jessica, Joanne, Kathleen R., Dr. Allen Killam, Dr. Valerie King, Dr. Donna Kirz, Dr. Margaret Nusbaum, Marion McCartney CNM, Dr. Susan Porto, Dr. Edward Quilligan, Joanne Saliba, Dr. Mark Sauer, Pam Spry CNM/Ph.D., Lisa Summers CNM/Dr.PH, Dr. David Walmer

American College of Nurse-Midwives (ACNM). *Highlights of Research Regarding Nurse-Midwifery Practice in the U.S.: Evidence-Based Health Care*. Washington, DC: July 1999.

Byrne JP, Crowther CA, Moss JR. A Randomized Controlled Trial Comparing Birth Centre with Delivery Suite Care in Adelaide, Australia. *Aust NZ J Obstet Gynaecol* 2000; 40(3): 268–74.

Devries R, Benoit C, Van Teijlingen ER, Wrede S, eds. *Birth by Design: Pregnancy, Maternity Care, and Midwifery in North America and Europe*. New York: Routledge, 2001.

Enkin M, Keirse MJ, Neilson J, Crowther C, Duley L,

Hodnett E, Hofmeyr J. *A Guide to Effective Care in Pregnancy and Childbirth* (3rd ed.). New York: Oxford University Press, 2000.

Enkin M, Keirse MJ, Renfrew M, Neilson J. *A Guide to Effective Care in Pregnancy and Childbirth* (2nd ed.). New York: Oxford University Press, 1995.

Hodnett ED. Caregiver support for women during childbirth (Cochrane Review). In *The Cochrane Library*, 1, 2001. Oxford: Update Software.

Hodnett ED. Home-like Versus Conventional Institutional Settings for Birth (Cochrane Review). In *The Cochrane Library* 1, 2001. Oxford: Update Software.

Klaus MH, Kennell JH, Klaus PH. *Mothering the Mother.* Reading, MA: Perseus Books, 1993.

Leiter G, Kranz R. *Everything You Need to Know to Have a Healthy Twin Pregnancy*. New York: Dell Publishing, 2000.

Luke B, Eberlein T. *When You're Expecting Twins, Triplets, or Quads*. New York: Harper Perennial, 1999.

McCartney M, van der Meer A. *The Midwife's Pregnancy and Childbirth Book*. New York: Harper Perennial, 1990.

Murphy PA, Fullerton J. Outcomes of Intended Home Births in Nurse-Midwifery Practice: A Prospective Descriptive Study. *Obstet Gynecol* 1998; 92:461–470.

Noble E. *Having Twins*. Boston: Houghton Mifflin Company, 1991.

Olsen O, Jewel MD. Home Versus Hospital Birth (Cochrane Review). In *The Cochrane Library*, 1, 2001. Oxford: Update Software.

Rooks JP. *Midwifery and Childbirth in America*. Philadelphia: Temple University Press, 1997.

Rooks JP, Weatherby NL, Ernst EK. The National Birth Center Study. Part III—Intrapartum and Immediate Postpartum and Neonatal Complications and Transfers, Postpartum and Neonatal care, Outcomes, and Client Satisfaction. *J Nurse Midwifery* 112 Nov–Dec; 37(6):361–97.

Rooks JP, Weatherby NL, Ernst EKM, Stapelton S, Rosen D, Rosenfeld A. Outcomes of Care in Birth Centers: The National Birth Center Study. *N Engl J Med* 1989; 321:1804–11.

Rosenblatt RA, Dobie SA, Hart LG, Schneeweiss R, Gould D, Raine TR, et al. Interspecialty Differences in the Obstetric Care of Low-Risk Women. *Am J Public Health* 1997; 387:344–52.

Rothman BK. *In Labor: Women and Power in the Birthplace.* New York: W.W. Norton and Company, 1991.

Scott KD, Klaus PH, Klaus MH. The Obstetrical and Postpartum Benefits of Continuous Support During Childbirth. *J Women's Health Gend Based Med* 1999; 8(10):1257–64.

Simkin P, Whalley J, Keppler A. *Pregnancy, Childbirth, and the Newborn.* New York: Meadowbrook Press, 1991.

Turnbull D, Holmes A, Shields N, Cheyne H, Twaddle S, Gilmore WH, et al. Randomized, Controlled Trial of Efficacy of Midwife-Managed Care. *Lancet* 1996; 248:213–18.

Waldenstrom U, Nilsson CA. Experience of Childbirth in Birth Center Care. A Randomized Controlled Study. *Acta Obstet Scand* 1994; 73(7):547–54.

Waldenstrom U, Nilsson CA, Winbladh B. The Stockholm Birth Centre Trial: Maternal and Infant Outcome. *Br J Gynaecol* 1997; 104(4):410–18.

Wiegers TA, Keirse MJ, van der Zee J, Berghs GA. Outcome of Planned Home and Planned Hospital Births in Low Risk Pregnancies: Prospective Study in Midwifery Practices in the Netherlands. *BMJ* 1996; 313:1309–13.

Part Three: Getting Pregnant
Chapter 5: The Good News

• • •

Personal interviews (taped) with: Dr. Margaret Bates, Dion, Dr. Mark Dwight, Dr. Margaret Nusbaum, Dr. Mark Sauer, Dr. David Walmer, Anna, Auben, Holly, Claudia, Cheryl, Kathleen R., Joanne, Jennifer, Jessica, Marsh, Rhonda, Sarah, Sharlene, Sharon, Reyn.

Abma JC, Chandra A, Mosher WD, Peterson LS, Piccinino LJ. Fertility, Family Planning, and Women's Health: New Data From the 1995 National Survey of Family Growth. *Vital and Health Statistics*. U.S. Department of Health and Human Services. Series 23, No. 19. May 1997.

Angell M. New Ways to Get Pregnant. Editorial. *New Engl J Med* 1990; 323(17):1200–1.

Curtin SC, Martin JA. Births: Preliminary Data for 1999. *National Vital Statistics Reports* August 8, 2000; 48(14).

Kearney B. *High-Tech Conception*. New York: Bantam Books, 1998.

Marrs R, Bloch LF, Silverman KK. *Dr. Richard Marrs' Fertility Book*. New York: Delacorte Press, 1997.

National Center for Chronic Disease Prevention and Health Promotion. 1998 Assisted Reproductive Technology Success Rates: National Summary and Fertility Clinic Reports. *CDC's Reproductive Health Information Source. (www2.cdc.gov/nccdphp/drh/art98)*

Sauer MV. Extending Reproductive Potential in the Older Woman. In *Treatment of the Postmenopausal Woman: Basic and Clinical Aspects*, Lobo RA, ed. New York: Raven Press, Ltd., 1994.

Sauer MV, Paulson RJ. Human Oocyte and Preembryo Donation: An Evolving Method for the Treatment of Infertility.

Am J Obstet Gynecol 1990; 163(5):1421–4.

Sauer MV, Paulson RJ, Ary BA, Lobo RA. Three Hundred Cycles of Oocyte Donation at the University of Southern California: Assessing the Effect of Age and Infertility Diagnosis on Pregnancy and Implantation Rates. *Journal of Assisted Reproduction and Genetics* 1994; 11(2):92–5.

Ventura SJ, Martin JA, Curtin SC, Mathews TJ. Report of Final Natality Statistics, 1996. *Monthly Vital Statistics Report* (Suppl.) June 30, 1998; 46(11).

Ventura SJ, Martin JA, Curtin SC, Mathews TJ, Park MM. Births: Final Data for 1998. *National Vital Statistics Report* March 28, 2000; 48(3).

Ventura SJ, Martin JA, Curtin SC, Menacker F, Hamilton BE. Births: Final Data for 1999. *National Vital Statistics Reports* April 17, 2001; 49(1).

Winkelman CF. "The Fertility Gods." *Southern Exposure*, Summer 1996.

Winkelman CF. "The Fertility Gods: Making Babies." *The Chapel Hills News*, 25 June 1995.

Winkelman CF. "Science Outstrips Meaning of the Name 'Mom.'" *The Chapel Hill News*, 30 June 1995.

Chapter 6: Your Odds for Successful Midlife Pregnancy

* * *

Personal interviews (taped) with: Dr. Margaret Bates, Dr. Alice Domar, Dr. Jamie Grifo, Dr. Allen Killam, Leda, Dr. Mark Sauer, Stacy, Dr. David Walmer

Abma JC, Chandra A, Mosher WD, Peterson LS, Piccinino LJ. Fertility, Family Planning, and Women's Health: New Data From the 1995 National Survey of Family Growth. *Vital and Health Statistics*. U.S. Department of Health and Human Services: Centers for Disease Control and National Center for

Health Statistics. Series 23, No. 19. May 1997.

American Society for Reproductive Medicine (ASRM). *NEWS*, February 2, 1999.

American Society for Reproductive Medicine (ASRM). *Researchers Make Advances in Freezing Ovarian Tissue.* ASRM Conference 1999. Toronto, Ontario, Canada, September 25–30, 1999.

ASRM. *Media Fact Sheet on Infertility.* American Society for Reproductive Medicine, 1999.

Aytoz A, Camus M, Tournaye H, Bonduelle M, Van Steirteghem A, Devroey P. Outcome of Pregnancies after Intracytoplasmic Sperm Injection and the Effect of Sperm Origin and Quality on this Outcome. *Fertil Steril* 1998; 70:500–5.

CDC. *1998 Assisted Reproductive Technologies Success Rates.* National Summary and Fertility Clinic Reports. *CDC's Reproductive Health Information Source. (www.cdc.gov/nccdphp/drh/art98/section1.htm)*

Curtin SC, Martin JA. Births: Preliminary Data for 1999. *National Vital Statistics Reports* August 2000; 48(14).

Domar AD, Clapp D, Slawsby EA, Dusek J, Kessel B, Freizinger M. Impact of Group Psychological Interventions on Pregnancy Rates in Infertile Women. *Fertil Steril* 2000; 73:805–12.

Grifo J, Liu H, Zhang J, Krey L. "GV Transfer and Maternal Age." Paper presented at an annual meeting of the American Society of Reproductive Medicine, 1996.

Hill, JA. Recurrent Pregnancy Loss. In *Obstetrics: Normal and Problem Pregnancies* (3rd ed.). Gabbe SJ, Niebyl JR, Simpson JL, eds. Philadelphia: Churchill Livingstone, 1996.

Kearney B. *High-Tech Conception.* New York: Bantam Books, 1998.

Liu H, Wang CW, Grifo JA, Krey LC, Zhang J.

"Reconstruction of Mouse Oocytes by Germinal Vesicle Transfer: Maturity of Host Oocyte Eytoplasm Determines Meiosis." *Human Reproduction.* 1999; 14(9):2357–61.

National Center for Chronic Disease Prevention and Health Promotion: *1998 Assisted Reproductive Technology Success Rates: National Summary and Fertility Clinic Reports.* CDC's Reproductive Health Information Source. *(www2.cdc.gov/nccdphp/drh/art98)*

Pantos K, Meimeti-Damianaki T, Vaxevanoglou T, Kapetanakis E. Oocyte Donation in Menopausal Women Aged over 40 Years. *Human Reproduction* 1993; 8(3):488–91.

Sauer MV. Extending Reproductive Potential in the Older Woman. In *Treatment of the Postmenopausal Woman: Basic and Clinical Aspects*, Lobo RA, ed. New York: Raven Press, Ltd., 1994.

Sauer MV, Paulson RJ. Human Oocyte and Preembryo Donation: An Evolving Method for the Treatment of Infertility. *Am J Obstet Gynecol* 1990; 163(5):1421–4.

Sauer MV, Paulson RJ, Ary BA, Lobo RA. Three Hundred Cycles of Oocyte Donation at the University of Southern California: Assessing the Effect of Age and Infertility Diagnosis on Pregnancy and Implantation Rates. *Journal of Assisted Reproduction and Genetics* 1994; 11(2):92–5.

Sauer MV, Paulson RJ, Lobo RA. Reversing the Natural Decline in Human Fertility. *JAMA* 1992; 268:1275–9.

Scott JR. Immunotherapy for Recurrent Miscarriage (Cochrane Review). In *The Cochrane Library*, 1, 2001. Oxford: Update Software.

Simpson JL. Fetal Wastage. In *Obstetrics: Normal and Problem Pregnancies* (3rd ed.). Gabbe SJ, Niebyl JR, Simpson JL, eds. Philadelphia: Churchill Livingstone, 1996.

Turiel JS. *Beyond Second Opinions.* Berkeley and Los Angeles: University of California Press, 1998.

Van Steirteghem AC, Nagy Z, Joris H, Liu J, Staessen C, Smitz J, et al. High Fertilization and Implantation Rates after Intracytoplasmic Sperm Injection. *Hum Reprod* 1993; 8:1061–6.

Ventura SJ, Martin JA, Curtin SC, Mathews TJ. Report of Final Natality Statistics, 1996. *Monthly Vital Statistics Report* (Suppl.) June 30, 1998; 46(11).

Ventura SJ, Martin JA, Curtin SC, Mathews TJ, Park MM. Births: Final Data for 1998. *National Vital Statistics Report* March 28, 2000; 48(3).

Ventura SJ, Martin JA, Curtin SC, Menacker F, Hamilton BE. Births: Final Data for 1999. *National Vital Statistics Reports* April 17, 2001; 49(1).

Winkelman CF. "The Fertility Gods." *Southern Exposure*, Summer 1996.

Winkelman CF. "The Fertility Gods: Making Babies." *The Chapel Hills News,* 25 June 1995.

Winkelman CF. "Science Outstrips Meaning of the Name 'Mom.'" *The Chapel Hill News,* 30 June 1995.

Wisot A, Meldrum D. *Conceptions & Misconceptions: A Guide Through the Maze of In Vitro Fertilization and Other Assisted Reproduction Techniques.* Vancouver: Hartley & Marks, 1997.

Chapter 7: The "Drugs of Pregnancy": Making Informed Choices about Fertility Drugs and Progesterone

• • •

Personal interviews (taped) with: Dr. Gertrude Berkowitz, Dr. Howard Bern (1995), Dr. Louise Brinton, Dr. Luis Cibils, Dr. Mary Croughan-Minihane, Dr. Richard Hajeck, Dr. Patricia Hartge, Dr. Arthur Herbst, Dr. Lovell Jones, Dr. Louis Keith, Dr. Allen Killam, Dr. Arthur Kohrman, Dr. Gideon Koren,

Leda, Dr. Baruch Modan, Dr. Brooks Ranney, Dr. Elaine Ron, Dr. Mary Anne Rossing, Dr. Mark Sauer, Stacy, Dr. David Walmer, Debra Weiner MPH, Dr. Alice Whittemore

From previous interviews from "The Fertility Gods" in *The Chapel Hill News*: Dr. Richard Marrs, Dr. Arthur Caplan, Dr. Bruce Stadel, Dr. Bernadine Healy

American Society for Reproductive Medicine (ASRM). Multiple Pregnancy Associated with Infertility Therapy. *A Practice Committee Report: An Educational Bulletin.* November 2000.

American Society for Reproductive Medicine (ASRM). Researchers Make Advances in Freezing Ovarian Tissue. ASRM Conference 1999. Toronto, Ontario, Canada, September 25–30, 1999.

Artini PG, Fasciani A, et al. Fertility Drugs and Ovarian Cancer. *Gynecol Endocrinology* 1997; 11(1):59–68.

BBC News. *Health: Ovarian Cancer Link to Infertility Probed.* BBC Online Network *(news.bbc.co.uk/hi/english/health/news)*

Beltsos AN, Odem RR. Ovulation Induction and Ovarian Malignancy. *Semin Reprod endocrinol* 1996; 14(4):367–74.

Berger GS, Goldstein M, Fuerst M. *The Couple's Guide to Fertility.* New York: Doubleday, 1994.

Chitkara U, Berkowitz RL. Multiple Gestations. In *Obstetrics: Normal and Problem Pregnancies*, Gabbe SJ, Niebyl JR, Simpson JL, eds. Philadelphia: Churchill Livingstone, 1996.

Croughan-Minihane, MS. *The Risk of Ovarian Cancer Associated with Infertility and Infertility Treatments, Abstract.* Presented at the 2001 meeting of the American Society for Reproductive Medicine.

Crowther CA. Hospitalization and Bed Rest for Multiple Pregnancy (Cochrane Review). In *The Cochrane Library* 1, 2001. Oxford: Update Software.

Cunha GR, Taguchi O, Namikawa R, et al. Teratogenic Effects of Clomiphene, Tamoxifen, and Diethystilbestral on the Developing Human Female Genital Tract. *Human Pathology.* 1987(18).

Curtin SC, Martin JA. Births: Preliminary Data for 1999. *National Vital Statistics Reports* 2000; 48(14).

Dutton DB. *Worse Than the Disease: Pitfalls of Medical Progress.* Cambridge: Cambridge University Press, 1988.

Enkin M, Keirse MJ, Neilson J, Crowther C, Duley L, Hodnett E, Hofmeyr J. *A Guide to Effective Care in Pregnancy and Childbirth* (3rd ed.). New York: Oxford University Press, 2000.

FDA. *FDA Talk Paper.* January 13, 1993.

Herbst AL, Bern HA, eds. *Developmental Effect of Diethystilbestral (DES) in Pregnancy.* New York: Thieme Stratton, 1981.

Hoescht MR. *Prescribing Information as of February 1996: CLOMID.* The Pharmaceutical Company of Hoescht, 1996.

Hughes E, Collins J, Vandekerckhove P. Clomiphene Citrate for Ovulation Induction in Women with Oligo-amenorrhoea (Cochrane Database System). In *The Cochrane Library,* rev. 2000. Oxford: Update Software.

InterNational Council on Infertility Information Dissemination (INCIID). Overview of Injectable Fertility Drugs. *INCIID Fact Sheet. www.inciid.org,* 1999.

InterNational Council on Infertility Information Dissemination (INCIID). CLOMID Use and Abuse. *INCIID Fact Sheet. www.inciid.org,* 1997.

Johnson JWC, Jones G, King TM. Correspondence. *New Engl J Med.* March 11, 1976: 615.

Jones KL. Effects of Therapeutic, Diagnostic, and Environmental Agents. In *Obstetrics: Normal and Problem Pregnancies* (3rd ed.), Gabbe SG, Niebyl JR, Simpson JL, eds.

Philadelphia: Churchill Livingstone, 1996.

Jones LA. Longterm Effects of Neonatal Administration of Estrogen and Progesterone, Alone and in Combination, on Male BALBc and BALB/cFC3H Mice. *Proceed Soc Exper Med Biol* 1980; 165:17.

Jones LA, Bern HA. Cervicovaginal and Mammary Gland Abnormalities in Balb/cCrgl Mice Treated Neonatally with Progesterone and Estrogen, Alone or in Combination. *Cancer Research* 1979; 39:2560.

Jones LA, Bern HA, Wong L. Cervicovaginal and Mammary Gland Abnormalities in Old BALB/cCrgl Mice Treated Neonatally with Progesterone. *J Toxicol Environ Health* 1977; 3:360–1.

Jones LA, Pacillas-Verjan RP. Transplantability and Sex Steroid Dependence of Cervicovaginal Tumors Derived from Female BALB/cCrgl Mice Neonatally Treated with Ovarian Steroids. *Cancer Research* 1979; 39:2591.

Kearney B. *High-Tech Conception.* New York: Bantam Books, 1998.

Kohrman R, Jones L, Bern H. Correspondence, March 11, 1976. *N Engl J Med*: 614.

Lerner-Geva L, Blumstein T, Modan B. Cohort of Infertile Women, *Israel J Obstet Gynecol* 1997; 8(3).

Luke B, Eberlein T. *When You're Expecting Twins, Triplets, or Quads.* New York: Harper Perennial, 1999.

Marrs RP. Ovarian Stimulation Drugs and Ovarian Cancer: What *Are* the Risks? Comments. Commissioned by the American Fertility Society (now the American Society for Reproductive Medicine), January, 1993.

Marrs R, Bloch LF, Silverman KK. *Dr. Richard Marrs' Fertility Book.* New York: Delacorte Press, 1997.

Modan B, Ron E, Lerner-Geva L, Blumstein T, Menczer J, Rabinovici J, et al. Cancer Incidence in a Cohort of Infertile

Women. *Am J Epidemiol* 1998; 147:1038–42.

Motherisk *(www.motherisk.com)*

National Cancer Institute. Fertility Drugs as a Risk Factor for Ovarian Cancer. *Cancer Facts*. National Cancer Institute, National Institutes of Health, March 3, 1995.

Noble E. *Having Twins*. Boston: Houghton Mifflin Company, 1991.

Paulson RJ, Sachs J. *Rewinding Your Biological Clock*. New York: WH Freeman and Company, 1998.

Paulson RJ, Sauer MV, Lobo RA. In Vitro Fertilization in Unstimulated Cycles: A New Application. *Fertil Steril* 1989; 51:1059.

Physicians' Desk Reference (Edition 54). Montvale, NJ: Medical Economics Company, Inc., 2000.

Ron E, Lunenfeld B, Menczer J, et al. Cancer Incidence in a Cohort of Infertile Women. *Am J Epidemiol* 1997; 125:780–90.

Rosen B, Irvine J, et al. The Feasibility of Assessing Women's Perceptions of the Risks and Benefits of Fertility Drug Therapy in Relation to Ovarian Cancer Risk. *Fertil Steril* 1997; 68(1):90–4.

Rossing MA, Daling JR. Complexity of Surveillance for Cancer Risk Associated with In-vitro Fertilisation. *Lancet,* Nov 6, 1999; 354(9190).

Rossing MA, Daling JR, Weiss NS. Ovarian Tumors in a Cohort of Infertile Women. *The New Engl J Med* 1994; 331:771–6.

Shushan A, Elchalal U, Paltiel O, et al. Human Menopausal Gonad Otropin and the Risk of Epithelial Ovarian Cancer. *Fertil Steril* 1996; 16.

Simpson JL. Fetal Wastage. In *Obstetrics: Normal and Problem Pregnancies* (3rd ed.). Gabbe SJ, Niebyl JR, Simpson JL, eds. Philadelphia: Churchill Livingstone, 1996.

Spirtas R, Kaufman S, Alexander NJ. Fertility Drugs and Ovarian Cancer: Red Alert or Red Herring? *Fertil Steril* 1993; 59(2): 291–3.

Turiel JS. *Beyond Second Opinions.* Berkeley and Los Angeles: University of California Press, 1998.

Unkila-Kallio L, Leminen A. Malignant Tumors of the Ovary or the Breast in Association with Infertility: A Report of Thirteen Cases. *Acta Obstet Gynecol Scand* 1997; 76(2):89–95.

Venn A, Watson L, Bruinsma F, Giles G, Healy D. Risk of Cancer after Use of Fertility Drugs with In Vitro Fertilization. *Lancet,* Nov 6, 1999; 354(9190).

Ventura SJ, Martin JA, Curtin SC, Menacker F, Hamilton BE. Births: Final Data for 1999. *National Vital Statistics Reports* 2001; 49(1).

Ventura SJ, Martin JA, Curtin SC, Mathews TJ, Park MM. *Births: Final Data for 1988. National Vital Statistics Report 2000;* 48(3).

Whittemore A. The Risk of Ovarian Cancer After Treatment for Infertility. Editorial. *N Engl J Med* 1994; 331(12).

Whittemore AS, Harris R, Itnyre J, the Collaborative Ovarian Cancer Group. Charcteristics Relating to Ovarian Cancer Risk: Collaborative Analysis of Twelve U.S. Case-Control Studies. II. Invasive Epithelial Ovarian Cancers in White Women. *Am J Epidemiol* 1992; 136:1184–1203.

Whittemore, AS, Harris R, Itnyre J, Halpern J, the Collaborative Ovarian Cancer Group. Characteristics Relating to Ovarian Cancer Risk: Collaborative Analysis of Twelve US Case-Control Studies. I. Methods. *Am J Epidemiol* 1992; 136:1175–83.

Winkelman, CF. "Cancer Risk a Concern, Doctors Told." *The Chapel Hill News,* 28 July 1995.

Winkelman CF. "The Fertility Gods." *Southern Exposure*, Summer 1996.

Winkelman CF. "The Fertility Gods: Making Babies." *The Chapel Hills News,* 25 June 1995.

Winkelman CF. "Science Outstrips Meaning of the Name 'Mom.'" *The Chapel Hill News,* 30 June 1995.

Winkelman, CF. "UNC Fertility Clinic Toughens Cancer Warning." *The Chapel Hill News,* 11 February 1996.

Winkelman, CF. "UNC's Egg Donor Clinic: Are Doctors Playing Down the Cancer Risk?" *The Chapel Hill News,* 28 June 1995.

Wisot A, Meldrum D. *Conceptions and Misconceptions: A Guide Through the Maze of In Vitro Fertilization and Other Assisted Reproduction Techniques.* Vancouver: Hartley & Marks, 1997.

Chapter 8: Overcoming Age-Related Obstacles to Pregnancy: Fibroids, Endometriosis, Fallopian Tube Problems

❖ ❖ ❖

Personal interviews (taped) with: Dr. Margaret Bates, Dr. Watson Bowes Jr., Dr. Mark Dwight, Dr. Robert Israel, Joanne, Kathleen, Dr. Allen Killam, Dr. Susan Porto, Dr. Mark Sauer, Dr. David Walmer

Kearney B. *High-Tech Conception.* New York: Bantam Books, 1998.

Marrs R, Bloch LF, Silverman KK. *Dr. Richard Marrs' Fertility Book.* New York: Delacorte Press, 1997

Northrup C. *Women's Bodies, Women's Wisdom: Creating Physical and Emotional Health and Healing.* New York: Bantam Books, 1998.

Simpson JL. Fetal Wastage. In *Obstetrics: Normal and Problem Pregnancies,* Gabbe SJ, Niebyl JR, Simpson JL, eds.

Philadelphia: Churchill Livingstone, 1996.

Part Four: You're Pregnant! Nutrition, Exercise, and Environmental Health
Chapter 9: Fitness for the Long Haul

❖ ❖ ❖

Personal interviews (taped) with: Amanda, Dr. Raul Artal Mittelmark, Dr. Watson Bowes Jr., Jessica, Joanne, Dr. Donna Kirz, Miriam, Dr. Susan Porto, John Rogers Ph.D., Dr. Katherine Shaw

Abrams B, Pickett KE. Maternal Nutrition. In *Maternal-Fetal Medicine* (4th ed.). Creasy RK, Resnik R, eds. Philadelphia: W.B. Saunders Company.

Artal Mittelmark R, Wiswell RA, Drinkwater BL, eds. *Exercise in Pregnancy*. Baltimore: Williams & Wilkins, 1991.

Colborn T, Dumanoski D, Meyers JP. *Our Stolen Future*. New York: Dutton, 1996.

Eisenberg A, Murkoff HE, Hathaway SE. *What to Eat When You're Expecting*. New York: Workman Publishing, 1986.

FDA. *All About Eating for Two*. FDA Consumer. U.S. Food and Drug Adminstration, April 1990.

FDA. *Healthy Pregnancy, Healthy Baby*. FDA Consumer, March–April 1999. *(www.cfsan.fda.gov)*

Fuchs A-R, Fuchs F. Physiology and Endocrinology of Parturition. In *Obstetrics: Normal and Problem Pregnancies*, Gabbe SG, Niebyl JR, and Simpson JL, eds. New York: Churchill Livingstone, 1996.

Goldbeck N, Goldbeck D. *American Wholefoods Cuisine*. New York: Plume, 1983.

Institute of Medicine. *Nutrition During Pregnancy*. Washington, DC: National Academy Press, 1990.

Johnson TRB, Walker MA, Niebyl JR. Preconception and Prenatal Care. In *Obstetrics: Normal and Problem Pregnancies*, (3rd ed.). Gabbe SG, Niebyl JR, and Simpson JL, eds. New York: Churchill Livingstone, 1996.

Katz VL, McMurray R, Cephalo R. Aquatic Exercise During Pregnancy, Exercise in Pregnancy. In *Exercise in Pregnancy*. Baltimore: Williams & Wilkins, 1991.

Kramer MS. Regular Aerobic Exercise During Pregnancy (Cochrane Review). In *The Cochrane Library*, 1, 2001. Oxford: Update Software.

Motherisk. *(www.motherisk.com)*

OTIS. *(www.otispregnancy.org)*

Reece AE, Hobbins JC, Mahoney MJ, Petrie RH. *Handbook of Medicine of the Fetus and Mother*. Philadelphia: J.B. Lippincott Company, 1995.

Sever LE, Mortensen ME. Teratology and the Epidemiology of Birth Defects: Occupational and Environmental Perspectives. In *Obstetrics: Normal and Problem Pregnancies* (3rd ed.). Gabbe SG, Niebyl JR, and Simpson JL, eds. New York: Churchill Livingstone, 1996.

Simkin P, Whalley J, Keppler A. *Pregnancy, Childbirth, and the Newborn*. New York: Meadowbrook Press, 1991.

Chapter 10: Pregnant at Work

* * *

Personal interviews (taped) with: Amanda, Dr. Margaret Bates, Dr. Watson Bowes Jr., Cindy, Dr. Alice Domar, Holly, Jennifer, Dr. Allen Killam, Dr. Gideon Koren, Meg, Dr. Susan Porto, Dr. John Rogers, Sarah, Stacy

Jewell D, Young G. Interventions for Nausea and Vomiting in Early Pregnancy (Cochrane Review). In *The Cochrane Library*, 1, 2001. Oxford: Update Software.

Johnson TRB, Walker MA, Niebyl JR. Preconception and Prenatal Care. In *Obstetrics: Normal and Problem Pregnancies*, (3rd ed.). Gabbe SG, Niebyl JR, and Simpson JL, eds. New York: Churchill Livingstone, 1996.

Motherisk. *(www.motherisk.org)*

OSHA. *(www.osha.gov)*

Reece AE, Hobbins JC, Mahoney MJ, Petrie RH. *Handbook of Medicine of the Fetus and Mother*. Philadelphia: J.B. Lippincott Company, 1995.

Sever LE, Mortensen ME. Teratology and the Epidemiology of Birth Defects: Occupational and Environmental Perspectives. In *Obstetrics: Normal and Problem Pregnancies* (3rd ed.). Gabbe SG, Niebyl JR, and Simpson JL, eds. New York: Churchill Livingstone, 1996.

Simkin P, Whalley J, Keppler A. *Pregnancy, Childbirth, and the Newborn*. New York: Meadowbrook Press, 1991.

Part Five: Preventing and Managing Potential Problems
Chapter 11: Who Is High Risk?

* * *

Personal interviews (taped) with: Amanda, Anna, Dr. Howard Bern, Dr. Gertrude Berkowitz, Dr. Watson Bowes Jr., Dr. Murray Enkin, Laraine Guyette CNM/Ph.D., Dr. Murph Goodwin, Dr. Lovell Jones, Dr. Allen Killam, Dr. Donna Kirz, Dr. Susan Porto, Rhonda, Dr. Katherine Shaw, Dr. Mark Sauer, Michelle Trant

Abrams R, Cooper N, Coustan D, Hollander P, Jovanovic-Peterson L, Lorber D, Metzger B, Wason C. *Gestational Diabetes: What to Expect* (3rd ed.). Alexandria, VA: American Diabetes Association, 1997.

Berkowitz GS, Skovron ML, Lapinski RH, Berkowitz RL. Delayed Childbearing and the Outcome of Pregnancy. *N Engl J Med* 1990; 322:659–64.

Bianco A, Stone J, Lynch L, Lapinski R, Berkowitz G, Berkowitz R. Pregnancy Outcome at Age 40 and Older. *Obstet Gynecol* 1996; 87:917–22.

Bobrowski RA, Bottoms SF. Underappreciated Risks of the Elderly Multipara. *Am J Obstet Gynecol* 1995; 172:1764–70.

Buehler JW, Kaunitz AM, Hogue CJ, Hughes JM, Smith JC, Rochat RW. Maternal Mortality Aged 35 Years or Older: United States. *JAMA* 1986; 255:53–7.

Czeizel A. Maternal Mortality, Fetal Death, Congenital Anomalies and Infant Mortality at an Advanced Maternal Age. *Maturitas* (Suppl.) 1988; 1:73–81.

Dildy GA, Jackson GM, Fowers GK, Oshiro BT, Varner MW, Clark SL. Very Advanced Maternal Age: Pregnancy after Age 45. *Am J Obstet Gynecol* 1996; 175:668–74.

Enkin M, Keirse MJ, Neilson J, Crowther C, Duley L, Hodnett E, Hofmeyr J. *A Guide to Effective Care in Pregnancy and Childbirth* (3rd ed.). New York: Oxford University Press, 2000.

Enkin M, Keirse MJ, Renfrew M, Neilson J. *A Guide to Effective Care in Pregnancy and Childbirth* (2nd ed.). New York: Oxford University Press, 1995.

Forman RF, Meirik O, Berendes HW. Delayed Childbearing in Sweden, *JAMA* 1984; 252:3135–9.

Goer H. *Obstetrics Myths Versus Research Realities.* Westport, CT: Bergin & Garvey, 1995.

Goldbeck N, Goldbeck D. *American Wholefoods Cuisine.* New York: Plume, 1983.

Gonik B, Bobrowski RA. Medical Complications of Labor and Delivery. In *Management of Labor and Delivery* (4th ed.). Creasy RK, ed. Boston: Blackwell Science, 1997.

Gordon D, Milberg J, Daling J, Hickok D. Advanced Maternal Age as a Risk Factor for Cesarean Delivery. *Obstet and Gynecol* 1991; 77(4).

Herbst AL, Bern HA, eds. *Developmental Effect of Diethystilbestrol (DES) in Pregnancy.* New York: Thieme Stratton, 1981.

Hill, JA. Recurrent Pregnancy Loss. In *Obstetrics: Normal and Problem Pregnancies* (3rd ed.). Gabbe SJ, Niebyl JR, Simpson JL, eds. Philadelphia: Churchill Livingstone, 1996.

Hollander D, Breen JL. Pregnancy in the Older Gravida: How Old Is Old? Review. *Obstetrical and Gynecological Survey* 1990; 45(2):106–11.

Katz Rothman B. *The Tentative Pregnancy.* New York: W.W. Norton, 1993.

Kirz DS, Dorchester W, Freeman RK. Advanced Maternal Age: The Mature Gravida. *Am J Obstet Gynecol* 1985; 152:7–12.

Landon MB. Diabetes Mellitus and Other Endocrine Diseases. In *Obstetrics: Normal and Problem Pregnancies,* (3rd ed.). Gabbe SJ, Niebyl JR, Simpson JL, eds. Philadelphia: Churchill Livingstone, 1996.

Lavin ER, Wood SH. *The Essential Over 35 Pregnancy Guide.* New York: Avon Books, 1998.

Lehmann DK, Chism J. Pregnancy Outcome in Medically Complicated and Uncomplicated Patients Aged 49 Years or Older. *Am J Obstet Gynecol* 1987; 157:738–42.

Martel MM, Wacholder S, Lippman A, Brohan J, Hamilton E. Maternal Age and Primary Cesarean Section Rates: A Multivariate Analysis. *Am J Obstet Gynecol* 1987; 156:305–8.

McCartney M, van der Meer A. *The Midwife's Pregnancy and Childbirth Book.* New York: Harper Perennial, 1990.

Moore TR. Diabetes in Pregnancy. In *Obstetrics: Normal and Problem Pregnancies* (3rd ed.). Gabbe SJ, Niebyl JR, Simpson JL, eds. Philadelphia: Churchill Livingstone, 1996.

Narayan H, Buckett W, McDougall W, Cullimore J. Pregnancy after Fifty: Profile and Pregnancy Outcome in a Series of Elderly Multigravidae. *European Journal of Obstetrics and Gynecology and Reproductive Biology* 1992; 47:47–51.

Prysak M, Lorenz RP, Kisley A. Pregnancy Outcome in Nulliparous Women 35 Years and Older. *Obstet Gynecol* 1995; 85:65–70.

Reece AE, Hobbins JC, Mahoney MJ, Petrie RH, eds. *Handbook of Medicine of the Fetus and Mother*. Philadelphia: J.B. Lippincott Company, 1995.

Resnick R. Editorial. The "Elderly Primigravida" in 1990. *N Eng J Med* 1990; 322:693–4.

Roberts JM. Pregnancy-Related Hypertension. In *Obstetrics: Normal and Problem Pregnancies* (3rd ed.), Gabbe SJ, Niebyl JR, Simpson JL, eds. Philadelphia: Churchill Livingstone, 1996.

Sibai BM. Hypertension in Pregnancy. In *Obstetrics: Normal and Problem Pregnancies* (3rd ed.). Gabbe SJ, Niebyl JR, Simpson JL, eds. Philadelphia: Churchill Livingstone, 1996.

Simkin P, Whalley J, Keppler A. *Pregnancy, Childbirth, and the Newborn*. New York: Meadowbrook Press, 1991.

Simpson JL. Fetal Wastage. In *Obstetrics: Normal and Problem Pregnancies* (3rd ed.). Gabbe SJ, Niebyl JR, Simpson JL, eds. Philadelphia: Churchill Livingstone, 1996.

Ventura SJ, Martin JA, Curtin SC, Mathews TJ, Park MM. Births: Final Data for 1998. *National Vital Statistics Report* March 28, 2000; 48(3).

Ventura SJ, Martin JA, Curtin SC, Menacker F, Hamilton BE. Births: Final Data for 1999. *National Vital Statistics Reports* April 17, 2001; 49(1).

Chapter 12: Genetic Testing, Genetic Counseling, and Other Forms of Prenatal Diagnosis

* * *

Personal interviews (taped) with: Anna, Dr. Murph Goodwin, Holly, Connie, Joanne, Kathleen R., Dr. Allen Killam, DeeDee Lafayette, Rhonda, Dr. Susan Porto, Dr. Katherine Shaw, Michelle, Melissa.

Alfirevic Z. Early Amniocentesis Versus Transabdominal Chorion Villus Sampling for Prenatal Diagnosis (Cochrane Review). In The *Cochrane Library*, 1, 2001. Oxford: Update Software.

Enkin M, Keirse MJ, Neilson J, Crowther C, Duley L, Hodnett E, Hofmeyr J. *A Guide to Effective Care in Pregnancy and Childbirth* (3rd ed.). New York: Oxford University Press, 2000.

Gibbs RS, Sweet RL. Maternal and Fetal Infectious Disorders. In *Maternal-Fetal Medicine* (4th ed.). Creasy RK, Resnik R, eds. Philadelphia: W.B. Saunders Company.

Katz Rothman, B. *The Tentative Pregnancy*. New York: W.W. Norton and Company, Inc., 1993.

Neilson, JP. Ultrasound for Fetal Assessment in Early Pregnancy (Cochrane Review). In *The Cochrane Library*, 1, 2001. Oxford: Update Software.

Reece AE, Hobbins JC, Mahoney MJ, Petrie RH. *Handbook of Medicine of the Fetus and Mother*. Philadelphia: J.B. Lippincott Company, 1995.

Scioscia AL. Prenatal Genetic Diagnosis. In *Maternal-Fetal Medicine* (4th ed.). Creasy RK, Resnik R, eds. Philadelphia: W.B. Saunders Company.

Simpson JL. Genetic Counseling and Prenatal Diagnosis. In *Obstetrics: Normal and Problem Pregnancies* (3rd ed.). Gabbe SJ, Niebyl JR, Simpson JL, eds. Philadelphia:

Churchill Livingstone, 1996.

Chapter 13: Coping with Pregnancy Loss

• • •

Personal interviews (taped) with: Anna, Holly, Dr. Allen Killam, Leda, Rhonda, Susan

Curtis GB. *Your Pregnancy After 30*. Tucson, AZ: Fischer Books, 1996.

Kitzinger, S. *The Complete Book of Pregnancy and Childbirth*. New York: Alfred A. Knopf, 1997.

Luke B, Eberlein T. *When You're Expecting Twins, Triplets, or Quads*. New York: Harper Perennial, 1999.

Noble E. *Having Twins*. Boston: Houghton Mifflin Company, 1991.

Reece AE, Hobbins JC, Mahoney MJ, Petrie RH, eds.. *Handbook of Medicine of the Fetus and Mother*. Philadelphia: J.B. Lippincott Company, 1995.

Simpson JL. Fetal Wastage. In *Obstetrics: Normal and Problem Pregnancies* (3rd ed.). Gabbe SJ, Niebyl JR, Simpson JL, eds. Philadelphia: Churchill Livingston, 1996.

Part Six: Pregnancy with Twins, Triplets, and More

Chapter 14: The Ups and Downs of Pregnancy, Birth, and Parenthood with Multiples

• • •

Personal interviews (taped) with: Dr. Stan Beyler (from 1995 newspaper series, "The Fertility Gods"), Dr. Watson Bowes Jr., Cheryl, Dion, Dr. Mark Dwight, Jean, Dr. Allen Killam, Dr. Louis Keith, Dr. David Meldrum, Dr. Susan Porto, Dr. Mark Sauer, Sharon, Dr. Katherine Shaw, Sharon, Stacy, Dr. David Walmer

Agnew CL, Kelin AH, Ganon JA. *Twins! Pregnancy Birth and the First Year of Life*. New York: Harper Perennial, 1997.

American Society for Reproductive Medicine (ASRM). Multiple Pregnancy Associated with Infertility Therapy. *A Practice Committee Report: An Educational Bulletin*. November 2000.

Benirschke K. Multiple Gestation: Incidence, Etiology, and Inheritance. In *Obstetrics: Normal and Problem Pregnancies* (3rd ed.). Gabbe SJ, Niebyl JR, Simpson JL, eds. Philadelphia: Churchill Livingstone, 1996.

Chitkara U, Berkowitz RL. Multiple Gestations. In *Obstetrics: Normal and Problem Pregnancies* (3rd ed.). Gabbe SJ, Niebyl JR, Simpson JL, eds. Philadelphia: Churchill Livingstone, 1996.

Crowther, CA. Caesarean Delivery for the Second Twin (Cochrane Review). In *The Cochrane Library*, 1, 2001. Oxford: Update Software.

Crowther CA. Hospitalization and Bed Rest for Multiple Pregnancy (Cochrane Review). In *The Cochrane Library*, 1, 2001. Oxford: Update Software.

Curtin SC, Martin JA. Births: Preliminary Data for 1999. *National Vital Statistics Reports* 2000; 48(14).

Enkin M, Keirse MJ, Neilson J, Crowther C, Duley L, Hodnett E, Hofmeyr J. *A Guide to Effective Care in Pregnancy and Childbirth* (3rd ed.). New York: Oxford University Press, 2000.

Enkin M, Keirse MJ, Renfrew M, Neilson J. *A Guide to Effective Care in Pregnancy and Childbirth* (2nd ed.). New York: Oxford University Press, 1995.

Kearney B. *High-Tech Conception*. New York: Bantam Books, 1998.

Leiter, G, Kranz R. *Everything You Need to Know to Have a Healthy Twin Pregnancy*. New York: Dell Publishing, 2000.

Luke B, Eberlein T. *When You're Expecting Twins, Triplets, or Quads.* New York: Harper Perennial, 1999.

Noble E. *Having Twins.* Boston: Houghton Mifflin Company, 1991.

Reece AE, Hobbins JC, Mahoney MJ, Petrie RH, eds. *Handbook of Medicine of the Fetus and Mother.* Philadelphia: J.B. Lippincott Company, 1995.

Simpson L, D'Alton ME. Multiple Pregnancy. In *Management of Labor and Delivery* (4th ed.). Creasy RK, ed. Boston: Blackwell Science, 1997.

Ventura SJ, Martin JA, Curtin SC, Mathews TJ. Report of Final Natality Statistics, 1996. *Monthly Vital Statistics Report* (Suppl.) 1998; 46(11).

Ventura SJ, Martin JA, Curtin SC, Mathews TJ, Park MM. Births: Final Data for 1998. *National Vital Statistics Report.* 2000, 48(3).

Ventura SJ, Martin JA, Curtin SC, Menacker F, Hamilton BE. Births: Final Data for 1999. *National Vital Statistics Reports* 2001; 49(1).

Winkelman CF. "The Fertility Gods." *Southern Exposure,* Summer 1996.

Winkelman CF. "The Fertility Gods: Making Babies." *The Chapel Hills News,* 25 June 1995.

Winkelman CF. "Science Outstrips Meaning of the Name 'Mom.'" *The Chapel Hill News,* 30 June 1995.

Winkelman, CF. "UNC's Egg Donor Clinic: Are Doctors Playing Down the Cancer Risk?" *The Chapel Hill News,* 28 June 1995.

Wisot A, Meldrum D. *Conceptions and Misconceptions: A Guide Through the Maze of In Vitro Fertilization and Other Assisted Reproduction Techniques.* Vancouver: Hartley & Marks, 1997.

Part Seven: Giving Birth
Chapter 15: Preparing for Childbirth

* * *

Personal interviews (taped) with: Cecilia Bacom, Elizabeth Bing, Michell Brill, Kathleen Gray Farthing, Holly, Kathleen R., Dr. Allen Killam, Linda-Carol, Marion McCartney CNM, Sharlene

Balaskas J. *Active Birth: The New Approach to Giving Birth.* Cambridge, MA: Harvard Common Press, 1992.

Bing, Elizabeth. *Six Practical Lessons for an Easier Childbirth* (3rd rev. ed.). New York: Bantam Books, 1994.

Bradley, R. *Husband-Coached Childbirth.* New York: Harper & Row, 1981.

Dick-Read G. Childbirth Without Fear: *The Original Approach to Natural Childbirth* (5th ed.). New York: Harper Collins, 1987.

Enkin M, Keirse MJ, Neilson J, Crowther C, Duley L, Hodnett E, Hofmeyr J. *A Guide to Effective Care in Pregnancy and Childbirth* (3rd ed.). New York: Oxford University Press, 2000.

Enkin M, Keirse MJ, Renfrew M, Neilson J. *A Guide to Effective Care in Pregnancy and Childbirth* (2nd ed.). New York: Oxford University Press, 1995.

Fanagan M. Antenatal Preparation for Labor. In *Management of Labor and Delivery* (4th ed.). Creasy RK, ed. Boston: Blackwell Science, 1997.

Goldman L. "The Use of Hypnosis in Obstetrics," *Psychiatric Medicine* 1992; 10(4).

Hathaway M, Hathaway J, and Bek S, eds. *The Bradley Method Student Workbook.* Sherman Oaks, CA: American Academy of Husband-Coached Childbirth, 1989.

Kitzinger S. *The Complete Book of Pregnancy and*

Childbirth. New York: Alfred A. Knopf, 1997.

Klaus MH, Kennell JH, Klaus PH. *Mothering the Mother*. Reading, MA: Perseus Books, 1993.

Leboyer F. *Birth Without Violence*. New York: Knopf, 1975.

Lieberman AB. *Easing Labor Pain*. Boston: The Harvard Common Press, 1992.

McCartney M, van der Meer A. *The Midwife's Pregnancy and Childbirth Book*. New York: Harper Perennial, 1990.

Scott KD, Klaus PH, Klaus MH. The Obstetrical and Postpartum Benefits of Continuous Support During Childbirth. *J Womens Health Gend Based Med* 1999; 8(10).

Simkin P. *The Birth Partner*. Boston: The Harvard Common Press, 1989.

Simkin P, Whalley J, Keppler A. *Pregnancy, Childbirth, and the Newborn*. New York: Meadowbrook Press, 1991.

Chapter 16: Creating a Birth Plan

• • •

Personal interviews (taped) with: Anna, Holly, Kathleen R., Dr. Allen Killam, Dr. Donna Kirz, Sharlene, Penny Simkin

Hathaway M, Hathaway J, and Bek S, eds. *The Bradley Method Student Workbook*. Sherman Oaks, CA: American Academy of Husband-Coached Childbirth, 1989.

Simkin P. *The Birth Partner*. Boston: The Harvard Common Press, 1989.

Chapter 17: Exploring Your Options

• • •

Personal interviews (taped) with: Elizabeth Bing, Michelle Brill MPH, Carla, Nancy Wainer Cohen, Dr. Murray Enkin, Kathleen R., Kathleen Gray Farthing, Laraine Guyette

CNM/Ph.D., Dr. Allen Killam, Dr. Donna Kirz, Dr. Louise Kirz, Marion McCartney CNM, Louise Aucott CNM, Dr. Edward Quilligan, Paula, Dr. Susan Porto, Dr. Edward Quilligan, Sharlene, Penny Simkin, Mary Sommers, Pam Spry CNM/Ph.D., Thelma

American College of Nurse-Midwives (ACNM). *Highlights of Research Regarding Nurse-Midwifery Practice in the U.S.: Evidence-Based Health Care.* Washington, DC.

Arms S. *Immaculate Deception II: Myth, Magic and Birth.* Berkeley: Celestial Arts, 1996.

Enkin M, Keirse MJ, Neilson J, Crowther C, Duley L, Hodnett E, Hofmeyr J. *A Guide to Effective Care in Pregnancy and Childbirth* (3rd ed.). New York: Oxford University Press, 2000.

Enkin M, Keirse MJ, Renfrew M, Neilson J. *A Guide to Effective Care in Pregnancy and Childbirth* (2nd ed.). New York: Oxford University Press, 1995.

Ferguson WG. Management of Labor and Delivery in Low-Risk Patients. In *Management of Labor and Delivery* (4th ed.). Creasy, ed. Boston: Blackwell Science, 1997.

Goer Henci. Obstetric Myths Versus Research Realities: *A Guide to the Medical Literature.* London: Bergin & Garvey, 1995.

Goings JR. The Impact of Midwifery Care, Childbirth Preparation, and Labor Support on Cesarean Section Rates. In *Cesarean Section: Guidelines for Appropriate Utilization,* Flamm BL, Quilligan EJ, eds. New York: Springer-Verlag, 1995.

Harper B. *Gentle Birth Choices.* Rochester, VT: Healing Arts Press, 1994.

Hodnett ED. Caregiver Support for Women During Childbirth (Cochrane Review). In *The Cochrane Library,* 1, 2001. Oxford: Update Software.

Kitzinger S., ed. *The Midwife Challenge*. London: Pandora Press, 1991.

Kitzinger S. *The Complete Book of Pregnancy and Childbirth*. New York: Alfred A. Knopf, 1997.

Klaus MH, Kennell JH, Klaus PH. *Mothering the Mother*. Reading, MA: Perseus Books, 1993.

Korte D. *The VBAC Companion*.

Korte D, Scaer R. *A Good Birth. A Safe Birth*. New York: Bantam, 1984.

MacDorman MF, Singh GK. Midwifery Care, Social and Medical Risk Factors, and Birth Outcomes in the USA. *J Epidemiol Community Health,* 1998; 52:310–17.

McCartney M, van der Meer A. *The Midwife's Pregnancy and Childbirth Book*. New York: Harper Perennial, 1990.

Murphy PA, Fullerton J. Outcomes of Intended Home Births in Nurse-Midwifery Practice: A Prospective Descriptive Study. *Obstet Gynecol* 1998; 92:461–70.

Rooks JP. *Midwifery and Childbirth in America*. Philadelphia: Temple University Press, 1997.

Rooks JP, Weatherby NL, Ernst EK. The National Birth Center Study. Part III—Intrapartum and Immediate Postpartum and Neonatal Complications and Transfers, Postpartum and Neonatal Care, Outcomes, and Client Satisfaction. *J Nurse Midwifery* 112 Nov–Dec; 37(6):361–97.

Rooks JP, Weatherby NL, Ernst EKM, Stapelton S, Rosen D, Rosenfeld A. Outcomes of Care in Birth Centers: The National Birth Center Study. *New England Journal of Medicine* 1989; 321:1804–11.

Rosenblatt RA, Dobie SA, Hart LG, Schneeweiss R, Gould D, Raine TR, et al. Interspecialty Differences in the Obstetric Care of Low-Risk Women. *Am J Public Health* 1997; 387:344–52.

Rothman BK. *In Labor: Women and Power in the*

Birthplace. New York: W.W. Norton and Company, 1991.

Scott KD, Klaus PH, Klaus MH. The Obstetrical and Postpartum Benefits of Continuous Support During Childbirth. *J Women's Health Gend Based Med* 1999; 8(10):1257–64.

Simkin P, Whalley J, Keppler A. *Pregnancy, Childbirth, and the Newborn.* New York: Meadowbrook Press, 1991.

Turnbull D, Holmes A, Shields N, Cheyne H, Twaddle S, Gilmore WH, et al. Randomized, Controlled Trial of Efficacy of Midwife-Managed Care. *Lancet* 1996; 248:213–18.

Ventura SJ, Martin JA, Curtin SC, Menacker F, Hamilton BE. Births: Final Data for 1999. *National Vital Statistics Reports* April 2001; 49(1).

Wiegers TA, Keirse MJNC, van der Zee J, Berghs GAH. Outcome of Planned Home and Planned Hospital Births in Low Risk Pregnancies: Prospective Study in Midwifery Practices in the Netherlands. *BMJ* 1996; 313: 1309–13.

Chapter 18: Due Dates: Preterm and Postterm Births

* * *

Personal interviews (taped) with: Amanda, Dr. Gertrude Berkowitz, Dr. Watson Bowes Jr., Dr. Murray Enkin, Dr. Allen Killam, Pam Spry CNM/Ph.D.

Alfirevic Z. Oral Misoprostol for Induction of Labour (Cochrane Review). In *The Cochrane Library*, 1, 2001. Oxford: Update Software.

Boulvain M, Irion O. Stripping/Sweeping the Membranes for Inducing Labour or Preventing Post-term Pregnancy (Cochrane Review). In *The Cochrane Library*, 1, 2001. Oxford. Update Software.

Boylan PC. General Principles of Labor Management. Creasy RK, ed. Boston: Blackwell Science, 1997.

Creasy RK. Normal Labor and Delivery. In *Management of*

Labor and Delivery (4th ed.). Creasy RK, ed. Boston: Blackwell Science, 1997.

Creasy RK. Preterm Delivery. In *Management of Labor and Delivery*, Creasy RK, ed. Boston: Blackwell Science, 1997.

Creasy RK, Iams JD. Preterm Labor and Delivery. In *Obstetrics: Normal and Problem Pregnancies* (3rd ed.). Gabbe SJ, Niebyl JR, Simpson JL, eds. Philadelphia: Churchill Livingstone, 1996.

Crowley, P. Interventions for Preventing or Improving the Outcome of Delivery at or Beyond Term (Cochrane Review). In *The Cochrane Library*, 1, 2001. Oxford: Update Software.

Enkin M, Keirse MJ, Neilson J, Crowther C, Duley L, Hodnett E, Hofmeyr J. *A Guide to Effective Care in Pregnancy and Childbirth* (3rd ed.). New York: Oxford University Press, 2000.

Enkin M, Keirse MJ, Renfrew M, Neilson J. *A Guide to Effective Care in Pregnancy and Childbirth* (2nd ed.). New York: Oxford University Press, 1995.

Glantz JC, Woods JR Jr. Significance of Amniotic Fluid Meconium. In *Obstetrics: Normal and Problem Pregnancies* (3rd ed.). Gabbe SJ, Niebyl JR, Simpson JL, eds. Philadelphia: Churchill Livingstone, 1996.

Goer H. *Obstetrics Myths Versus Research Realities: A Guide to the Medical Literature.* London: Bergin & Garvey, 1995.

Hofmeyr GJ. Amnioinfusion for Meconium-Stained Liquor in Labour (Cochrane Review). In *The Cochrane Library*, 1, 2001. Oxford: Update Software.

Hofmeyr GJ, Gulmezoglu AM. Vaginal Misoprostol for Cervical Ripening and Induction of Labour (Cochrane Review). In *The Cochrane Library*, 1, 2001. Oxford: Update Software.

Reece AE, Hobbins JC, Mahoney MJ, Petrie RH, eds.

Handbook of Medicine of the Fetus and Mother. Philadelphia: J.B. Lippincott Company, 1995.

Resnik R, Calder A. Post-Term Pregnancy. In *Obstetrics: Normal and Problem Pregnancies* (3rd ed.). Gabbe SJ, Niebyl JR, Simpson JL, eds. Philadelphia: Churchill Livingstone, 1996.

Smith CA, Crowther CA. Acupuncture for Induction of Labour (Cochrane Review). In *The Cochrane Library*, 1, 2001. Oxford: Update Software.

Solomon JE, D'Alton ME. Induction of Labor. In *Management of Labor and Delivery* (4th ed.). Creasy RK, ed. Boston: Blackwell Science, 1997.

Tan BP, Hannah ME. Oxytocin for Prelabour Rupture of Membranes at or Near Term (Cochrane Review). In *The Cochrane Library*, 1, 2001. Oxford: Update Software.

Chapter 19: What Is Labor?

❋ ❋ ❋

Personal interviews (taped) with: Leah Albers CNM, Anna, Auben, Louise Aucott CNM, Dr. Gertrude Berkowitz, Michelle Brill, Dr. Margaret Bates, Dr. Watson Bowes Jr., Carla, Cathy, Claudia, Dr. Mark Dwight, Dr. Murray Enkin, Laraine Guyette, Dr. Murph Goodwin, Holly, Jennifer, Kathleen R., Kevin, Dr. Allen Killam, Dr. Donna Kirz, Lucy, Marion McCartney, Pete, Dr. Susan Porto, Dr. Edward Quilligan, Dr. Brooks Ranney, Rhonda, Sharlene, Penny Simkin, Mary Sommers, Pam Spry CNM, Lisa Summer CNM/Ph.D.

Albers LL. The Duration of Labor in Healthy Women. *J Perinatol* 1999; 19(2):114–9.

Albers LL, Schiff M, Gorwoda JG. The length of Active Labor in Normal Pregnancies. *Obstet Gynecol* 1996; 87(3):355–9.

Bowes WA. Clinical Aspects of Normal and Abnormal

Labor. In *Obstetrics: Normal and Problem Pregnancies* (3rd ed.). Gabbe SJ, Niebyl JR, Simpson JL, eds. Philadelphia: Churchill Livingstone, 1996.

Creasy RK. Normal Labor and Delivery. In *Management of Labor and Delivery* (4th ed.). Creasy RK, ed. Boston: Blackwell Science, 1997.

Enkin M, Keirse MJ, Neilson J, Crowther C, Duley L, Hodnett E, Hofmeyr J. *A Guide to Effective Care in Pregnancy and Childbirth* (3rd ed.). New York: Oxford University Press, 2000.

Enkin M, Keirse MJ, Renfrew M, Neilson J. *A Guide to Effective Care in Pregnancy and Childbirth* (2nd ed.). New York: Oxford University Press, 1995.

Ferguson WGL. Management of Labor and Delivery in Low-Risk Patients. In *Management of Labor and Delivery* (4th ed.), Creasy RK, ed. Boston: Blackwell Science, 1997.

Friedman EA. Dystocia and "Failure to Progress" in Labor. In *Cesarean Section: Guidelines for Appropriate Utilization*, Flamm BL, Quilligan EJ, eds. New York: Springer-Verlag, 1995.

Garite TJ. Premature Rupture of the Membranes. In *Obstetrics: Normal and Problem Pregnancies* (3rd ed.). Gabbe SJ, Niebyl JR, Simpson JL, eds. Philadelphia: Churchill Livingstone, 1996.

Glantz JC, Woods JR Jr. Significance of Amniotic Fluid Meconium. In *Obstetrics: Normal and Problem Pregnancies* (3rd ed.). Gabbe SJ, Niebyl JR, Simpson JL, eds. Philadelphia: Churchill Livingstone, 1996.

Guttmacher AF, Kaiser IH. *Pregnancy, Birth, and Family Planning*. New York: Penguin, 1987.

Hofmeyr GJ, Gulmezoglu AM. Vaginal Misoprostol for Cervical Ripening and Induction of Labour (Cochrane Review). In *The Cochrane Library*, 1, 2001. Oxford:

Update Software.

Katz VL, Bowes WA. Meconium Aspiration Syndrome: Reflections on a Murky Subject. *Am J Obstet Gynecol* 1992; 166:171.

Kitzinger S. *The Complete Book of Pregnancy and Childbirth*. New York: Alfred A. Knopf, 1997.

McCartney M, van der Meer A. *The Midwife's Pregnancy and Childbirth Book*. New York: Harper Perennial, 1990.

O'Brien WF, Cefalo RC. Labor and Delivery. In *Obstetrics: Normal and Problem Pregnancies* (3rd ed.). Gabbe SJ, Niebyl JR, Simpson JL, eds. Philadelphia: Churchill Livingstone, 1996.

Reece AE, Hobbins JC, Mahoney MJ, Petrie RH, eds. *Handbook of Medicine of the Fetus and Mother*. Philadelphia: J.B. Lippincott Company, 1995.

Rooks JP. *Midwifery and Childbirth in America*. Philadelphia: Temple University Press, 1997.

Simkin P, Whalley J, Keppler A. *Pregnancy, Childbirth, and the Newborn*. New York: Meadowbrook Press, 1991.

Solomon JE, D'Alton ME. Induction of Labor. In *Management of Labor and Delivery* (4th ed.). Creasy RK, ed. Boston: Blackwell Science, 1997.

Tan BP, Hannah ME. Oxytocin for Prelabour Rupture of Membranes at or Near Term (Cochrane Review). In *The Cochrane Library*, 1, 2001. Oxford: Update Software.

Thacker SB, Stroup DF. Continuous Electronic Heart Rate Monitoring for Fetal Assessment During Labor (Cochrane Review). In *The Cochrane Library*, 1, 2001. Oxford: Update Software.

Zeisler H, Tempfr C, Mayerhofer K, Barrada M, Husslein P. Influence of Acupuncture on the Duration of Labor. *Gynecol Obstet Invest* 1998; 46:22–5.

Chapter 20: Maternal Positions for Labor and Birth

● ● ●

Personal interviews (taped) with: Auben, Leah Albers, Louise Aucott, Carla, Michelle Brill, Dr. Murray Enkin, Nancy Wainer Cohen, Lucy, Marion McCartney, Mary, Laraine Guyette, Dr. Susan Porto, Pam Spry

Albers LL, et al. Factors Related to Perineal Trauma in Childbirth. *J Nurse Midwifery* 1996; 41(4):269–76.

Enkin M, Keirse MJ, Neilson J, Crowther C, Duley L, Hodnett E, Hofmeyr J. *A Guide to Effective Care in Pregnancy and Childbirth* (3rd ed.). New York: Oxford University Press, 2000.

Enkin M, Keirse MJ, Renfrew M, Neilson J. *A Guide to Effective Care in Pregnancy and Childbirth* (2nd ed.). New York: Oxford University Press, 1995.

Gupta, JK, Nikodem VC. Woman's Position During Second Stage of Labour (Cochrane Review). In *The Cochrane Library*, 1, 2001. Oxford: Update Software.

Hofmeyr GJ, Kulier R. Hands/Knees Posture in Late Pregnancy or Labour for Fetal Malposition (Lateral or Posterior) (Cochrane Review). In *The Cochrane Library*, 1, 2001. Oxford: Update Software.

Kitzinger S. *The Complete Book of Pregnancy and Childbirth*. New York: Alfred A. Knopf, 1997.

Lieberman AB. *Easing Labor Pain*. Boston: The Harvard Common Press, 1992.

McCartney M, van der Meer A. *The Midwife's Pregnancy and Childbirth Book*. New York: Harper Perennial, 1990.

Simkin P. *The Birth Partner*. Boston: The Harvard Common Press, 1989.

Simkin P, Whalley J, Keppler A. *Pregnancy, Childbirth, and the Newborn*. New York: Meadowbrook Press, 1991.

Chapter 21: Birth and Bonding

* * *

Personal interviews (taped) with: Auben, Louise Aucott CNM, Carla, Cathy, Dr. Murray Enkin, Laraine Guyette CNM/Ph.D., Holly, Joanne, Kathleen R., Kevin, Dr. Donna Kirz, Dr. Louise Kirz, Leslie, Linda-Carol, Lucy, Miriam, Marion McCartney CNM, Peter, Reyn, Rhonda, Pam Spry CNM/Ph.D.

Enkin M, Keirse MJ, Neilson J, Crowther C, Duley L, Hodnett E, Hofmeyr J. *A Guide to Effective Care in Pregnancy and Childbirth* (3rd ed.). New York: Oxford University Press, 2000.

Enkin M, Keirse MJ, Renfrew M, Neilson J. *A Guide to Effective Care in Pregnancy and Childbirth* (2nd ed.). New York: Oxford University Press, 1995.

Fanagan M. Antenatal Preparation for Labor. In *Management of Labor and Delivery* (4th ed.). Creasy RK, ed. Boston: Blackwell Science, 1997.

Guttmacher AF, Kaiser IH. *Pregnancy, Birth, and Family Planning*. New York: Penguin, 1987.

Kitzinger S. *Breastfeeding Your Baby*. New York: Alfred A. Knopf, 1998.

Kitzinger S. *The Complete Book of Pregnancy and Childbirth*. New York: Alfred A. Knopf, 1997.

Klaus MH, Klaus PH. *Your Amazing Newborn*. Reading, MA: Perseus Books, 1998.

McCartney M, van der Meer A. *The Midwife's Pregnancy and Childbirth Book*. New York: Harper Perennial, 1990.

Riggs JW, Blanco JD. "The Puerperium." In *Management of Labor and Delivery* (4th ed.). Creasy RK, ed. Boston: Blackwell Science, 1997.

Sikorski J, Renfrew MJ. Support for Breastfeeding Mothers

(Cochrane Review). In *The Cochrane Library*, 1, 2001. Oxford: Update Software.

Chapter 22: Pain Relief in Childbirth

● ● ●

Personal interviews (taped) with: Auben, Carla, Cathy, Dr. Z. J. Chen, Kathleen R., Dr. Allen Killam, Dr. Louise Kirz, Lucy, Miriam, Dr. Yi Pan, Dr. Susan Porto, Sharlene, Stacy

Chestnut DH, et al. Does Early Administration of Epidural Affect Obstetric Outcome in Nulliparous Women Who Are in Spontaneous Labor? *Anesthesiology* 1994; 80(6):1201–8.

Chestnut DH. Does Epidural Analgesia During Labor Affect the Incidence of Cesarean Delivery? *Reg Anest* 1997; 22(6):495–9.

Chestnut DH. Epidural Anelgesia and the Incidence of Cesarean Section: Time for Another Close Look. *Anesthesiology* 1997 September; 87(3):472–476.

Enkin M, Keirse MJ, Neilson J, Crowther C, Duley L, Hodnett E, Hofmeyr J. *A Guide to Effective Care in Pregnancy and Childbirth* (3rd ed.). New York: Oxford University Press, 2000.

Enkin M, Keirse MJ, Renfrew M, Neilson J. *A Guide to Effective Care in Pregnancy and Childbirth* (2nd ed.). New York: Oxford University Press, 1995.

Ferguson WGL. Management of Labor and Delivery in Low-Risk Patients. In *Management of Labor and Delivery* (4th ed.), Creasy RK, ed. Boston: Blackwell Science, 1997.

Hawkins JL, Chestnut DH, Gibbs CP. Obstetric Anesthesia. In *Obstetrics: Normal and Problem Pregnancies* (3rd ed.). Gabbe SJ, Niebyl JR, Simpson JL, eds. Philadelphia: Churchill Livingstone, 1996.

Howell CJ. Epidural Versus Non-Epidural Analgesia for

Pain Relief in Labour (Cochrane Review). In *The Cochrane Library*, Issue 3, 1999. Oxford: Update Software.

Kitzinger S. *The Complete Book of Pregnancy and Childbirth*. New York: Alfred A. Knopf, 1997.

McCartney M, van der Meer A. *The Midwife's Pregnancy and Childbirth Book*. New York: Harper Perennial, 1990.

Renfrew MJ, Lang S, Wollridge MW. Early Versus Delayed Initiation of Breastfeeding (Cochrane Review). In *The Cochrane Library*, 1, 2001. Oxford: Update Software.

Russell R, Reynolds F. Pain Relief and Anesthesia During Labor. In *Management of Labor and Delivery*. Creasy RK, ed. Boston: Blackwell Science, 1997.

Sears W, Sears M. *The Birth Book*. Boston: Little, Brown, and Company, 1994.

Simkin P, Whalley J, Keppler A. *Pregnancy, Childbirth, and the Newborn*. New York: Meadowbrook Press, 1991.

Vinant RD Jr, Chestnut DH. Epidural Analgesia During Labor. *Am Fam Physician* 1998;58(8):1,743–4,1,746.

Part Eight: Childbirth Interventions, Variations, and Complications
Chapter 23: Inducing Labor, Suppressing Labor, and Other Medical Interventions in Childbirth

* * *

Personal interviews (taped) with: Leah Albers CNM/Dr. PH., Dr. Gertrude Berkowitz, Dr. Watson Bowes Jr., Dr. Z. J. Chen, Dr. Murray Enkin, Laraine Guyette CNM, Kevin, Dr. Allen Killam, Dr. Donna Kirz, Marion McCartney CNM, Dr. Susan Porto, Dr. Brooks Ranney, Pam Spry CNM

Albers LL. The Duration of Labor in Healthy Women. *J Perinatol* 1999; 19(2):114–9.

Albers LL, Schiff M, Gorwoda JG. The Length of Active Labor in Normal Pregnancies. *Obstet Gynecol* 1996; 87(3):355–9.

Creasy RK. Normal Labor and Delivery. In *Management of Labor and Delivery* (4th ed.). Creasy RK, ed. Boston: Blackwell Science, 1997.

Enkin M, Keirse MJ, Neilson J, Crowther C, Duley L, Hodnett E, Hofmeyr J. *A Guide to Effective Care in Pregnancy and Childbirth* (3rd ed.). New York: Oxford University Press, 2000.

Enkin M, Keirse MJ, Renfrew M, Neilson J. *A Guide to Effective Care in Pregnancy and Childbirth* (2nd ed.). New York: Oxford University Press, 1995.

Garite TJ. Premature Rupture of the Membranes. In *Obstetrics: Normal and Problem Pregnancies* (3rd ed.). Gabbe SJ, Niebyl JR, Simpson JL, eds. Philadelphia: Churchill Livingstone, 1996.

Glantz JC, Woods JR Jr. Significance of Amniotic Fluid Meconium. In *Obstetrics: Normal and Problem Pregnancies*, Gabbe SJ, Niebyl JR, Simpson JL, eds. Philadelphia: Churchill Livingstone, 1996.

Hofmeyr GJ, Gulmezoglu AM. Vaginal Misoprostol for Cervical Ripening and Induction of Labour (Cochrane Review). In *The Cochrane Library*, 1, 2001. Oxford: Update Software.

Katz VL, Bowes WA Jr. Meconium Aspiration Syndrome: Reflections on a Murky Subject. *Am J Obstet Gynecol* 1992; 166:171.

Kitzinger S. *The Complete Book of Pregnancy and Childbirth*. New York: Alfred A. Knopf, 1997.

Resnick R, Calder A. Post-Term Pregnancy. *Maternal-Fetal Medicine* (4th ed.). Creasey, Resnick, eds. Philadelphia: W.B. Saunders Company, 1999.

Simkin P, Whalley J, Keppler A. *Pregnancy, Childbirth, and the Newborn.* New York: Meadowbrook Press, 1991.

Solomon JE, D'Alton ME. Induction of Labor. *Management of Labor and Delivery* (4th ed.). Creasy RK, ed. Boston: Blackwell Science, 1997.

Tan BP, Hannah ME. Oxytocin for Prelabour Rupture of Membranes at or Near Term (Cochrane Review). In *The Cochrane Library*, 1, 2001. Oxford: Update Software.

Thacker SB, Stroup DF. Continuous Electronic Heart Rate Monitoring for Fetal Assessment During Labor (Cochrane Review). In *The Cochrane Library*, 1, 2001. Oxford: Update Software.

Ventura SJ, Martin JA, Curtin SC, Menacker F, Hamilton BE. Births: Final Data for 1999. *National Vital Statistics Reports* April 2001; 49(1).

Zeisler H, Tempfr C, Mayerhofer K, Barrada M, Husslein P. Influence of Acupuncture on the Duration of Labor. *Gynecol Obstet Invest* 1998; 46:22–5.

Chapter 24: Augmenting Labor

* * *

Personal interviews (taped) with: Leah Albers CNM/Dr. PH, Dr. Watson Bowes Jr., Dr. Z. J. Chen, Laraine Guyette, Holly, Kathleen, Dr. Allen Killam, Dr. Donna Kirz, Marion McCartney CNM, Dr. Susan Porto, Dr. Brooks Ranney, Sharlene, Pam Spry CNM, Connie Banack (ICAN)

Albers LL. The Duration of Labor in Healthy Women. *J Perinatol* 1999; 19(2):114–9.

Albers LL, Schiff M, Gorwoda JG. The Length of Active Labor in Normal Pregnancies. *Obstet Gynecol* 1996; 87(3):355–9.

Alfirevic Z. Oral Misoprostol for Induction of Labour (Cochrane Review). In *The Cochrane Library*, 1, 2001. Oxford:

708 • The Complete Guide to Pregnancy after 30

Update Software.

Enkin M, Keirse MJ, Neilson J, Crowther C, Duley L, Hodnett E, Hofmeyr J. *A Guide to Effective Care in Pregnancy and Childbirth* (3rd ed.). New York: Oxford University Press, 2000.

Enkin M, Keirse MJ, Renfrew M, Neilson J. *A Guide to Effective Care in Pregnancy and Childbirth* (2nd ed.). New York: Oxford University Press, 1995.

Freidman EA. Dystocia and "Failure to Progress" in Labor. In *Cesarean Section: Guidelines for Appropriate Utilization*, Flamm BL, Quilligan EJ, eds. New York: Springer-Verlag, 1995.

Gleicher N, Demir RH, Novas JB, Myers SA. "Methods for Safe Reduction of Cesarean Section Rates. *Cesarean Section: Guidelines for Appropriate Utilization*, Flamm BL, Quilligan EJ, eds. New York: Springer-Verlag, 1995.

Gupta, JK, Nikodem VC. Woman's Position During Second Stage of Labour (Cochrane Review). In *The Cochrane Library*, 1, 2001. Oxford: Update Software.

Hofmeyr GJ, Gulmezoglu AM. Vaginal Misoprostol for Cervical Ripening and Induction of Labour (Cochrane Review). In *The Cochrane Library*, 1, 2001. Oxford: Update Software.

Kitzinger S. *The Complete Book of Pregnancy and Childbirth*. New York: Alfred A. Knopf, 1997.

McCartney M, van der Meer A. *The Midwife's Pregnancy and Childbirth Book*. New York: Harper Perennial, 1990.

Simkin P, Whalley J, Keppler A. *Pregnancy, Childbirth, and the Newborn*. New York: Meadowbrook Press, 1991.

Smith, CA, Crowther CA. Acupuncture for Induction of Labour (Cochrane Review). In *The Cochrane Library*, 1, 2001. Oxford: Update Software.

Solomon JE, D'Alton ME. Induction of Labor. In *Management of Labor and Delivery* (4th ed.). Creasy RK, ed. Boston: Blackwell Science, 1997.

Tan BP, Hannah ME. Oxytocin for Prelabour Rupture of Membranes at or Near Term (Cochrane Review). In *The Cochrane Library*, 1, 2001. Oxford: Update Software.

Zeisler H, Tempfr C, Mayerhofer K, Barrada M, Husslein P. Influence of Acupuncture on the Duration of Labor. *Gynecol Obstet Invest* 1998; 46:22–5.

Chapter 25: When Instrumental Assistance Is Necessary: Forceps and Vacuum Deliveries

Personal interviews (taped) with: Dr. Watson Bowes Jr., Cathy, Holly, Kevin, Dr. Donna Kirz, Dr. Susan Porto, Dr. Edward Quilligan, Rhonda, Dr. Manuel Spiegel, Pam Spry CNM

Barbieri RL. Editorial. *Current Prob Obstet Gynecol Fertil* May/June 1994; XVII(3).

Bowes WA Jr. Clinical Aspects of Normal and Abnormal Labor. In *Obstetrics: Normal and Problem Pregnancies*, Gabbe SJ, Niebyl JR, Simpson JL, eds. Philadelphia: Churchill Livingstone, 1996.

Bowes WA Jr., Katz VL. Operative Vaginal Delivery: Forceps and Vacuum Extractor. *Curr Prob Obstet Gynecol Fertil* 1994; 17:83.

Enkin M, Keirse MJ, Neilson J, Crowther C, Duley L, Hodnett E, Hofmeyr J. *A Guide to Effective Care in Pregnancy and Childbirth* (3rd ed.). New York: Oxford University Press, 2000.

Enkin M, Keirse MJ, Renfrew M, Neilson J. *A Guide to Effective Care in Pregnancy and Childbirth* (2nd ed.). New York: Oxford University Press, 1995.

Johanson RB, Menon BKV. Vacuum Extraction Versus Forceps for Assisted Vaginal Delivery (Cochrane Review). In *The Cochrane Library*, 1, 2001. Oxford: Update Software.

Keane DP. Operative Procedures. In *Management of Labor and Delivery* (4th ed). Creasy RK, ed. Boston: Blackwell Science, 1997.

O'Brien WF, Cefalo RC. Labor and Delivery. In *Obstetrics: Normal and Problem Pregnancies* (3rd ed.). Gabbe SJ, Niebyl JR, Simpson JL, eds. Philadelphia: Churchill Livingstone, 1996.

Chapter 26: Big Babies, Difficult Births: Cephalopelvic Disproportion and Fetopelvic Disproportion

• • •

Personal interviews (taped) with: Anna, Auben, Dr. Watson Bowes Jr., Cathy, Laraine Guyette CNM/Ph.D., Rhonda, Sharlene, Pam Spry CNM/Ph.D.

Bowes WA Jr. Dystocia. In *Management of Labor and Delivery* (4th ed.). Creasy RK, ed. Boston: Blackwell Science, 1997.

Enkin M, Keirse MJ, Neilson J, Crowther C, Duley L, Hodnett E, Hofmeyr J. *A Guide to Effective Care in Pregnancy and Childbirth* (3rd ed.). New York: Oxford University Press, 2000.

Enkin M, Keirse MJ, Renfrew M, Neilson J. *A Guide to Effective Care in Pregnancy and Childbirth* (2nd ed.). New York: Oxford University Press, 1995.

Freidman EA. Dystocia and "Failure to Progress" in Labor. In *Cesarean Section: Guidelines for Appropriate Utilization*, Flamm BL, Quilligan EJ, eds. New York: Springer-Verlag, 1995.

Gupta, JK, Nikodem VC. Woman's Position During Second Stage of Labour (Cochrane Review). In *The Cochrane Library*, 1, 2001. Oxford: Update Software.

Irion O, Boulvain M. Induction of Labour for Suspected Fetal Macrosomia (Cochrane Review). In *The Cochrane Library*, 1, 2001. Oxford: Update Software.

Winn HN, Hobbins JC. Fetal Macrosomia. In *Cesarean Section: Guidelines for Appropriate Utilization*, Flamm BL, Quilligan EJ, eds. New York: Springer-Verlag, 1995.

Chapter 27: "Several Times a Rare Thing Is Still a Rare Thing"

• • •

Personal interviews (taped) with: Dr. Margaret Bates, Dr. Watson Bowes Jr., Dr. Mark Dwight, Dr. Allen Killam, Dr. Donna Kirz, Leda, Dr. Susan Porto, Sharlene, Susan

Bendetti TJ. Obstetric Hemorrhage. In *Obstetrics: Normal and Problem Pregnancies* (3rd ed.). Gabbe SJ, Niebyl JR, Simpson JL, eds. Philadelphia: Churchill Livingstone, 1996.

Clark SL. Placenta Previa and Abruptio Placentae. In *Maternal-Fetal Medicine* (4th ed.). Creasy RK, Resnik R, eds. Philadelphia: W.B. Saunders Company, 1999.

Enkin M, Keirse MJ, Neilson J, Crowther C, Duley L, Hodnett E, Hofmeyr J. *A Guide to Effective Care in Pregnancy and Childbirth* (3rd ed.). New York: Oxford University Press, 2000.

Enkin M, Keirse MJ, Renfrew M, Neilson J. *A Guide to Effective Care in Pregnancy and Childbirth* (2nd ed.). New York: Oxford University Press, 1995.

Herbst AL, Bern HA, eds. *Developmental Effect of Diethystilbestrol (DES) in Pregnancy*. New York: Thieme Stratton, 1981.

Reece AE, Hobbins JC, Mahoney MJ, Petrie RH. *Handbook of Medicine of the Fetus and Mother*. Philadelphia: J.B. Lippincott Company, 1995.

Chapter 28: Cesarean Section and Vaginal Birth after Cesarean (VBAC)

• • •

Personal interviews (taped) with: Anna, Dr. Margaret Bates, Connie Banack, Dr. Gertrude Berkowitz, Dr. Watson Bowes Jr., Michelle Brill, Dr. Luis Cibils, Kathy Gray Farthing, Laraine Guyette CNM, Jessica, Dr. Allen Killam, Dr. Donna Kirz, Dr. Louise Kirz, Leslie, Marion McCartney, Dr. Susan Porto, Dr. Edward Quilligan, Rhonda, Sarah, Sharon

Alfirevic Z. Oral Misoprostol for Induction of Labour (Cochrane Review). In *The Cochrane Library*, 1, 2001. Oxford: Update Software.

American College of Obstetricians and Gynecologists (ACOG). Vaginal Birth After Previous Cesarean Delivery. *Clinical Management Guidelines for Obstetrician-Gynecologists. ACOG PRACTICE BULLETIN* October 1998; No. 2.

American College of Obstetricians and Gynecologists (ACOG). Vaginal Birth After Previous Cesarean Delivery. *Clinical Management Guidelines for Obstetrician-Gynecologists. ACOG PRACTICE BULLETIN* July 1999; No. 5.

Berkowitz GS, Skovron ML, Lapinski RH, Berkowitz RL. Delayed Childbearing and the Outcome of Pregnancy. *N Engl J Med* 1990: 322:659–64.

Broadhead TJ, James DK. Worldwide Utilization of Cesarean Section. In *Cesarean Section: Guidelines for Appropriate Utilization*, Flamm BL, Quilligan EJ, eds. New York: Springer-Verlag, 1995.

Crowther CA. Caesarean Delivery for the Second Twin (Cochrane Review). In *The Cochrane Library*, 1, 2001. Oxford: Update Software.

Enkin M, Keirse MJ, Neilson J, Crowther C, Duley L, Hodnett E, Hofmeyr J. *A Guide to Effective Care in Pregnancy and Childbirth* (3rd ed.). New York: Oxford University Press, 2000.

Enkin M, Keirse MJ, Renfrew M, Neilson J. *A Guide to*

Effective Care in Pregnancy and Childbirth (2nd ed.). New York: Oxford University Press, 1995.

Flamm BL. Cesarean Delivery in the United States: A Summary of the Past 20 Years. In *Cesarean Section: Guidelines for Appropriate Utilization,* Flamm BL, Quilligan EJ, eds. New York: Springer-Verlag, 1995.

Flamm BL. Introduction. In *Cesarean Section: Guidelines for Appropriate Utilization,* Flamm BL, Quilligan EJ, eds. New York: Springer-Verlag, 1995.

Flamm BL. Once a Cesarean, Always a Controversy. *Obstet Gynecol* 1997; 90(2):312–15.

Flamm BL. The Patient Who Demands Cesarean Delivery. In *Cesarean Section: Guidelines for Appropriate Utilization,* Flamm BL, Quilligan EJ, eds. New York: Springer-Verlag, 1995.

Flamm BL. Vaginal Birth After Cesarean Section. In *Cesarean Section: Guidelines for Appropriate Utilization,* Flamm BL, Quilligan EJ, eds. New York: Springer-Verlag, 1995.

Flamm BL, Berwick DM, Kabcenell A. Reducing Cesarean Section Rates Safely: Lessons from a "Breakthrough Series" Collaborative. *Birth* 1998; 25:117–24.

Goer H. *A Thinking Woman's Guide to a Better Birth*. New York: Penguin Putnam Inc, 1999.

Goings JR. The Impact of Midwifery Care, Childbirth Preparation, and Labor Support on Cesarean Section Rates. In *Cesarean Section: Guidelines for Appropriate Utilization,* Flamm BL, Quilligan EJ, eds. New York: Springer-Verlag, 1995.

Gregory KD, Korst LM, Cane P, Platt LD, Kahn K. Vaginal Birth after Cesarean and Rupture Rates in California. *Obstet Gynecol* 1999; 94(6):985–9.

Hale, RW, American College of Obstetricians and Gynecologists. Letter to the Editor. In Correspondence, *The New England Journal of Medicine*, February 27, 1997; 336(9).

Healthy People 2000. National Health Promotion and

Disease Prevention Objectives: Full Report with Commentary. (DHHS publication no. (PHS)91-50212). Washington, DC: Government Printing Office, 1990:378.

Healthy People 2001 Web site *(www.health.gov/ healthypeople)*.

Hofmeyr GJ, Gulmezoglu AM. Vaginal Misoprostol for Cervical Ripening and Induction of Labour (Cochrane Review). In *The Cochrane Library*, 1, 2001. Oxford: Update Software.

Hofmeyr GJ, Hannah ME. Planned Caesarean Section for Term Breech Delivery (Cochrane Review). In *The Cochrane Library*, 1, 2001. Oxford: Update Software.

Keane DP. Operative Procedures. In *Management of Labor and Delivery* (4th ed.). Creasy RK, ed. Boston: Blackwell Science, 1997.

Korte D. *The VBAC Companion*. Boston: The Harvard Common Press, 1997.

Kirz D. Advanced Maternal Age: The Mature Gravida.

McMahon MJ, Luther ER, Bowes WA Jr., Olshan AF. Comparison of a Trial of Labor with an Elective Second Cesarean Section. *N Engl J Med* 1996; 335:689–95.

Paul RH. Toward Fewer Cesarean Sections—The Role of a Trial of Labor. *N Engl J Med* 1996; 335:735–6.

Phelan JP. Cesarean Delivery: A Medical-Legal Perspective. In *Cesarean Section: Guidelines for Appropriate Utilization*, Flamm BL, Quilligan EJ, eds. New York: Springer-Verlag, 1995.

Plaut MM, Schwartz ML, Lubarsky SL. Uterine Rupture Associated with the Use of Misoprostol in the Gravid Patient with a Previous Cesarean Section. *Am J Obstet Gynecol* 1999; 180:1535–42.

Puza S, Roth N, Macones GA, Mennuti A, Morgan M. Does Cesarean Section Decrease the Incidence of Major Birth Trauma? *J Perinatol* 1998; 189:9–12.

Ravasia DJ, Wood SL, Pollard JK. Uterine Rupture During

Induced Trial of Labor Among Women with Previous Cesarean Delivery. *Am J Obstet Gynecol* 2000; 183(5):1176–9.

Sandmire HF, Demott RK. The Green Bay Cesarean Section Study IV: The Physician Factor as a Determinant of Cesarean Birth Rates for the Large Fetus. *Am J Obstet Gynecol* 1996; 174:1557–64.

Simkin P, Whalley J, Keppler A. *Pregnancy, Childbirth, and the Newborn*. New York: Meadowbrook Press, 1991.

Thorp, JA. Malpresentations and Special Situations. In *Management of Labor and Delivery* (4th ed.). Creasy RK, ed. Boston: Blackwell Science, 1997.

Zelop CM, Shipp TD, Repke JT, Cohen A, Caughey AB, Lieberman E. Uterine Rupture During Induced or Augmented Labor in Gravid Women with One Prior Cesarean Delivery. *Am J Obstet Gynecol* 1999; 181(4).

Chapter 29: Breech and Malpresentation

● ● ●

Personal interviews (taped) with: Dr. Watson Bowes Jr., Dr. Z. J. Chen, Dr. Luis Cibils, Connie, Dr. Mark Dwight, Dr. Murray Enkin, Dr. Murph Goodwin, Laraine Guyette, Eileen Hutton CNM, Dr. Allen Killam, Dr. Donna Kirz, Dr. Margaret Nusbaum, Dr. Yi Pan, Dr. Susan Porto, Dr. Edward Quilligan, Dr. Brooks Ranney, Dr. Katherine Shaw, Sharlene

Bowes WA Jr. Clinical Aspects of Normal and Abnormal Labor. In *Obstetrics: Normal and Problem Pregnancies* (3rd ed.). Gabbe SJ, Niebyl JR, Simpson JL, eds. Philadelphia: Churchill Livingstone, 1996.

Broadhead TJ, James DK. Worldwide Utilization of Cesarean Section. In *Cesarean Section: Guidelines for Appropriate Utilization*, Flamm BL, Quilligan EJ, eds. New York: Springer-Verlag, 1995.

Cardini F, Weixin H. "Moxibustion for Correction of Breech Presentation: A Randomized Controlled Trial." *JAMA* 1999; 282(214):1329.

Cibils LA. Breech Presentation. In *Cesarean Section: Guidelines for Appropriate Utilization*, Flamm BL, Quilligan EJ, eds. New York: Springer-Verlag, 1995.

Collea JV, Chein C, Quilligan EJ. The Randomized Management of Term Frank Breech Presentation: A Study of 208 Cases. *Am J Obstet Gynecol* 1980; 137:235–244.

Enkin M, Keirse MJ, Neilson J, Crowther C, Duley L, Hodnett E, Hofmeyr J. *A Guide to Effective Care in Pregnancy and Childbirth* (3rd ed.). New York: Oxford University Press, 2000.

Enkin M, Keirse MJ, Renfrew M, Neilson J. *A Guide to Effective Care in Pregnancy and Childbirth* (2nd ed.). New York: Oxford University Press, 1995.

Goer H. *A Thinking Woman's Guide to a Better Birth*. New York: Penguin Putnam Inc, 1999.

Hannah ME, Hannah WJ, Hewson SA, Hodnett ED, Saigal S, Willan AR. Planned Caesarean Section Versus Planned Vaginal Birth for Breech Presentation at Term: A Randomized Multicentre Trial. Term Breech Collaborative Group. *Lancet* 2000; 356(9239):1369–70.

Hofmeyr GJ. External Cephalic Version for Breech Presentation Before Term (Cochrane Review). In *The Cochrane Library*, 1, 2001. Oxford: Update Software.

Hofmeyr GJ, Hannah ME. Planned Caesarean Section for Term Breech Delivery (Cochrane Review). In *The Cochrane Library*, 1, 2001. Oxford: Update Software.

Hofmeyr GJ, Kulier R. Cephalic Version by Postural Management for Breech Presentation. *Cochrane Database Systemic Reviews* 2000; (2):CD000051.

Hofmeyr GJ, Kulier R. External Cephalic Version for

Breech Presentation at Term (Cochrane Review). In *The Cochrane Library*, 1, 2001. Oxford: Update Software.

Hutton EK, Hannah MEE, Amankwah K, Kaufman K, Hodnett ED. External Cephalic Version (ECV) and the Early ECV Trial. *J Soc Obstet Gynecol Can* 1999; 21(14): 1316–26.

Ranney B. The Gentle Art of External Cephalic Version. *Am J Obstet Gynecol* 1973; 116:239–41.

Roman J, Bakos O, Cnattingius S. Pregnancy Outcomes by Mode of Delivery Among Term Breech Births: Swedish Experience 1987–1993. *Obstet Gynecol* 1998; 92:945–50.

Seeds JW, Walsh M. Malpresentations. In *Obstetrics: Normal and Problem Pregnancies* (3rd ed.). Gabbe SJ, Niebyl JR, Simpson JL, eds. Philadelphia: Churchill Livingstone, 1996.

Smith C, Crowther C, Wilinson C, Pridmore B, Robinson J, Knee-Chest Postural Management for Breech at Term: A Randomized Controlled Trial. *Birth* 1999; 26(2):71–5.

Thorp JA. Malpresentations and Special Situations. In *Management of Labor and Delivery* (4th ed.). Creasy RK, ed. Boston: Blackwell Science, 1997.

van Loon AJ, Mantingh A, Serlier EK, Kroon G, Mooyaart EL, Huisjes HJ. Randomized Controlled Trial of Magnetic-Resonance Pelvimetry in Breech Presentation at Term. *Obstet Gynecol Survey* 1998; 53:276–7.

Part Nine: Motherhood
Chapter 30: The Transition Period: Uncharted Territory

• • •

Personal interviews (taped) with: Anna, Auben, Cathy, Eileen, Holly, Jennifer, Jessica, Joanne, Kathleen R., Katie,

Kevin, Leda, Leslie, Linda, Lucy, Mary, Miriam, Pete, Dr. Susan Porto, Reyn, Dr. Mark Sauer, Sharlene

Davis-Floyd, R. *Birth as an American Rite of Passage.* Berkeley, CA: University of California University Press, 1993.

Pryor G. *Nursing Mother, Working Mother.* Boston, MA: The Harvard Common Press, 1997.

Riggs JW, Blanco JD. The Puerperium. *In Management of Labor and Delivery* (4th ed.). Creasy RK, ed. Boston: Blackwell Science, 1997.

Roan, Sharon L. *Postpartum Depression: Every Woman's Guide to Diagnosis, Treatment and Prevention.* Holbrook, MA: Adams Media Corporation, 1997.

Chapter 31: Coping with Motherhood and Career

• • •

Personal interviews (taped) with: Auben, Cathy, Eileen, Holly, Jennifer, Jessica, Joanne, Kathleen R., Leslie, Lucy, Miriam, Dr. Susan Porto, Rhonda, Stacy

Kitzinger S. *Breastfeeding Your Baby.* New York: Alfred A. Knopf, 1998.

Kitzinger S. *The Complete Book of Pregnancy and Childbirth.* New York: Alfred A. Knopf, 1997.

Klaus MH, Klaus PH. *Your Amazing Newborn.* Reading, MA: Perseus Books, 1998.

McCartney M, van der Meer A. *The Midwife's Pregnancy and Childbirth Book.* New York: Harper Perennial, 1990.

Pryor G. *Nursing Mother, Working Mother.* Boston: The Harvard Common Press, 1997.

Rosenberg, JP. *A Question of Balance. Artists and Writers on Motherhood.* Watsonville, CA: Papier-Mache Press, 1995.

Sikorski J, Renfrew MJ. Support for Breastfeeding Mothers

(Cochrane Review). In *The Cochrane Library*, 1, 2001. Oxford: Update Software.

Chapter 32: Child Care

✵ ✵ ✵

Personal interviews (taped) with: Amanda, Caroline Butler MA, Cathy, Eileen, Holly, Jennifer, Miriam, Dr. Susan Porto

Internet Sources: see Resource List.

Resource List

Obstetricians
American College of Obstetricians and Gynecologists
P.O. Box 96920
Washington, DC 20090-6920
202-638-5577
www.acog.org
A resource for finding a physician; offers pregnancy and child-birth educational materials.

Midwives
American College of Nurse-Midwives (ACNM)
818 Connecticut Avenue, NW
Suite 900
Washington, DC 20006
202-728-9860
888-MIDWIFE
www.midwife.org
Provides information on how to find a nurse-midwife as well as information on the role of a nurse-midwife.

Midwives Alliance of North America (MANA)
4805 Lawrenceville Highway, Suite 116–279
Lilburn, GA 30047
President, Ina May Gaskin
888-932-6262
www.mana.org
e-mail: *info@mana.org*
Provides information on the midwife option for childbirth, home birth, certification, and training programs for midwives.

Doulas and Childbirth Educators

American Academy of Husband-Coached Childbirth (The Bradley Method)
Box 5224
Sherman Oaks, CA 91413-5224
800-4-A-BIRTH
www.bradleybirth.com
Offers courses in preparation for "natural childbirth."

Association of Labor Assistants and Childbirth Educators (ALACE)
P.O. Box 390436
Cambridge, MA 01239
888-222-5223
e-mail: *ALACEHQ@aol.com*
This organization trains doulas and childbirth educators.

Birthworks
P.O. Box 2045
Medford, NJ 08055
888-TO-BIRTH

e-mail: *mailroom@birthworks.org*
www.birthworks.org
For online newsletter contact: *debram@birthworks.org*
Seeks to give women confidence in their ability to give birth and
to physically and emotionally prepare women for birth. The
organization provides birthing classes, doulas, and doula training.

Childbirth and Postpartum Professional Association (CAPPA)
800-548-3672
www.childbirthprofessionals.com
An international organization that provides training and certification to childbirth educators, labor doulas, postpartum doulas,
and lactation educators. It also helps parents locate these professionals.

Doulas of North America (DONA)
206-324-5440
fax: 206-325-047
www.dona.com
Provides information on doulas—how to find one or become
one—and offers book lists and education regarding childbirth
options.

International Childbirth Education Association (ICEA)
P.O. Box 20048
Minneapolis, MN 55420
952-854-8660
fax: 952-854-8772
www.icea.org
e-mail: *info@icea.org*
Offers a mail-order book center and certificate programs for
doulas, childbirth educators, postnatal educators, and perinatal
fitness educators.

Lamaze International
(formerly the American Society for Psychoprophylaxis in Obstetrics, ASPO Lamaze)
2025 M Street
Suite 800
Washington, DC 20036
202-857-1128
800-368-4404
www.lamaze.org
e-mail: *lamaze@dc.sba.com*
Offers childbirth classes that promote "normal . . . healthy and fulfilling childbearing experiences for women and their families."

Mothercare
6009 54 A Avenue
Camrose
Alberta
Canada T4V4G7
www.mother-care.ca
e-mail: *info@mother-care.ab.ca*
Provides childbirth information and an online bookstore with books on pregnancy, birth, and the newborn.

National Association of Postpartum Care Services (NAPCS)
800 Detroit Street
Denver, Colorado 80206
800-45-DOULA
fax: 303-321-4058
www.napcs.org
e-mail: *DoulaCare@aol.com*
This organization trains postpartum doulas (doulas who assist mothers in the first weeks or months after the birth and who provide education and breastfeeding support). NAPCS also

provides referral lists of postpartum doulas in your area.

Birthing Centers

National Association of Childbearing Centers (NACC)
3123 Gottschall Road
Perkiomenville, PA 18074-9546
215-234-8068
fax: 215-234-8829
www.birthcenters.org
e-mail: *reachnacc@birthcenters.org*
Designed to help women find a birth center in their area, to educate women and their families about birthcenters and midwives, and to celebrate birth.

Cesarean Section and VBAC

International Cesarean Awareness Network (ICAN)
1304 Kingsdale Avenue
Redondo Beach, CA 90278
310-542-6400
fax: 310-542-5368
www.ICAN-online.org
e-mail: *info@ICAN-online.org*
Offers information on the myths and realities of cesarean section and VBAC. The goal of this organization is to lower the rising cesarean section rate in the United States.

Infertility (Alternative and Conventional Treatments)

American Society for Reproductive Medicine (ASRM)
1209 Montgomery Highway

Birmingham, AL 53216-2809
205-978-5000
fax: 205-978-5005
www.asrm.com
main e-mail: *asrm@asrm.org*

Institute for Reproductive Health
Georgetown University Medical Center
3800 Reservoir Rd, NW, 3PHC
Washington, DC 20007
202-687-1392
fax: 202-687-6846
www.irh.org
e-mail: *irhinfo@georgetown.edu*
This group focuses on natural family planning and fertility awareness. Its goal is to make natural methods easy to learn and use and
to help people make informed family planning decisions.

International Council on Infertility Information Dissemination
(INCIID)
P.O. Box 6836
Arlington, Virginia 22206
703-379-9178
www.inciid.org
e-mail: *inciidinfo@inciid.org*
A large consortion of infertility experts on the Internet. Look
for the Fertility after 40 forum and the Pregnancy after 40
forum.

Mind/Body Center for Women's Health
(associated with Harvard University)
Alice Domar, Ph.D.
The Mind/Body Institute

Beth Israel Deaconess Hospital
Harvard Medical Center
Boston, MA
617-632-9530
The Center offers ten-week support groups and mind/body groups for women who are having difficulty getting pregnant.

Niravi Payne, M.S.
Whole Person Fertility Program
200 Periwinkle Way
Suite B217
Sanibel, Florida 33957
800-666-HEALTH
941-472-7792
fax: 941-472-6904
www.niravi.com
e-mail: *niravi@aol.com*
Ms. Payne uses psychotherapy to address the mind/body issues that may create obstacles to becoming pregnant.

RESOLVE
1310 Broadway
Somerville, MA 02144
Help line: 617-623-0744 (helpline hours are: Monday through Friday 9 A.M.–12 P.M., 1–4 P.M., (EST), Monday evenings 5–9 P.M.
www.resolve.org
e-mail: *resolveinc@aol.com*
An organization that provides support and information to people who are experiencing infertility.

Women's Health Interactive Infertility Center
970-282-9437
fax: 970-282-0023

www.womens-health.com/health_center/infertility
e-mail: *whi@womens-health.com*
Provides information to couples experiencing infertility.

Bed Rest/Minimal Activity Support/High-Risk Pregnancy Support

Confinement Line Care of Childbirth Education Association
P.O. Box 1609
Springfield, VA 22151
703-941-7183

Pregnancy Bed Rest: Information and Support for Families and Caregivers
http://armstrong.son.wisc.edu/˜son/bedrest/faq/faq.html
Information and support for women on bed rest and their families.

Sidelines
P.O. Box 1808
Laguna Beach, CA 92652
contact: Candace Hurley 714-497-2265
High-risk pregnancy information and telephone support.

Hypnosis for Childbirth and Pain Management

American Society of Clinical Hypnosis (ASCH)
139 East Elm Court
Suite 201
Roselle, IL 60172-2000
630-980-4740
fax: 630-351-8490
e-mail: *info@asch.net*

Milton Erickson Foundation
3606 North 24th Street
Phoenix, Arizona 85016
602-956-6196
www.erickson-foundation.org

New York Milton Erickson Society for Pyschotherapy and Hypnosis
212–873-6459
fax: 212-874-6148
info@nyseph.org
These hypnosis groups can refer you to licensed hypnotherapists who do hypnosis for childbirth.

Acupuncture
www.ACUPUNCTURE.com
This comprehensive Web site provides lists of acupuncturists in your area and describes their training and their areas of specialty.

Breastfeeding Information, Support Groups, Consultation
La Leche League International
P.O. Box 4079
Schaumberg, IL 60168-4079
voice mail: 847-519-7730
fax: 847-519-0035
order department: 847-519-9585
www.lalecheleague.org
e-mail: *LLLHQ@llli.org*
llli@llli.org
The organization provides breastfeeding information and

support and has breastfeeding support groups throughout the United States.

Medela
Breastfeeding National Network
800-435-8316
815-363-1166
www.medela.com
Medela sells breastfeeding products and offers lactation consultation and online breastfeeding chat sessions with a lactation consultant.

Breast Pumps and Related Equipment

Hollister Incorporated
800-323-4060 (Hollister Consumer Services)
www.hollister.com
Hollisters sells (and sometimes rents) breast pumps and also offers products and information related to breastfeeding.

Medela, Inc.
800-435-8316
815-363-1166
www.medela.com
e-mail: *customer.service@medela.com*
The company sells breast pumps and breastfeeding products, nursing bras, and so on.

Child Care

AuPair in America
American Institute of Foreign Study
River Plaza

9 West Broad Street
Stamford, CT 06902-3788
800-727-2437
www.aupairinamerica.com
e-mail: *aupair.info@aifs.com*
The organization provides au pairs by recruiting from forty different countries. Au pairs are between eighteen to twenty-six years of age. The au pair stays with the family for a year; the fee is approximately $260 per week.

Child Care Aware
1319 F Street NW
Suite 606
Washington, DC 20004
800-424-2246
www.childcareaware.org
An organization that provides lists of available child care—and information on how to evaluate child care centers. The organization is part of the Child Care Bureau, Administration for Children and Families, U.S. Department of Health and Human Services.

Single Mothers
National Organization of Single Mothers (NOSM)
P.O. Box 68
Midland, NC 28107
704-888-KIDS

Single Mothers Online
www.singlemothers.org
Provides information on everything from adoption to custody. Offers support groups and newsletter.

Parents Without Partners, Inc.
1650 South Dixie Hwy
Suite 510
Boca Raton, FL 33432
561-391-8833
e-mail: *pwp@jti.net*

At-home Mothers

Mothers At Home
9493-C Silver King Court
Fairfax, VA 22031
703-352-1072
800-783-4666
www.mah.org
e-mail: *mah@mah.org*
Provides support and information.

Working Mothers

Families and Work Institute
330 Seventh Avenue, 14th Floor
New York, NY 10001
212-465-2044
fax: 212-465-8637
www.familiesandwork.org
e-mail: *ebrownfield@familiesandwork.org*
Conducts research into the changing family, the changing work-force, and how children feel about working families.

Mothers & More: The Network for Sequencing Mothers
P.O. Box 31
Elmhurst, IL 60126

630-941-3553
fax: 630-941-3551
www.mothersandmore.org
e-mail: *nationaloffice@mothersandmore.org*
Supports "sequencing" women who alter their career paths to care for children at home or women who move in and out of paid employment. It suggests options for flex time and other options for women who are leaving or reentering the workforce.

New Ways to Work
785 Market Street
Suite 950
San Francisco, CA 94103
415-995-9860
fax: 415-995-9867
www.nww.org
e-mail: *info@nww.org*
Offers written materials and resources on job sharing and flexibility in the workplace.

Nine to Five: National Association of Working Women
1430 West Peachtree Street
Suite 610
Atlanta, GA 30309
800-522-9025

Job Survival Hotline: 800-522-0925
www.9to5.org
e-mail: *hotline9to5@igc.org*
The hotline offers job information that women can use to approach their employers about more flexible or child-friendly working arrangements.

The Women's Bureau Publications
(regarding laws on family leave)
U.S. Department of Labor
800-827-5335
11:00 A.M.–4:00 P.M., Monday–Friday
Provides information on working women's rights, pregnancy and age discrimination, and safe, affordable child care.

Work at Home Moms (WAHM online)
www.wahm.com/contact.html
Online magazine that provides information on home businesses.

Postpartum Depression

Depression After Delivery (DAD)
Information request line: 800-944-4PPD
For brochure, contact:
Depression After Delivery
P.O. Box 278
Belle Mead, NJ 08502
908-575-9121
e-mail: *dt@infotrail.com*

National Institute of Mental Health
Information Request Line
D/ART (Depression/Awareness, Recognition, and Treatment)
800-421-4211
301-443-4513
www.nimh.nih.gov

Postpartum Resource Center
109 Udall Road
West Islip, NY 11795

631-422-2255
fax: 631-422-1643
e-mail: *postpartum@aol.com*
A worldwide umbrella organization for individuals and groups dedicated to the emotional well-being of pregnant women and mothers, the group addresses depression during pregnancy as well as postpartum depression.

Postpartum Support International
927 North Kellogg Avenue
Santa Barbara, CA 93111
805-967-7636
fax: 805-967-0608
www.postpartum.net
e-mail: *jhorikman@earthlink.net*

Maternal and Women's Health

National Asian Women's Health Organization (NAWHO)
250 Montgomery Street
Suite 900
San Francisco, CA 94104
415-989-9747
fax: 415-989-9758
www.nawho.org
Offers information on reproductive health of Asian American women and families.

National Women's Health Network (NWHN)
514 10th Street NW, Suite 400
Washington, DC 20004
Administrative: 202-347-1140
For health information: 202-628-7814

fax: 202-347-1168
www.womenshealthnetwork.org
NWHN is a non-profit health advocacy organization that advocates for better federal policy on women's health issues.

Teratology Society
1767 Business Center Drive, Suite 302
Reston, VA 20190
703-438-3104
fax: 703-438-3113
e-mail: *tshq@teratology.org*
Provides information on herbs and drugs in order to help prevent birth defects.

DES Mothers, Daughters, Sons, Granddaughters

DES Action
610 16th Street
Suite 301
Oakland, CA 94612
800-DES-9288
fax: 510-465-4815
510-465-4011
www.desaction.org
e-mail: *desaction@earthlink.net*
DES action provides a newsletter, information, and support to mothers and children exposed to DES.

DES 3rd Generation
Box 328
Mahwah, NJ 07430

Infant Health

Allergy and Asthma Network
Mothers of Asthmatics, Incorporated
2751 Prosperity Avenue
Suite 150
Fairfax, VA 22031
703-641-9595
800-878-4403
fax: 703-573-7794
www.aanma.org
Aims to educate parents about asthma and allergies and to provide community outreach and research.

Circumcision Resource Center
P.O. Box 232
Boston, MA 02133
617-523-0088
www.circumcision.org
Informs the public and professionals about circumcision.

Disease Information
Group B Streptococcal Disease (GBS)
Centers for Disease Control
www.cdc.gov/ncidod/dbmd/gbs/index.htm

Group-B Strep Association (GBSA)
Chapel Hill, NC
919-932-3657
fax: 919-932-3657
www.groupbstrep.org
Resources for preventing and screening for Strep B infections
(that may be transmitted from mother to child during birth).

Motherisk—The Hospital for Sick Children
555 University Avenue

Toronto, Ontario, Canada M5G 1X8
416-813-6780
www.motherisk.org
A source for evidence-based information about the safety or
risk of drugs, chemicals, and diseases during pregnancy.

National SIDS Resource Center
2070 Chain Bridge Road
Suite 450
Vienna, VA 22182
703-821-8955
www.circsol.com/SIDS
e-mail: *dis@circsol.com*

National SIDS Support Center
1314 Bedford Avenue
Suite 205 B
Baltimore, MD 21208
800-638-7437
410-415-6628
fax: 410-415-5093
www.sids-id-psc.org
e-mail: *sds62@aol.com*

REPROTOX (Reproductive Toxicology Center)
www.reprotox.org
e-mail: *reprotox@reprotox.org*
Offers information on potentially harmful effects of environmental
chemicals and toxins on reproduction and fetal development.

Parents of Twins and Multiples
Center for Loss in Multiple Birth (CLIMB)

c/o Jean Kollantai
P.O. Box 91377
Anchorage, AK 99509
907-222-5321
www.climb-support.org
e-mail: *climb@pobox.alaska.net*
newsletter@climb-support.org

Center for the Study of Multiple Birth
Dr. Louis Keith
333 E. Superior Street
Room 464
Chicago, IL 60611
312-266-9093
www.multiplebirth.com
e-mail: *lgk395@nwu.edu*
Provides information and research on multiples.

International Twins Association (ITA)
c/o Lynn Long or Lori Stewart
6898 Channel Road
Minneapolis, MN 55432
612-571-3022
612-571-2910

National Organization of Mothers of Twins Club, Inc.
P.O. Box 438
Thompson Station, TN 37179
877-540-2200
www.nomotc.org
The organization provides information on local twins support
groups, referrals, research materials, and information.

Triplet Connection
P.O. Box 99571
Stockton, CA 95209
209-474-0885
fax: 209-474-9243
www.tripletconnection.org
e-mail: *tc@tripletconnection.org*
A national support and information networking organization offering a large database as well as information packets for parents of twins and triplets.

Twin Services
P.O. Box 10066
Berkeley, CA 94709
510-524-0863
www.twinservices.org
Information on multiple birth plus links to international organizations with information and research relevant to pregnancy with twins, triplets, and more. Access to *www.Twinslist.org* resources for multiple birth.

Children with Special Needs or Birth Abnormalities

National Down Syndrome Society (NDSS)
666 Broadway
New York, NY 10012-2317
212-460-9330
www.ndss.org
A comprehensive online resource about Down's syndrome.

National Information Center for Children and Youth with Disabilities (NICHCY)

P.O. Box 1492
Washington, DC 20013-1492
800-695-0285
202-884-8200 (voice)
www.nichcy.org
e-mail: *nichcy@aed.org*
A national information referral resource that provides information on disabilities in children and youth.

Parents Support Groups
National Child Abuse Hotline
800-4-A-CHILD (800-422-4453)

Pregnancy Loss and Support
The Bereavement and Loss Center of New York
170 East 83rd Street
New York, NY 10028
212-879-5655
A nonsectarian professional counseling service that specializes in loss and grief related to infertility, miscarriage, children, mates, siblings, and so on. The center also provides referrals outside of New York.

Pregnancy-Loss Peer-Support Program
National Council of Jewish Women
212-687-5030

SHARE
Share-Pregnancy and Infant Loss Support, Inc.
300 1st Capitol Drive
St. Joseph's Health Center

St. Charles, MO 63301
800-821-6819
636-947-6164
www.nationalshareoffice.com
e-mail: *share@nationalshareoffice.com*
A nondenominational organization offering support for parents
who have lost a baby and providing emotional support, publications, and national listings for support organizations in your area.

Web Sites with Information on Medical Care During Pregnancy and Childbirth

The Cochrane Library
www.cochrane.org
A resource for evidence-based medical studies.

Pub Med
www.pubmedcentral.nih.gov
Free access to Medline abstracts of medical studies.

Index

• • •

About the Author

Carol Winkelman is an award-winning medical writer specializing in medicine and women's health. She has taught writing at the University of California at Irvine, the University of North Carolina at Chapel Hill, and Duke University. Currently, she gives workshops in medical and scientific writing at universities and federal agencies.